DOCTORS OF DECEPTION

DOCTORS OF DECEPTION

What They Don't Want You to

Know about Shock Treatment

LINDA ANDRE

RUTGERS UNIVERSITY PRESS

New Brunswick, New Jersey, and London

Library of Congress Cataloging-in-Publication Data

Andre, Linda, 1959–
Doctors of deception : what they don't want you to know about shock
treatment / Linda Andre.

   p. ; cm.

   Includes bibliographical references and index.

   ISBN 978–0–8135–4441–0 (hardcover : alk. paper)

   1. Shock therapy.   2. Electroconvulsive therapy.   I. Title.

   [DNLM: 1. Electroconvulsive Therapy—adverse effects.   2. Electroconvulsive
Therapy—ethics.   3. Electroconvulsive Therapy—history.   4.   Informed Consent.
5. Mental Disorders—therapy.   6. Treatment Outcome. WM 412 A555d 2009]

   RC485.A53 2009

   616.89′12—dc22   2008014124

A British Cataloging-in-Publication record for this book is available from the British Library.

Visit our Web site: http://rutgerspress.rutgers.edu

Manufactured in the United States of America

For Fred Pfeil

1949–2005

This dark book is dedicated,
with light, and hope,
and much love always

I don't mean to say that these policies were ever written down or even necessarily known to the persons and organizations who have been actors in the drama, but they are detectable in the sweep of events and the rationalizations of the actors.

—Marilyn Rice

Contents

Acknowledgments — ix
Notes on Terminology — xi

1   The Trouble with Time — 1

2   Eugenic Conceptions I: Ticking Time Bombs — 13

3   Eugenic Conceptions II: Useless Eaters — 28

4   A Little Brain Pathology — 44

5   Informed Consent and the Dawn of the
Public Relations Era — 67

6   The American Psychiatric Association Task Force — 86

7   The Making of an American Activist — 107

8   The ECT Industry Cows the Media — 124

9   Long Strange Trip: ECT at the Food and
Drug Administration — 138

10   The Committee for Truth in Psychiatry — 156

11   Anecdote or Evidence? — 170

12   Shaming Science — 189

13   The Lie That Won't Die — 212

14   Erasing History — 231

15   The Triumph of Public Relations over Science — 253

16   Should ECT Be Banned? The Moral Context — 267

17   Where Do We Go from Here? — 287

Epilogue — 302

Appendix: Letters from
FDA Docket No. 82P-0316 — 306
Notes — 316
Resources — 349
Index — 351

Acknowledgments

I would not, could not have written this book if I hadn't had the good fortune to have known Marilyn Rice (1923–1992) and to have inherited her voluminous archives of published and unpublished material on shock. To find all this material on my own would have been impossible; to have it already collected for me was a scholar's dream. As well, Marilyn was the one person I could call at 3 A.M. to talk about all this stuff.

I am grateful to Tom and Louise Krause for permission to reproduce material from Marilyn's archives. Others who provided help and support on my long and often lonely journey from conception to finished book are Leonard Frank, Juli Lawrence of www.ect.org, Bob Whitaker, Sue Kemsley, and Laura Ziegler. Fred Pfeil was and is my inspiration for everything I do, and Tim Wooten gave me a much-needed push in the right direction. On a lighter note, the forums at www.newyorksurf.com and www.nynjsurf.com provided frequent and essential distraction and comic relief while working on this sad book.

In a sense, I have been writing this book for over twenty years. And the story continues.

Notes on Terminology

The words we use have tremendous power to shape our perceptions and our reality. Nowhere is this truer than in the field of psychiatry. Here words affect our very sense of who we are and, by making our choices seem limited, can have real and sometimes disastrous effects on our lives.

I would have prefered to use quotation marks for every occurrence of the terms "mental health," "mental illness," or "mentally ill" in order to avoid granting even subliminal credibility to the medical model I discuss in Chapter Two. For editorial reasons the quotes have been omitted, but please read the words as if they were in quotes.

When it comes to speaking about people with psychiatric labels, including myself, none of the currently fashionable terms, such as "psychiatric survivor," "recipient," "client," or "person with a psychiatric disability" is broad enough to apply to such a diverse group of people, and "consumer" has connotations of choice that are simply wishful. Whether we came into contact with psychiatry voluntarily or involuntarily, we were all once mental patients. Plus, everyone understands that term. Therefore I have chosen to use "mental patient."

DOCTORS OF DECEPTION

1   *The Trouble with Time*

Imagine you wake up tomorrow with your past missing. Although you look and feel the way you always have, and although everyone around you acts as if nothing's wrong, you slowly become aware that you don't have the most vital information about who you are. You may not recognize your home or know where your bank accounts are or what you are supposed to do for a living. You can't remember your wedding, or your college education. Every day you discover more about how much of your life is gone. You're like a detective trying to find out about the person who was once you. Eventually you realize that years of your life have been erased, never to return. Worse, you find that your daily memory and mental abilities aren't what they were before. You are somehow slower, less sharp, less able or unable to resume your former work. With the integrity of your life destroyed, you no longer know who you are.

When you say what happened, no one believes you.

See? You can't imagine. You can't believe this happened to me.

The most obvious thing needs to be said first. Your memory is not a component of your self, like your hair color or temperament. You don't lose it like you lose a suitcase. Your memory—the sum total of all you have ever thought, seen, smelled, heard, learned, and done in your life—*is* your self. When it is gone, you are a diminished person, and if enough of it is gone, you are a different person.

Even this way of talking about it—lost—is not accurate. Something lost, after all, may be recovered; a lost object can still be imagined, even if you don't know where it is; the fact that it ever existed at all is not lost to you. When you lose your suitcase, you still know its shape, color, and size, and exactly what was in it.

The memory "loss" that happens with shock treatment is really memory erasure. A period of time is wiped out as if it never happened. Unlike memory loss associated with other conditions such as Alzheimer's, which come on gradually and allow patients and families to anticipate and prepare for the loss to some extent, the amnesia associated with electroconvulsive therapy or ECT is sudden, violent, and unexpected. Your life is essentially unlived. You never wrote that article, made that friend, took that trip, read that book, gave birth to that child.

You didn't just lose your suitcase; you can't say where you got it, what it looks like, what you packed in it, what trips you've taken it on. You don't know that you ever had it.

Here is what I know: I was born in Ohio to a working-class family. I was such a good student that by second grade I was known as "The Brain" and shunned by my peers. Straight A's couldn't win me the approval of an abusive mother. I was bored and miserable in school, but I knew I had to go to college even though no one in my family ever had. Looking back now, I see how my every choice in life—from how I spent my time to who my friends were—was governed by the simple fact of my intelligence, and how my personality and my habits evolved to nurture and protect it. At seventeen, I was awarded a National Merit Scholarship to New York University. I became a photographer, exhibiting at a major New York City gallery at the age of twenty, and discovered a talent for writing photographic theory and criticism. Before I graduated, I published scholarly articles in professional journals. I had a group of like-minded friends, and was very happy. That's as much as I remember about my life up to age twenty-five, but I've seen documents that tell me that when I was twenty-three, I was accepted into NYU's graduate school, and that the next year I received a prestigious National Endowment for the Arts critical writing grant in the amount of $5,000. By the time I was twenty-four, I had published eight articles. I know because I have copies of them.

Here is what I don't know: when, why, or how I apparently stopped being happy and began feeling bad, the kind of bad that gets you labeled depressed and can lead to shock treatment. I've been told that I worried out loud to a friend that I might undermine my successful career because I'd internalized my mother's messages about how worthless I was. She suggested a kind of proactive psychotherapy; not because anything was wrong, but as a kind of preventive measure. Her brand of therapy (a radical, unproven type involving roleplaying) backfired. I became convinced that I did not deserve my success and was miserable. This is as close as I have been able to come to reconstructing my six-month period of depression.

I know I had no idea at the time that a psychiatrist could lock you up without warning, keep you incarcerated without so much as a walk outside for a breath of fresh air for months or years, and force you to take drugs and have shock treatment. But that is what happened to me. My (now-estranged) brother became annoyed that I asked him for support during this period, and dragged me to a psychiatrist's office. Once there, the doors were locked, and I was not allowed to leave. It had been a setup. He had lied to the doctors, telling them I was suicidal so they would have legal pretext to detain me. Years later, he would tell me that he heard me screaming in outrage at his duplicity as he walked away.

I was never legally committed (a procedure in which the lawyers for a hospital go to court and ask a judge's permission to detain a patient against her will for a specified period of time; the hospital must prove the patient is so severely mentally ill as to meet the commitment standard in her state). Without a court order, a facility can detain a citizen for no more than seventy-two hours in most states. After that, threats and coercion are usually sufficient to force her to "sign in voluntarily." I later learned that the mere threat of commitment, repeated over and over, had worked to convince me I had no choice but to submit to whatever the doctors wanted, and that my estranged brother had been complicit, threatening me that he would sign the commitment petition. But there never was any such petition.

I have no memory of ever feeling depressed or of my one involuntary encounter with psychiatry. The shock treatment erased five years of my life: four before, one after.

Also known as electroshock, shock treatment (invented in 1938) is a controversial procedure used on persons with certain psychiatric labels, usually depression, schizophrenia, or mania. Nobody knows how many people get it, but some say it's as many as one to two million people worldwide each year. While that number may be exaggerated for public relations purposes, if only 100,000 people in the United States are shocked each year, at 2005 prices ECT brings in $5 billion annually in that country alone. My "procedure" cost $20,000 in 1984.

In each shock treatment, up to 200 volts of electricity are applied to the brain via electrodes placed on the head. The amount of electricity is usually many multiples of that required to override the brain's natural defense mechanisms and to elicit a grand mal epileptic seizure of thirty seconds or more. No one ever gets just one treatment. Patients get at least one series, which is usually an induced seizure every other day for three to four weeks. In recent years, doctors have begun to recommend that shock treatment once begun be continued for a lifetime, once a month. If patients can be convinced to accept it, that recommendation will multiply the $5 billion figure exponentially.

There is no doubt that electrically induced seizures dramatically affect mood, memory, and cognition. In a mental hospital, those changes are in the direction of producing docility and compliance in troubled and troubling patients, and are seen as improvement. The doctors who say ECT treats mental illness cannot explain why it works. Doctors who don't use it point out that the same effect of calmness and temporary euphoria is associated with any form of brain trauma. But ECT is unique in producing permanent amnesia greater than that seen in just about any other neurological insult or disease. Decades of life can be erased in routine clinical treatment, and if excessive amounts are given, an entire life can be obliterated.

When I found out I had been shocked, I questioned everyone who was around me at the time. I never got any real answers. The only person who knew what I was thinking and feeling was me, and those thoughts and feelings have been permanently erased from my memory. Words like "depression" and diagnostic codes cannot give me a clue. For the most part, I can't even know how much of the information I do have about that time in my life is true, and how much has been altered by people who have their own reasons for not telling me the truth. Nor is there anything in my hospital record that can explain what I was going through. What is clear is that with my health insurance about to run out after months of unsuccessful drug treatment, the doctors pressured me to have shock and the hospital lawyers threatened me that if I didn't sign for it I would never get out. I know now that the lawyers may have been bluffing about whether they would have sought a commitment order, and that even if they had gone that far they might not have succeeded. Most commitments are just rubber-stamped by judges, but I would have fought with all my strength for my freedom if I had known I could. But I didn't know, and I had no access to the outside world for information about my legal rights or about shock. Worn down by five months behind locked doors, I "consented."

Before shock, patients are specifically told by our doctors that we won't lose our memory, or that if we do, any permanent loss will be only for the time of the treatment itself, and that any other erased memories will come back. About permanent loss of cognitive abilities, doctors say nothing. Thus the double horror: having lives and abilities erased, not only without any warning, but after being assured that it *couldn't* happen. And then when it does, the same doctors just keep assuring you that it *didn't* happen.

As if we were so crazy that we don't even know what we remember and don't remember. I guess that's what they think.

Here's what was erased: most of the knowledge and skills accumulated during my college education, my college graduation, a graduation party no one else who attended it will ever forget, my entire relationship with the love of my life, the other important relationships in my life in whole or in part, my career as a writer and scholar, two foreign countries, trips to California, Vermont, Massachusetts, and possibly any number of other states, the reason for the end of a friendship with someone I do remember loving very much, the death of a friend's brother, the location and contents of a safe deposit box to which I still hold the key, and more, much more than I will ever know.

For the most part, the effect of shock is like rewinding a videotape, then deleting the rest of it, although random islands of shadowy images and feelings may remain. The tape is your life. Although it takes a long time to live a life, it takes only a short time to delete it. Years and even decades of life can be erased in less than an hour. Each shock treatment takes only a couple of minutes.

The amount of life unlived is impossible to predict and different for everyone. The thing that's the same for everyone is that the weeks, months, years, or decades unlived are the most recent ones. This is the opposite of normal forgetting. To call shock memory erasure "forgetting" is to normalize something in order to speak about it at all, but like "loss," "forgetting" fails to convey the character of the shock experience. Shock bears about as much relation to gentle and gradual normal human forgetting as being killed in a war does to dying of old age. Shock kills memories blindly and randomly. It makes no difference how important the memory was in the first place, or whether it was a bad or good memory. You can't get your memories back by tricks like going to the place where they happened. They don't come back, ever.

Shock doesn't make you forget things; it makes you never have known them. It's not like the memories are still stored in your brain but you can't access them, as often happens with old information like the name of your third-grade teacher. After shock, the memories no longer exist. You wouldn't recognize the name of your teacher if you saw it, just as if you never knew it. You might not know you had ever gone to college, let alone what grades you got. You wouldn't have any emotional connection to past events in your life. They would seem to have happened to someone else. That's because they did.

Even that common word "memory" seems inadequate to describe what is erased by shock. We tend to think of our memory as a timeline, with markers set out for discrete events—moved to New York, 1977; met Fred, 1982. But memory encompasses no less than everything we think, feel, and learn every day of our lives. Memory is not just a string of events but *processes* that happen over time, and that involve long-term intellectual and emotional effort and investment. Your relationship to the person you call your spouse is part of your memory, as is all the accumulated learning that allows you to pick up a highly technical book in your area of expertise and understand it. When some or all of that time period when you built the relationship or amassed the knowledge is erased, so is the relationship and so is the knowledge. What are relationships *but* shared time and history? Erase the time, and you have only two people who don't know each other—or worse, one person who knows the history of a relationship and feels its tug on her heart, and one who doesn't.

You can find yourself married to a stranger. You can find yourself holding a job you have no idea how to perform.

One of the saddest things frequently said about survivors of ECT is that someone is "just never the same again." There's even a name for this in the literature: the "taming effect." Whether or not it is possible to define exactly what's missing, something essential to one's humanity and personality—some part of one's birthright—has been destroyed. Creativity is especially vulnerable. Shocked artists no longer create, musicians can no longer play. Spatial, mechanical, and mathematical abilities can be compromised. Each person will be most affected by the loss of what she valued most highly.

I had studied piano for a dozen years before shock. Afterwards, I struggled but could never again play at the level I had achieved before. It took me forever to learn anything, and I completely lost the ability to play from memory. Every time I play I can't help but be reminded of how much I've lost.

After shock, I no longer had the desire to create photographs. I remembered how much I loved photography, but I felt none of that now. The only thing sadder than losing one of the things in life that had brought me the most joy and recognition would have been going through the motions of doing it just because I knew I used to. I never photographed again seriously. My very fine camera lies in a box in my closet because it's too painful to look at it, too heartbreaking to sell it. Nothing in the world short of shock could have made me put it away forever.

My life was stolen. No words can really describe it. Memory. Loss. Forgetting. None of them even come close.

Those of us who have experienced the erasure of our lives due to shock have a terrible secret, impossible to tell, impossible not to know. We know that time doesn't always and only go forward. It can go backward with a push of a button. It becomes necessary to dissemble, to try to "pass" as someone with an intact memory and a history that can be told in narrative fashion, so that relations with other humans don't break down in incomprehension. They ask, "What do you mean you can't remember your college education?" the way they'd ask, "What do you mean there's no gravity?"

What survivors of shock need is for time to stop, so we can try to rebuild, relearn, or start over. When we lose years of knowledge and experience, we need as many years to try to get back to where we were. But time won't stop for us. It keeps going forward even as we try to recover and rebuild. There is no getting back, ever, to where we would have been had shock not intervened.

There is also a way in which electroshock alters the meaning and import of those lives that came before and that come after. You know those books about time travel? Change one thing in history, and you change all of history. Wipe out one person's life, and you affect everyone else's. Shock never, ever affects just one person.

My mother's mother came to America in 1906. She was twenty-four years old, alone, and had fourteen dollars in her pocket. I can hardly imagine the courage it took to make that journey. I like to think she was hoping for the opportunity to give her children and grandchildren a better life than she'd had. My mother, for all practical purposes a single parent, worked long hours and took out a second mortgage to help pay for my college education. Maybe they should not have struggled so for my sake; it would be all the same now.

In college, I was the one in the library until 3 a.m. On vacations, I'd bring a stack of books to read and study while my friends were partying. It's not that I didn't want to have fun, but a question of priorities. I had a fierce intellect to nurture. At all times in my life I knew one thing for certain: my fine mind was not a gift, but a responsibility. I navigated my entire life by that certain knowledge.

I might just as well have spent my college years in bed watching MTV or the Home Shopping Network. My work and dedication have been reduced to nothing, or worse: to a cruel joke on me. Were it possible to regain my education, I would still be behind by all the years it would take me to relearn what I once knew. But I can't regain what I lost, because shock took away my abilities as well as my memories.

July 14, 1988, is a date that breaks my life into two, unrelated pieces. That is the day I had proof that electroshock permanently damaged my brain. I'd finally had a neuropsychological evaluation, the whole battery of tests to see how you think, learn, reason, and remember. On that day, I was handed the report that said my IQ was now 118. Because I had had the same IQ test about ten years earlier, I expected the report to say what it had said then: 156. I had lost 38 points. And notwithstanding the controversy over what IQ testing does and does not measure, or whether the tests are culturally biased, there can be no doubt that such a huge decline in one individual means something devastating had happened.

The tests of the many different mental abilities that go into an IQ score, as well as the other tests designed by neuroscientists to assess specific areas of brain function and detect brain damage, confirmed my worst fears. Previously, although I knew I was unable to think as I had before, to write as I had before, and to learn as I always had, I took solace in the words of some of my fellow ECT survivors. They too struggled with the knowledge that they were impaired, the inability to quantify what they had lost, the shame they felt, and the desperate hope that they were somehow wrong about their deficits. "We're still intelligent," they'd say bravely, and then add a qualifier that seemed to explain what they couldn't do, like, "We just can't *use* our intelligence." And prior to 11 a.m. that morning in July, I really had no better words to describe what I could no longer do. I clung to the hope that psychiatrists who say ECT doesn't cause permanent brain damage were right.

Mostly, people who have had ECT are terrified to have an evaluation done. I was. We don't want to have everything down in black and white, so that there is no hiding, no pretending, no hoping that, somehow, someday we'll be whole again. Now, I couldn't hide. *Deficits in executive function, cognitive flexibility, abstract thinking, planning. . . . Difficulties with higher level cognitive processes. . . . Significant decreases in her attentional and organizational abilities . . . severe enough to undermine her ability to work. . . . Results clearly indicative of brain injury secondary to ECT. . . .*

Put together like that—*brain injury*—there are not two more terrifying words in the English language.

I was careful not to cry in front of the neuropsychologist, who handed me the report very callously, saying, "Any questions?"

I left the office quickly. I felt I could not go forward. I was hungry but felt too confused to go to a restaurant. At that moment I couldn't even make the small decision of what to eat. How could I live without a fourth of my intelligence? How would I relate to other people, when the only way I had ever done it was through shared intellectual interests? In the language of the neuropsychological report, I didn't know how to shift cognitive set. I hadn't heard that phrase before, and although it was based on my performance on a test involving sorting cards with patterns on them, there was no denying it was true. I had no idea how to modify my mental problem-solving strategies to reflect the situation at hand. Put more simply, I no longer knew who I was. I could go to a restaurant and still prefer ketchup to mustard on my hamburger; things like that hadn't changed. It was only the most important parts of my self, the ones that made me *me*, that were missing.

Later, I would come to learn about brain damage and how the tests can diagnose it even if a person doesn't have prior test scores for comparison. People don't normally have gaping holes in their intellects. Their scores on tests of intellectual ability don't career wildly, from the top percentiles on subtests of abilities that have been largely spared, to the bottom percentiles where they've been decimated. That is what happens with brain damage, with the end result being an overall lowering of cognitive ability.

Nevertheless, if you meet someone who has been brain damaged by ECT, she likely won't immediately appear to you to be mentally deficient. That's because those of us shocked in adulthood, often after considerable achievement, usually retain much of our storehouse of information about the world (what's known as "semantic memory"), our vocabulary, and the habits and values of intelligent, educated persons. This is arguably to our advantage, but it is also a source of unending pain and frustration. What once came easily to me is now extremely difficult when it's not impossible, and takes much more time and effort. There is no way I can come anywhere close to what I was able to achieve before.

There was some relief in finally having the words to say what happened to me: brain injury. I wanted to tell my friends that now that we could name this thing, we could handle it, we could get past it. The only words we had before were treatment, therapy; words that named it the opposite of what it was. I was cured, the doctors had said. So why couldn't I remember? Why couldn't I work? Why couldn't I carry on an intelligent conversation? If my friends believed the doctors, then I had to be lazy, crazy, or lying.

Now, I wanted to tell them, "see, that's not true." But it had taken too long—four years—to find the term. They couldn't wait around. I had lost everyone.

It has now been more than two decades, and I still can't get used to being this brain-damaged person. Unable to calculate my change or balance my checkbook, I'll argue that I've been shortchanged with the passionate certainty that I'm absolutely right. Then I feel the now-familiar sinking feeling, and I realize I am wrong and the other person—the bank teller or delivery person—is right. I am reminded yet again, although I still do not and probably never will *feel* different, that I cannot trust my brain. I learned to trust my brain so early, I can't unlearn it. Now I'm always thinking I can do things I can't, wanting to be something I can't be.

Sometimes for a few moments in the morning when I wake up, I think I'm still me.

Who can understand this? The Olympic skier who lost a leg and now skis on one foot, the paralyzed diver who becomes a chess champion? What's the refrain of every person who acquires a physical disability? Thank God, I've still got my brain. As Christopher Reeve used to say: "Thank God, I'm still me."

Shock "memory loss" is really a chain of losses that don't lessen but compound over time. Because I no longer knew who I was, I couldn't build new relationships. Because I lost my knowledge and skills, I could no longer work. Because I couldn't work, I became financially and socially marginal. Without work, friends, or identity, I lost my place in the world. Because I have no place in the world, my son has no place. And so on, in a slow social death that can last a lifetime.

Those of us who've had electroshock are among the bravest people in the world. The most everyday, ordinary acts—just getting up and getting through every day as if it *mattered*—are a bold act of faith, for how do we know that today won't be taken away, too? We don't. We know that our days can disappear like footsteps in wet sand, as if they were never lived. We know that our psychiatric history which includes ECT means that our days, months, and years are considered disposable and are likely to be disposed of again should we have another encounter with psychiatry. We never take for granted that what we know today, we'll remember tomorrow.

In the end, we just have to make the leap, living every day as if our efforts do matter. That's our simple act of boundless courage, our daily scaling of Everest. No one sees, no one knows; no one believes, unless they've had shock too.

For twenty-five years, I lived in a world where memory and intelligence were prized. Living in the same world for nearly twenty-five more years, I regularly experience cognitive dissonance so severe I feel almost paralyzed with contradiction. Sometimes I tune out: game shows where you get a million dollars for knowing the most; ads for herbal supplements that enhance memory, vocabulary tapes to make you smarter; a *New York Times* article calling prevention and treatment of memory loss "industry's next growth sector." And sometimes I just cannot get my mind to hold on to two contradictory facts at once. A psychiatrist who administers and actively promotes shock wrote a book about "how to prevent memory loss and enhance memory power." Duke University's medical center has a busy ECT clinic and is home to some of the shock industry's most prominent promoters, yet this same university hosts the National Center for Gifted Children, which seeks out children with high IQs. I can imagine one of those children someday having his intelligence electrically reduced at the same university where he once attended special courses to enrich his intellect.

How is it that the gift is nurtured on one hand, and thrown away on the other? Can a society that places such value on intact memory and rewards intellectual achievement countenance wholesale memory loss and brain damage? Or would it have to make up another story for what's going on with shock?

Why aren't patients told shock causes permanent amnesia and cognitive deficits? Why did no one warn me I could end up *brain damaged*? How long have doctors known this? How do they get away with lying to patients, destroying lives the way they did mine? Why doesn't anyone believe us when we say we've been harmed? Why doesn't anyone do anything about it?

Thank God, I hadn't lost my capacity for critical thinking. It turned out that this was exactly what I would need to answer these questions for myself.

2 *Eugenic Conceptions I*

I'd lost my whole world and gained a psychiatric label. Now I was thrust into a world I hadn't known existed, a kind of parallel universe. I was not prepared for what happened there. I didn't feel like a mental patient, had no memory or experience of any psychiatric treatment or symptoms, and never went near a psychiatrist again; yet I had become someone who could be treated in ways that would be unthinkable—even illegal—for someone without a label.

Whether in the schoolyard or the courtroom, calling someone crazy is the surest, fastest way of totally invalidating him or her as a person. If craziness is an illness, then it's not like other illnesses that affect only a body part or a function and leave the person otherwise intact. In what we call mental illness, the person *is* the illness, and the illness is the person. As activist lawyer Susan Stefan says, it becomes "the central, overwhelming aspect of the person's social identity in a way that does not permit any other part of that person's story to be told, the lens through which all accounts are viewed, the frame to every self-portrait."[1]

I was about to learn what it means to be considered crazy.

A Brief History of the Mental Patient Movement

Mental patients have, for nearly forty years, been building a civil rights movement just as blacks and gays have done, although our movement remains largely unknown, our goals unrealized. Nor have other marginalized groups joined us as allies.

In 1970 groups of former mental patients began to organize to protest the violations of human, legal, and civil rights within psychiatric institutions. They called themselves "ex-inmates" to emphasize that they had been held against their will and that there was nothing helpful about such "treatment." They rejected their pseudomedical psychiatric labels and the stigmatizing and blaming of one individual for what were often family or societal problems.

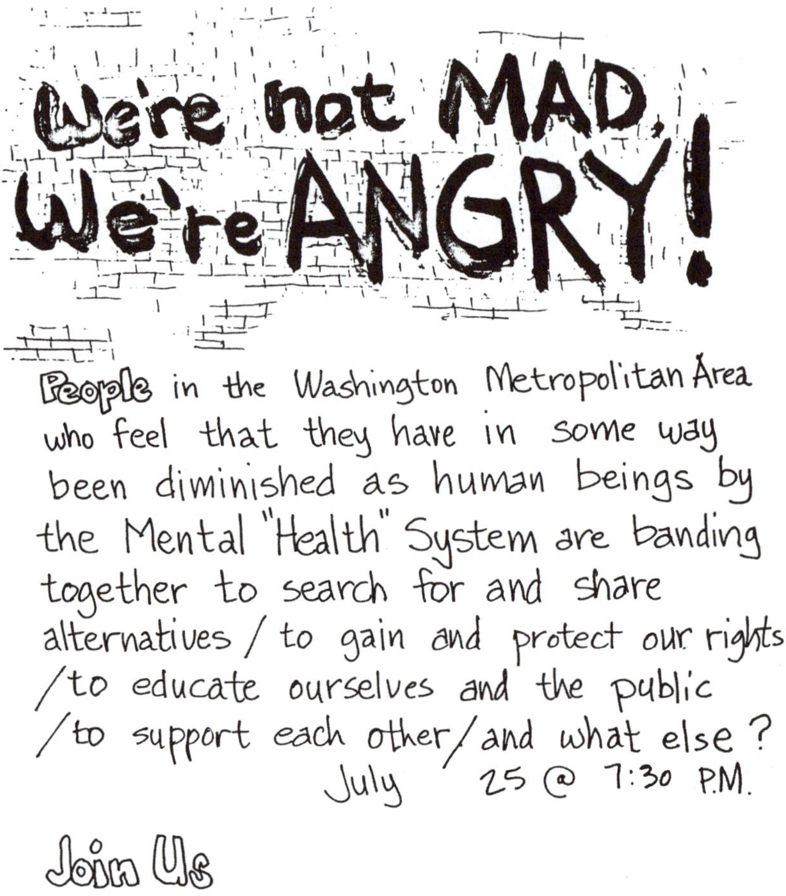

We're not MAD,
We're ANGRY!

People in the Washington Metropolitan Area who feel that they have in some way been diminished as human beings by the Mental "Health" System are banding together to search for and share alternatives / to gain and protect our rights /to educate ourselves and the public /to support each other/and what else ?
July   25 @ 7:30 P.M.

Join Us

Figure 1. The simple premises of the mental patients' rights movement, circa 1979. Flyer from the Washington Network for Alternatives to Psychiatric Dependency.

The ex-inmates' liberation movement started with the formation of the Insane Liberation Front in Portland, Oregon, followed by the Mental Patients' Liberation Front in Boston and the Mental Patients' Liberation Project in New York City. Then groups began forming everywhere. An annual Conference for Human Rights and Against Psychiatric Oppression began in 1973. Newspapers and newsletters sprang up. For many years, the voice of the movement was *Madness Network News*, published by a collective of mental patients in California. A 1974 anthology of articles from the newspaper put it this way:

> Maybe you tried to get help for your friend, husband, or child—or tried to help the person yourself. Maybe it was you who wanted help, or didn't want help, but got it anyway. If you wound up with professional "help," you may have seen how frequently the "help" is delivered through a syringe or a pill. If so, you have heard the underlying message delivered with the "treatment": The "patient"—you or someone you care about—is mad; no longer a valid, responsible individual, but an invalid, irresponsible one. You may also be aware that this kind of "help" can dog your mind and make you forget what you were trying to remember; it's "help" that attempts to stuff part of your self back inside of you and away from the rest of the world. You may also know that the role of people labeled crazy once the psychiatric system has a firm hold on them is really that of an acquiescent prisoner.

More than thirty years later, this statement is just as true and timely. While criticism of psychiatry, and particularly of electroshock, is dismissed by professionals as nothing more than a by-product of what one calls "the hippy-dippy sixties," this supposedly self-evident statement completely misses the point.[2] We who have experienced psychiatry are motivated by our own experiences, not by events that happened before we were born. Many of us can never forget the injustice of being locked up against our will when we had committed no crime, often on the basis of nothing but a lie by a family member, and then forced to submit to terrifying and damaging "treatment." Others came to psychiatry voluntarily, fully expecting (and paying for) help, but were swallowed up, dehumanized, and deeply harmed instead. We began to understand, through joining together, that these experiences were not unique. In fact, they were typical of the practice of psychiatry today, which is increasingly biological, and yet not based on science. In the reduction of all human problems to chemistry, based on an unproven theory of brain disease, there is in fact often no real help for many desperate people who don't get better or even experience toxic or deadly side effects from drugs or shock. Those of us who've had these experiences, and say so, find that the field brooks no criticism. Rather than addressing our concerns, it dismisses us as "antipsychiatry" or accuses us of being Scientologists. But we only want the same human and civil rights as everyone else. We don't want to be locked up when we have committed no crime, on the pretext that it's for our own good. It's not. Being deprived of liberty is inherently harmful, never helpful—except for the institutions, the professionals, the drug and shock machine companies, and everyone else who profits from locking us up.

We want the right to say no to drugs and shock treatment. We want fully informed consent—including complete disclosure of everything the doctors and companies know about risks and adverse effects—so that when pills and electricity are offered to us, we can make an informed decision. Of course, this is meaningless without the right to say no. In short, we want control over our own minds and bodies.

None of this sounds very radical. But to get it we have to fight a multibillion-dollar industry that stands to lose a great deal of its market if it can no longer employ deception, coercion, and force. And we have to fight hate and prejudice that's been around, it seems, for centuries.

By the early 1980s, there were two national mental patient organizations. These groups operated on little to no money. In 1986, the federal government cautiously began funding the most conservative mental patients' organizations, and this small amount of money, combined with other factors like the expansion of the mental health industry, has changed the character of our rights movement.

Some of us want to reform the mental health system, to make it deliver better services, perhaps by becoming professionals ourselves. Others don't believe that reforming a system based on coercion is possible, and want to abolish it. Some of us find professional help useful, if given choice and control over that help. But since any contact with the system involves a risk of being forced into treatment we don't want, many of us would prefer to be left alone or to turn to self-help groups if we ever experience extreme emotional states.

Today we may call ourselves psychiatric survivors, consumers, recipients, ex-patients, or persons with psychiatric disabilities. Whatever name we choose, the fundamental principle of the mental patients' movement has always been self-determination. We speak for ourselves. No one speaks for us, especially not professionals, whose stake in the system is much different from ours. We want to have a voice in all policy decisions that affect our lives. Our unofficial slogan, "Nothing about us, without us," comes from the South African anti-apartheid movement by way of the disability rights movement.

There is one issue on which all of us agree. There is no such thing as "forced treatment"; if it's forced, it's social control for the benefit of others, not treatment. We want the right that every other competent adult patient and every person without a psychiatric label in America has: to refuse treatment—rationally or irrationally, for any reason or no reason—without that refusal being seen as proof of how much we need it.

Shock has always been high on the agenda of most mental patient organizations. Shock survivors have organized within larger groups and in smaller local or ad hoc groups with names like REJECT (Coalition for Responsible Education and Judgment on ECT), World Association of Electroshock Survivors, and CAEST (Coalition for the Abolition of Electroshock in Texas). Most of these groups feel that shock is harmful, immoral, and should be banned.[3]

One of the longest-established independent mental patient organizations, MindFreedom International (formerly Support Coalition International), adopted this policy on shock in 2001:

> The Board of Directors of Support Coalition International unanimously and strongly condemns the psychiatric procedure of electroshock ("electroconvulsive therapy," "ECT") as a serious human rights violation. It is our informed opinion, based on common sense, personal experience and scientific knowledge, that electroshock is a crime against humanity. It directly violates section 5 of the United Nations Universal Declaration of Human Rights which outlaws "cruel, degrading and inhumane treatment or punishment," and the UN Convention Against Torture. It is our informed opinion that electroshock constitutes cruel and unusual punishment. We also believe that virtually all electroshock is forcibly administered—that is, without genuine, fully informed consent.[4]

We've got a long way to go. Persons who have or are said to deserve a psychiatric label are the only Americans who can be forcibly detained and imprisoned without having committed any crime, without a hearing, and without due process. Every state also has the authority to force drugs and ECT on unwilling individuals by court order.

Becoming Crazy

In my personal life, and as I took on a public role as an activist for the rights of other psychiatrically labeled people, I quickly learned that few who haven't been labeled themselves care about mental patients. No one thinks we have anything of value to lose; no one who hasn't been through the system believes it could ever happen to them. More than that, people simply dismiss what we say as symptoms of our supposed mental illness.

Throughout history, medical experiments and unproven procedures have been performed on those whose lives were thought to be of less value simply because of the group they belonged to, and this was done not only without their consent but without their knowledge. The most well known example is the Tuskegee experiments performed beginning in the 1930s on black men who were denied treatment for syphilis so government researchers could study the course of the disease. But there are many other examples from the not-so-distant past: prisoners, mostly black, were used as guinea pigs by pharmaceutical and cosmetic companies who applied dioxin, among other toxic substances, to their skin, leaving them permanently damaged and disfigured.[5] Other inmates had radiation applied to their testicles by the U.S. Atomic Energy Commission to determine what dose would cause permanent damage.[6] Researchers from the Massachusetts Institute of Technology fed disabled and institutionalized children radioactive oatmeal, while telling their parents it was to improve their nutrition.[7]

From a safe distance, we now recognize these practices and the attitudes that gave rise to them as morally reprehensible and ethically wrong. But those attitudes and practices, while not extinct, are at least no longer acceptable. The Nuremberg code, informed consent laws, and institutional review boards (flawed and ineffective as they are) now exist for the purpose of protecting the rights of patients and research subjects. It's become possible to speak and write about things like the plutonium experiments performed by the government on unsuspecting citizens during the Cold War only because they are no longer happening. And only after public exposure and recognition of the injustice they had suffered were victims of some of the experiments able—decades later—to seek and receive compensation for their injuries.

But eugenic conceptions of mental patients are not only alive but highly socially acceptable, and shock treatment is an extremely lucrative practice championed and protected at the highest levels of society.

I thought I could redress my injuries and set a precedent for truthful informed consent for future patients by suing the hospital where I received my treatment, the doctor who administered it, and Mecta, the company that made the shock machine used on me. But I learned that not even my own lawyer would believe the word of a shock patient over that of her doctors. I did file a lawsuit, but after an eight-and-a-half-year struggle, I had to give up on it because I could not find an M.D. who would testify against the shock industry.[8] I tried to establish and enforce a child support order for my son. I tried for twelve years. But my son's father painted himself as the victim of a lying crazy woman, the judge sympathized, and he successfully argued his way out of paying even $25 a week.

Like most psychiatrically labeled women today, I was not even thought fit to raise a child. My mother, using my new label as her platform, sued me for custody of my son and easily convinced a judge I was dangerous. I was forced to settle the case when my lawyers told me I could not win custody of the child I had raised alone from birth.

I learned that whether, or how much, I was discriminated against had nothing to do with how I behaved or whether I saw a psychiatrist. Ironically, I was discriminated against more than most of the mental patients I knew who exhibited psychiatric symptoms but were segregated away in the mental patient world, meekly accepting their status as third-class citizens. The discrimination I faced was proportional to the degree to which I asserted my legal and civil rights. Had I never tried to enforce my right to sue for lack of informed consent, or my son's right to child support, my history of alleged craziness—about which I knew nothing—would have remained ancient history. Whether hatred of psychiatrically labeled people was used as a tool to discredit and devalue me had mostly to do with how much someone else had to gain.

Because of that, I came to see, there was nothing personal about it. The lawyer for New York Hospital, for instance, didn't even bother to look at me as he painted the potential jurors a picture of how pitifully crazy I was; he was just doing his job. The beauty of it was that he didn't have to add "she's lying about losing her memory"—that was just taken for granted. This kind of hate, nameless and universal, is used in the same impersonal way a carpenter might use a hammer: because it's there, because it's easy, because it gets the job done.

Eugenic Conceptions

It's easy to think that ECT's dark beginnings, which even the industry decries now as barbaric, are rooted in outdated attitudes. But like shock treatment, hatred and segregation of mental patients because of myths and fears about us are alive and well; they've just been repackaged.

In an era of patients' rights advocacy, coercion and compulsion in psychiatry are more widespread than ever. Forced psychiatric treatment has expanded into the community in the form of outpatient commitment, a concept virtually unheard of until the late 1980s. Anyone with a psychiatric label, even someone living independently, can, under certain conditions, be court-ordered to ingest psychiatric drugs against her will; if she does not, she can be committed to a psychiatric institution. Outpatient commitment laws have been passed in forty-three states. This was almost always a result of highly publicized incidents in which it was claimed that a person with a psychiatric label committed a violent crime because he was not taking his medications. In many cases there was no proof that the perpetrator was labeled or unmedicated. But no proof is necessary, because the public already believes that mental patients are dangerous.

This belief is one of many which Robert Whitaker, award-winning journalist and author of a history of psychiatric treatment in America, calls "eugenic conceptions" about persons with psychiatric labels.[9] They have to do with what we are thought to be capable or not capable of: shooting up schools, working, recovering, or raising children, for instance. What we as a society do *to* or *about* mental patients at any particular time in history is always motivated and said to be justified by these beliefs. As Whitaker says, they provide a baseline by which we judge psychiatric interventions. This was true in the 1930s when shock was invented, it was true in the 1950s when lobotomy was so popular, and it is true in the twenty-first century.

Today there is a strong forced-treatment lobby that didn't exist thirty years ago, in the form of the Treatment Advocacy Center (TAC), an organization created by board members of the National Alliance on Mental Illness (NAMI). TAC's sole purpose is to chip away at the legal right to refuse psychiatric treatment by creating stronger commitment laws. TAC board members regularly publish editorials and letters to the editor and appear on radio and television with the same sound-bite message: mental patients who aren't drugged are "ticking time bombs." An Internet search on this term as applied to "mental illness" yields over nine thousand hits, and TAC takes full credit. In a recent press release, it says, "TAC is now a force to be reckoned with in the national media, drawing coverage from national and local media outlets alike, its messages reaching an estimated 79 million people through the press in 2006 alone."[10]

Because of the lobbying efforts of organizations like TAC, as well as the drug companies themselves, there is increased public acceptance of the core—but unproven—beliefs that underlie the forced administration of drugs and shock. These include the belief that what we call mental illness has been proven to be a biological brain disease caused by a "chemical imbalance," and the correlate views that mental illness causes people to be dangerous and that treatment with drugs and shock somehow prevents people from committing harm to themselves or others.

The Medical Model

The theory that distressing or extreme emotional and cognitive states are symptoms of an actual physical disease is known as the medical model. This is one way of explaining emotional distress, but it's only one way. What's happened over the past couple of decades (thanks to the marketing efforts of the drug companies) is that it's been accepted as the *only* way—so much so that most anyone you ask can now spout the "chemical imbalance" theory without knowing where they heard it or why they believe it. According to this theory, persons labeled with depression have an imbalance of the neurotransmitters norepinephrine or serotonin, and those labeled with schizophrenia have an imbalance of the neurotransmitter dopamine. (Neurotransmitters are chemical compounds that transmit signals between nerve cells in the brain; however, these chemicals are found throughout the body, not just in the brain.)

But no one has shown that what we call mental illness is caused by an imbalance of brain chemicals. This is scientifically impossible, since there is no way to measure the levels of these chemicals in the brains of living beings. And even if this could be done, no one has any idea what a normal balance would be, or even if there is any such thing. In fact, there is no reason even to suspect that the brain functions as a hydraulic system in which there is any need for "balance" at all.

Even prominent psychiatrists who consult for the drug companies, such as David Healy (the author of many books on the history of psychiatry and an advocate of shock treatment), have acknowledged that the chemical imbalance theory is not only faulty but politically motivated. He writes, "The serotonin theory of depression is comparable to the masturbatory theory of insanity. Both have been depletion theories, both have survived in spite of the evidence, both contain an implicit message as to what people ought to do. In the case of these myths, the key question is whose interests are being served by a widespread promulgation of such views rather than how do we test this theory."[11]

And the president of the American Psychiatric Association (APA), when challenged in 2005, had to admit that the chemical imbalance theory was unproven and unprovable. After claiming it was based on neuroscience, he backed off and admitted, "We do not have a clean-cut lab test" to diagnose any such imbalance.[12] The chair of the APA's Committee on Public Affairs went on to clarify: "Chemical imbalance . . . it's a shorthand term really. We don't have tests because to do it, you'd probably have to take a chunk of brain out of someone . . . not a good idea, but I agree. There aren't any blood tests to determine a chemical imbalance."[13] Robert Whitaker says it even more plainly: "The story that people with mental disorders have known chemical imbalances—that's a lie. It's just something they say to help sell the drugs and help sell the biological model of mental disorders."[14]

Psychiatric drugs were developed by trial and error and weren't specifically intended for psychiatric patients. For instance, the laboratory that created what eventually became Thorazine, the first so-called wonder drug for schizophrenia, originally thought the compound would be useful as an anesthetic. Psychiatrists tried the drugs on patients and liked the results (no one asked whether the *patients* liked them), so they were marketed as antipsychotics or antidepressants. When it was discovered that these drugs affected neurotransmitters like serotonin and dopamine, psychiatrists reasoned backwards to come up with the theory that psychiatric patients had abnormally low levels of these neurotransmitters. It's like reasoning that if aspirin cures your headache, it must have been caused by an aspirin deficiency.[15]

Nor does the fact that depression and other mood states may cause changes that can be seen on brain scans prove that they are diseases of the brain. Studies have shown that exercise and psychotherapy also have effects on the brain that can be seen on scans. So, most likely, does anything else that has a powerful effect on the whole person.

The overwhelming public acceptance of the medical model, though not grounded in science, does have a major influence on how mental patients are perceived and on what can be done to us. The lack of any perceived alternative to biological treatment sells shock to desperate, vulnerable people. If drugs and shock are all that psychiatry currently has to offer, when the drugs don't help, people feel—and are told by their doctors—that shock is their only hope. They consent to shock because they really think they have no choice. But that's never true, because there are other ways of conceptualizing and treating even severe emotional states if you don't go down the dead-end road of the medical model.

How do we know this? At the beginning of the 1970s, the director of the National Institute for Mental Health's (NIMH) Center for Schizophrenia Studies funded a residential program called Soteria House where patients labeled schizophrenic were successfully treated without drugs. The results were published in major medical journals.[16] What happened? NIMH voted to shut the project down. It had worked so well that it undermined the very credibility of the biological theory of "mental illness." But successful programs modeled on Soteria House still exist in Europe. Since Soteria, both professionals and people with labels have contributed to the literature on effective alternative treatments for schizophrenia and major depression.[17]

The Perception of Violence

The widespread acceptance of the medical model has correlated with a rise in public perception that mental patients are dangerous and violent, including a rise in media depictions of so-called violent crazies. Studies have consistently shown that there is a relationship between belief in the "illness" model and negative attitudes toward people with psychiatric labels.[18] What has not been shown is that we are more violent than people without labels.

Because the topic hadn't been rigorously studied, a group of prominent researchers known as the MacArthur Research Network on Mental Health and the Law (created by the MacArthur Foundation) set out to examine the relationship between psychiatric labels and violence. Their study is the one you will often find quoted and misquoted in discussions of the topic, because anyone who makes a public claim about violent mental patients must take it into account one way or another. Previous studies had been confounded by methodological problems: How do you define violence? Do people get labeled mentally ill because they are violent instead of the other way around? How do you factor in the rate of violence in the community at large?

The study, published in the *Archives of General Psychiatry* in 1998, compared 1,136 discharged mental patients in three cities with a nondiagnosed control group living in the same communities. Researchers followed the groups for a year and found that discharged mental patients were no more likely to commit violence than anyone else. The study did not look at whether the mental patients were prescribed psychiatric drugs, or if so whether they took the drugs. Thus, it drew no conclusions about the effects of these drugs on violent behavior. It offers absolutely no support for the claim that treatment reduces or prevents violence.[19]

Other researchers and reports uphold the conclusions of the MacArthur group.[20] None of the research shows that psychiatric drugs prevent violence or dangerousness.

Shock is commonly forced upon people with the assertion that if they don't have it, they will kill themselves. Judges and family members take the word of doctors on this view. But there is no proof that shock prevents suicide, even in studies done by its promoters. There is, however, evidence that people who have had shock kill themselves more frequently than those who haven't had it. We will examine this research in a later chapter.

Laws curtailing the civil and legal rights of mental patients, like inpatient and outpatient commitment, are generally sold to the public with the implied promise that they will reduce violent behavior toward self or others. That is the trade-off the public is asked to make: fewer rights for some, more safety for all. But once the laws are in effect, no one wants to know whether the trade-off had the expected benefit. It's enough, it seems, that more allegedly crazy people can be forced into treatment, even without evidence that it benefits society. In a kind of bait and switch, *after* laws are passed, states that have implemented outpatient commitment will claim it is for the good of or helps the patient. That's because they don't have evidence that it results in the promised drop in violent crime rates. As a matter of fact, a study by a legal advocacy group in New York State found that its outpatient commitment law (named for Kendra Webdale, who'd been pushed to her death on the New York City subway tracks) wasn't even being used against people with a history of violence. Eighty-five percent of those subjected to outpatient commitment had not harmed anybody.[21]

But to sell forced treatment on the grounds that it is good for patients rather than the public wouldn't work because it would require that the public care about mental patients. As D. J. Jaffe, one of the architects of Kendra's Law, told NAMI members, public safety is what people care about. "So if you're changing your laws in your states, you have to understand that. Now once you understand that, it means you have to take the debate out of the mental health arena and put it in the criminal justice / public safety arena."[22]

The strategy has worked, but it is clear that it has cost persons with psychiatric labels a great deal while benefiting society very little or not at all. A 2005 review of the outcome literature on outpatient commitment concluded that "it is . . . difficult to conceive of another group in society that would be subject to measures to curtail the freedom of 85 people to avoid one admission to hospital or of 238 to avoid one arrest."[23]

Does anyone care? In 2007, *USA Today* published the results of a study that found that mental patients die, on average, *twenty-five years earlier* than other Americans.[24] The study looked at people who were treated in public mental health systems, who constitute the majority of mental patients. It found that serious and preventable conditions associated with psychiatric drugs, like diabetes and heart disease, contributed to the patients' early demises. And the fact that doctors often dismissed patients' reports of physical symptoms didn't help.

The story came and went. There was no outcry, no initiative on the part of any government agency to address the issue. The revelation that mental patients have a life expectancy of one-third less than the rest of the population seemed to concern few except the mental patients, who circulated the story among themselves on the Internet.

Human and Civil Rights for Mental Patients

You have to look beyond the headlines to see the argument for human and civil rights of mental patients. Chances are you've never heard of the National Council on Disability (NCD), or read an op-ed in which a spokesperson from that organization was quoted. It is a federal agency that makes recommendations to the president and Congress on disability policy. On January 20, 2000, it published a report called "From Privileges to Rights: Persons with Psychiatric Disabilities Speak for Themselves." The report took as its starting premise that "persons with psychiatric disabilities are, first and foremost, citizens who have the right to expect that they will be treated according to the principles of law that apply to all other citizens." Yet after many hours of testimony from persons with psychiatric labels that this is overwhelmingly not the case, it concluded, "The manner in which American society treats people with psychiatric disabilities constitutes a national emergency and a national disgrace. . . . People with psychiatric disabilities are routinely deprived of their most fundamental rights. . . . Practices that would be illegal if administered to people without disabilities are routinely used on people with psychiatric disabilities in the name of 'treatment.' Such practices should shock the conscience of all Americans." The report noted that the hearing it convened was "one of the few opportunities shock recipients have had to testify publicly to a government body about their experiences." The testimony was largely about lasting damage to memory.

The NCD report concluded with ten public policy recommendations. One of them was that "laws that allow the use of involuntary treatments such as forced drugging and inpatient and outpatient commitment should be viewed as inherently suspect, because they are incompatible with the principle of self-determination." Another core recommendation was that "public policy should move towards the elimination of electro-convulsive therapy and psychosurgery as unproven and inherently inhumane procedures."

Either people with psychiatric labels are full citizens with the same legal, civil, and human rights as everyone else, or we are not. There is, as we have seen, a division of opinion on this issue in America.

If we are, then we cannot be locked up without due process and without having committed any crime, and we cannot be forced to ingest drugs or submit to electric shock. If not, then laws that allow or mandate us to be treated as less than competent, less than rational, and less than human—as well as procedures that damage us—will proliferate.

Does a mental patient's no mean no, or does it mean yes? Do her words have meaning only when she agrees with those who claim to know what's in her best interest? Does she have the right to decide what happens to her brain and body? Can she ever be believed when she says she's been harmed by her doctor?

These are not academic or theoretical questions. They have the most profound consequences for the lives of millions of Americans. They have also had profound consequences for the way ECT has been developed, used, researched, promoted, and sold to the public.

3   *Eugenic Conceptions II*

USELESS EATERS

Within memory of those still alive today is a time when it was not only acceptable to speak of mental patients as worthless defectives and malignant growths, it was possible for those at the highest levels of society and within organized psychiatry to act on these beliefs.

The eugenics movement—advocating segregation, forced sterilization, and even the killing of mental patients—blossomed in America in the early to mid-twentieth century, thanks to funding from men with household names like Kellogg and Eastman.[1] And the movement's agenda was not carried out in secret, but was promoted by eminent scientists at some of America's top research universities.

Andrew Carnegie and John D. Rockefeller bankrolled the work of Harvard biologist Charles Davenport, the leading eugenics crusader in the United States at the turn of the twentieth century. In 1910, Davenport established the Eugenics Record Office in Cold Spring Harbor, New York, the epicenter of the American eugenics movement. Its purpose was to transform eugenic ideas into laws. In practical terms, this meant hiring workers to go into mental hospitals to compile data on "the burden which the unfit place upon their fellow-men."[2]

The Record Office pressed for the segregation of those considered insane in asylums, and for laws requiring that they be forcibly sterilized to further ensure they would not produce others like themselves. It was clear that the desired "permanent segregation" of mental patients was not for therapeutic purposes, but for the good of society.

Eugenicists tried to cloak their mission in science, turning out studies designed to prove that mental illness was inherited. In the 1920s, top scientists, including prominent psychiatrists like Adolf Meyer and American Psychiatric Association president Floyd Haviland, came together to found the American Eugenics Society. Its mission was to sell eugenics and promote sterilization laws to the American public. Its tools were textbooks, pamphlets, advertising campaigns, and even exhibits at state fairs—such as one that drew the passerby's attention with large type proclaiming: "Some People Are Born To Be A Burden On The Rest."[3]

By the 1930s, the chief of research at the New York State Psychiatric Institute wrote that "mankind would be much happier" if society could rid itself of schizophrenics, who were not "biologically satisfactory."[4] One eugenics advocate dismissed any opposition as follows: "It is the acme of stupidity to talk in such cases of individual liberty, of the rights of the individual. Such individuals have no rights. They have no right in the first instance to be born."[5] The *New York Times* opined in 1923 that mental defectives should not be allowed to marry, and, in fact, by 1933 there were no states in which those deemed insane could legally wed. In 1927 the U.S. Supreme Court ruled that forced sterilization was legal, making America, and not Germany, what historian Robert Whitaker calls "the first eugenic country" on earth.[6]

Not only did mainstream America (including major medical journals, the *New York Times*, and the American Public Health Association) support forced sterilization laws, but calls for killing defectives or "euthanasia" were made publicly and shamelessly in this country in the first decades of the century. For instance, Alexis Carrel, a Nobel Prize–winning physician at the Rockefeller Institute for Medical Research, proposed that the insane "should be humanely and economically disposed of in small euthanasic institutions supplied with proper gases." The year was 1935.[7]

By 1941, the popularity of eugenics among the American intelligentsia was at its peak. In May of that year, Foster Kennedy, a leading neurologist and a professor at Cornell University, spoke at the annual meeting of the American Psychiatric Association on "The Problem of Social Control of the Congenital Defective: Education, Sterilization, Euthanasia." The following year, Kennedy published his views in the country's most prestigious psychiatric journal, the *American Journal of Psychiatry*.[8] He advocated that "feebleminded" (a broad and ill-defined category that included those labeled with schizophrenia and manic-depression) children, "nature's mistakes," be killed upon reaching the age of five. For a safeguard, he proposed three medical examinations before "euthanasia." Only if doctors agreed would the "defective" be "relieved of the burden of living." He claimed that parents would want this execution.

His article was accompanied by a rebuttal, of sorts, by child psychiatrist Leo Kanner. Kanner's argument was that the lives of some mentally disabled persons had value, but not in and of themselves; only to the extent that they could be of service to the rest of society by doing dirty and menial tasks like digging ditches and shucking oysters. Therefore, they ought not to be killed, as long as they were "industrious."[9]

An anonymous editorial, written by one or more of the journal's editors, concluded the debate.[10] The problem with murder, according to these commentators, was the attitudes people had about it. In particular, the editors noted that parents might have sentimental attachments even to defective children and suggested that psychiatrists play a role in modifying those psychopathological attitudes "by exposure to mental hygiene principles." It noted that there was no disagreement between Kennedy and Kanner about forced sterilization; both were in favor of it. Their differences were thus not as great as they might seem. As historian of psychiatry Jay Joseph has pointed out, "The progression from sterilization to killing is 'logical' because, once it has been established that the state should actively participate in preventing the reproduction of 'genetically undesirable' people through compulsory sterilization, it eventually seems more 'efficient' to wipe out the alleged gene carriers themselves."[11]

Early Somatic Treatments

In the era when eugenics openly flourished, so did drastic somatic treatments for those considered mentally ill. If their lives didn't matter, what did it matter what was done to them? If they were to die, that was of small concern; perhaps their only value was as experimental animals, on which "anything that holds out hope should be tried."[12]

Some of the treatments included malarial-fever therapy, in which high fevers were induced by injecting people with blood from malaria patients; sleep therapy, in which patients were drugged to make them sleep for a week or more; forced inhalation of carbon dioxide; and, by the 1930s, the deliberate destruction of healthy brain tissue known as psychosurgery (and later lobotomy). These were not considered marginal or unscientific treatments–far from it; the inventors of fever therapy and psychosurgery won medicine's highest honor, the Nobel Prize, in 1927 and 1949.[13]

It was in this climate that shock treatment was invented.

The name "shock" didn't originally refer to electrical shock, but to the physical state of shock produced by critically low blood sugar (hypoglycemia). In 1927 Manfred Sakel, a Viennese physician, inadvertently induced a coma in a patient by injecting her with too much insulin. He observed that her mental state, said to be psychotic, seemed improved when she woke up. After that, he experimented on animals in his kitchen, determined that the comas could be terminated with glucose without killing them, and then started deliberately overdosing persons with schizophrenia.[14]

Massive amounts of insulin deprive the brain of energy, inducing spasms and seizures. Overdosed patients eventually lapse into coma and die, but in insulin treatment they are injected with intravenous glucose to terminate the coma after several hours or whenever the doctor decides it's been long enough. This is repeated, five days a week, for up to three months.

Brain damage and death were the known and expected possible consequences of insulin shock. In a 1941 manual, psychiatrists were told: "Clinical evidence of neurological disturbances complicating shock therapy is abundant. Such clinical signs of brain damage have been confirmed by laboratory findings, electroencephalographic findings, and through psychological performance tests. . . . It is not unlikely that injury to the brain, either reversible or irreversible, is the common change resulting from the shock therapies. . . . We think the possibility of permanent brain damage exists."[15]

If a doctor failed to terminate a patient's coma with glucose injections in time, the result was "not infrequently" fatal, according to this manual. But it went on to reassure clinicians that "recovered psychiatric cases often show dramatic improvement in their mental state."

Sakel was not trained as a scientist and could not explain why his treatment worked. His attempt to do so was, historian Elliott Valenstein writes, "so vaguely stated and so impossible to relate to any known—let alone measurable—biological process that it was all but incomprehensible."[16]

In 1936, the commissioner of the New York State Office of Mental Hygiene was so impressed with the "cure" that he brought Sakel to New York to teach the state's doctors to perform it. Insulin was touted by the media in the 1930s as a "miracle" and became widely used in the United States through the 1960s.[17] Many thousands of survivors of insulin shock are alive today.

Sakel was bitter about the later use of the term "shock treatment" for ECT, saying, "There is just one shock treatment, introduced by me in 1933. . . . Convulsions produced by whatever means is not a distinct 'shock' or a new treatment."[18]

Seizures as Therapy

The idea of inducing epileptic seizures to "cure" mental patients was based on the erroneous assumption that schizophrenia and epilepsy never co-occur. Hungarian psychiatrist Ladislas Meduna came to this conclusion after studying slides of epileptic brain tissue.

Having come to a wrong conclusion based on speculation, he proceeded to experiment on a human. The first convulsive treatment took place, according to one account, on January 23, 1934. The person selected for this experiment had been in the hospital for four years in a catatonic state. On that morning, he was injected with a solution of camphor in oil, which caused a seizure. Meduna found the whole process so distressing that he had to be supported by his nurses afterwards when returning to his room.[19] Yet he somehow found it in him to repeat the process four more times. After the fifth seizure, the patient got out of bed. He was eventually released from the hospital.

By all accounts, the patient forgot at least four years of his life; he knew nothing of having been in the hospital. But he hadn't died, and his symptoms abated, at least temporarily. The experiment was considered a success.

Camphor proved an unreliable way of inducing seizures, however, and was soon replaced by a synthetic camphor preparation called metrazol (its European name is cardiazol). A series of metrazol treatments involved twenty to forty closely spaced induced seizures. Because of the violence of the seizures, patients were at great risk of broken bones and teeth. It was undisputed that the treatment caused memory loss, and the pattern of amnesia and impaired memory ability—which increased with the number of treatments and was most dense for more recent memories—was the same as what was to emerge with electroshock. For example, a 1939 case study found that a patient who had excelled at Chinese checkers and badminton prior to treatment not only could no longer play them but had forgotten the rules. The researchers concluded that "metrazol acts in such a noxious manner as to destroy recently established neural patterns of the highest cerebral functions."[20]

Patients feared the treatment to such an extent that some doctors theorized that fear was actually the therapeutic element of the treatment.[21] Patients were conscious for the five to fifteen seconds it took for the seizure to occur after the metrazol injection. One described the treatment as "being roasted alive in a white hot furnace" and a psychiatrist observed that nearly all patients were "overwhelmed by fear of impending death."[22] The terror patients experienced before losing consciousness was described as like being thrown off a high building.[23]

Afterwards, metrazol produced a profound change in patients' behavior. As with insulin, patients who'd been shocked became childlike (to the point of regression), cooperative, and docile. They also frequently experienced permanent amnesia. Whether this was seen as "improvement" or brain damage depended on who was doing the seeing, and what value the person placed on the lives and brains of mental patients. Early research showed brain damage in autopsied animals and humans, as well as abnormalities of the electroencephalogram (EEG), which were dismissed as consistent with clinical improvement.[24] One metrazol apologist suggested that the patient's "readaption to normal life" came at the expense of a permanent lowering of intellectual functioning, but seemed sanguine about that possibility; the patient might, "in the language of chess, be sacrificing a piece to win the game."[25]

Early data were equivocal as to whether metrazol worked at all, with some doctors claiming good results, one hospital reporting no success at all in a group of 275 patients, and yet others reporting poorer outcomes than with no treatment.[26] But professional judgment was clearly in favor of the procedure; doctors were okay with sacrificing their patients' chess pieces, it seemed, whether they won the game or not. The press, as with insulin, uncritically praised the new shock treatment. Metrazol shock was soon widely adopted, and by 1940, all major mental hospitals in the United States used it.

Dogs, Hogs, and Human Guinea Pigs

Meanwhile, in fascist Italy, psychiatrists Ugo Cerletti and Lucio Bini were experimenting with convulsive treatments. Their work was funded by the fascist movement, and was informed by the same eugenic agenda as in the United States and Germany: they were looking for ways to lighten the financial and social burden mental patients unfairly placed on everyone else.

In the 1930s, Cerletti and Bini had developed the first apparatus for inducing seizures by use of electricity, and had been experimenting on dogs, killing large numbers of them. Their dogs died because the Italian researchers had placed the electrodes on the mouth and anus, and the electric current passed through the heart. They were afraid to place electrodes on the brain for fear of causing damage to it. That would have muddied the eventual results of their experiments, which were designed to investigate the effects of epilepsy on the brain. At the time, Cerletti said he never thought that these experiments would have any practical application.

Then Cerletti learned about Meduna's work; Meduna claimed it was he who first suggested to Cerletti and Bini that they try electricity as a means of inducing seizures in humans.[27] Cerletti pondered, "For the first time we were considering epileptic seizures not as a harmful and pernicious manifestation, but as a useful one in certain psychotic states."[28] But would electric shock kill the patients?

In a Rome slaughterhouse, Cerletti had a revelation. He saw pigs being shocked with electrodes on the sides of their heads. The shocks to the head didn't kill the animals, but stunned them so that they didn't squeal and struggle while they were butchered. "Very likely," Cerletti admitted in 1950, "except for this fortuitous and fortunate circumstance of pigs' pseudo-electrical butchery, electroshock would not have been born."[29]

With pigs as his research subjects, Cerletti then conducted the only pre-market clinical safety trials of electroshock that have ever been done. He described the results as follows:

> The animals rarely died, and then only when the duration of electric current flowed through the body and not the head. The animals that received the severest treatment remained rigid during the flow of the

electric current, then after a violent convulsive seizure they would lie on their sides for a while, sometimes for several minutes, and finally they would attempt to rise. After many attempts of increasing efficacy, they would succeed in standing up and making a few hesitant steps until they were able to run away. These observations gave me convincing evidence of the harmlessness of a few tenths of a second of application through the head of a 125-volt electric current, which was more than enough to ensure a complete convulsive seizure.[30]

"At this point," Cerletti said, "I felt we could venture to experiment on man." This was so even though his examinations of the brains of animals he killed after shock left little doubt that the procedure had caused many "undoubtedly pathological" changes, which he described in great detail.[31]

That the observation that shocked animals were able to run away from further treatment was all it took to convince the inventor of ECT that it was safe for humans is likely to stun the modern American conscience. We would like to believe that medical treatments have been rigorously tested. Even in an era of warning labels, we trust that they would not be allowed to be used if they had not been found to be reasonably safe. But this was the late 1930s, in a fascist country and an era when eugenicists in many countries openly advocated "euthanasia" of mental patients, and only a heartbeat away from the first planned, deliberate killings of patients by psychiatrists. There was no Food and Drug Administration evaluating Cerletti's homemade shock machine. There were no review boards deciding whether the research was safe. Not only was no one protecting the rights of human guinea pigs, there was no recognition that mental patients had any rights at all.

A Superstitious Notion

Clinical trials concluded, Cerletti set out to find a subject for the first application of ECT to a human, and found it in a vagrant who was picked up by police for loitering in a train station. The man, known in the literature only as S.E., was arrested on April 15, 1938, and brought to the hospital "for observation." He sought no psychiatric treatment, consented to no treatment, and was held against his will. Nothing was known of his past history. On April 18, 1938, Cerletti found him to be "lucid" and "well-oriented," but with "low affective reserves." A diagnosis of "schizophrenic syndrome" was made, and the experiment proceeded. The treatment was given in secret because of fears about what could happen.

At first, the machine was set to deliver only eighty volts of electricity, and it produced neither unconsciousness nor a seizure. Cerletti described what happened:

> Naturally, we, who were conducting the experiment, were under great emotional strain and felt that we had already taken quite a risk. Nevertheless, it was quite evident to all of us that we had been using a too low voltage. It was proposed that we should allow the patient to have some rest and repeat the experiment the next day. All at once, the patient, who evidently had been following the conversation, said clearly and solemnly, without his usual gibberish: "Not another one! It will kill me!" I confess that such explicit admonition under such circumstances, and coming from a person whose enigmatic jargon had until then been very difficult to understand, shook my determination to carry on with the experiment. But it was just this fear of yielding to a superstitious notion that caused me to make up my mind. The electrodes were applied again.[32]

Looking back at his invention, Cerletti admitted, "When I saw the patient's reaction, I thought to myself, This should be abolished! Ever since I have looked forward to the time when another treatment would replace electroshock."[33] Had Cerletti spoken or published his thoughts at the time, he could have unilaterally abolished electroshock at the outset. But he probably would have seen that as yielding to the superstitious notion that patients should have control over their brains and bodies.

Interestingly, a history of ECT written by contemporary proponents has cast doubt on all the previously published accounts of the first electroshock. They relate a different account, said to have been discovered in Bini's unpublished and untranslated notebook. According to these authors, Cerletti's first attempt to induce a seizure was unsuccessful, and the patient was allowed to leave the treatment room. The outcome of the second try on an unnamed woman is not specified, and not until the third try more than a week later did the procedure induce a grand mal seizure in the original patient, who was said to have recovered after ten more shocks. The authors conclude that "the creators of electroshock had been so eager to give the public a perfect story that they concealed a few weaknesses to their claims present in the record."[34]

If true, that was the earliest case of shock doctors managing concerns about ECT with public relations tactics, and it worked. The new shock therapies—insulin, metrazol, and electric—were adopted widely, quickly, and uncritically. Insulin, introduced in 1933, reached its peak use in 1938 when 54 percent of hospitals reported using it. Metrazol, introduced in 1935, peaked in 1939 with 65 percent of hospitals using it. Electroshock was adopted even more quickly and soon used more widely than either insulin or metrazol. In a survey conducted in 1941, 93 percent of state institutions and 74 percent of private institutions in the United States reported using one or more forms of shock treatment.[35]

The popular press of the time–*Newsweek, Time, Reader's Digest, Science Digest, Scientific American,* and others—played a major role in promoting the therapies, feeding the public's appetite for dramatic cures.[36] In addition, a veritable avalanche of favorable articles about shock treatment appeared in the major psychiatric journals. At last, the publicity suggested, psychiatry was really doing something scientific for its lost souls.

Animals in Human Form

But there remained the problem for psychiatry of the long-term, chronic patients who were not helped by the new somatic treatments. Germany was about to come up with a solution.

The idea that mental patients were "useless eaters" who ought to be killed for the good of all had been popularized by German psychiatrists Alfred Hoche and Karl Binding in their 1920 book *Permission for the Destruction of Lives Unworthy of Life.* In the 1920s, the German eugenics movement thrived thanks to substantial funding from Americans. The Rockefeller Foundation, for instance, gave the equivalent of millions of dollars in today's money to the Kaiser Wilhelm Institute, which became Germany's leading center for eugenics research. Charles Davenport's successor as president of the International Federation of Eugenic Organizations was German psychiatrist and director of the Kaiser Wilhelm Institute for Psychiatry Ernst Rudin—best remembered today as one of Hitler's henchmen.[37]

German psychiatrists began putting eugenic ideas into practice as early as 1938, starving psychiatric patients, including children, to death in asylums. Psychiatry embarked on this course on its own initiative, out of its own eugenic zeal, without any directive or mandate from Adolf Hitler. In 1939 leading German psychiatrists organized, not to debate or to protest the killing of mental patients, but to decide on the best method. After ruling out staged train crashes, they consulted with police toxicologists and settled on carbon monoxide gas. Historian Michael Burleigh describes the conversation that took place between a Nazi official and a chemist:

"Can the Criminal Technical Institute manufacture large quantities of poison?"
"For what? To kill people?"
"No."
"To kill animals?"
"No."
"What for, then?"
"To kill animals in human form: that means the mentally ill, whom one can no longer describe as human and for whom no recovery is in sight."[38]

In October 1939, the first "questionnaires" were distributed throughout the German mental hospital system. For each patient, a panel of psychiatrists would make a selection: + for life, − for death, ? if they weren't sure. Hitler's "Law on Euthanasia for the Incurably Ill" was drafted in 1940 in response to pressure from psychiatrists, and backdated to serve as justification for what the doctors were already doing.[39]

Gas chambers and crematoriums were set up within psychiatric institutions. The killing centers were under the control and administration of psychiatrists from 1939 to 1941. The organized killing of mental patients was code-named Operation T-4, after the name and number of the street where it was headquartered. Its official name, the one it used on its letterhead, was the Reich Association of Mental Hospitals. Hitler took over the control of T-4 late in 1941, in response to public protest by a prominent Catholic bishop.

Ostensibly, T-4 was shut down; actually, it simply became decentralized, and euthanasia was integrated into daily asylum routine. In fact, the T-4 program largely supported itself financially through fraudulent billings to insurance companies and welfare agencies.[40]

The enthusiastic use of shock treatment was an integral part of the T-4 plan. The plan called for drastically reducing the number of beds in German psychiatric hospitals by either "active therapy" (shock) or "euthanasia." The available statistics show a clear connection between the increased use of insulin or electric shock and a rise in inpatient deaths. When the use of insulin was forbidden because of wartime scarcity, the Führer's office and the Reich's commissioner for mental hospitals called the provision of electroshock equipment particularly "important to the war effort." By 1943, nearly all public hospitals had electroshock machines, thanks to the advocacy of the T-4 procurement adviser.[41]

Psychiatrists who had been in charge of the killing centers for mental patients went on to initiate the "Final Solution" for the Jews. Dr. Werner Heyde, who had been in charge of Operation T-4, led the commission of psychiatrists in charge of selecting people for death at Buchenwald, Ravensbruck, and Auschwitz. The original commandants and staff of the death camps at Treblinka, Belzec, and Sobibor were recruited from the T-4 program.

When the Germans tested the feasibility and practicality of mass killings on mental patients, they simply chose the path of least resistance. Some degree of complicity on the part of the public was necessary for the success of their enterprise. If the public had mobilized against the killing of mental patients, the holocaust of the Jews might not have taken place. The mental patient experiment showed that the public was, in fact, willing to accept mass killing as a solution to perceived social problems—at least, as long as the victims were devalued and seen as less than human.

At least 270,000 mental patients were killed between 1939 and 1946.[42]

Not So Far from There to Here:
The Genesis of the American Shock Industry

The ECT industry would not be what it is today without the psychiatrists of the Nazi era. Indeed, the most vocal shock proponents in the United

States. trace their training to a group of emigrés that played a role in the eugenics-based psychiatry of Europe. These few men in prestigious positions wielded enormous influence through their teaching and writing.

Lothar Kalinowsky (1899–1992) trained as a psychiatrist in Berlin, but lost his position in 1933 because he was half Jewish. That same year he was offered a job at Cerletti's hospital in Rome. On a trip to Vienna in 1936 he observed Meduna's metrazol shock, and reported back to Cerletti. Supposedly, according to Kalinowsky, Cerletti then asked, "Why didn't he use electricity?"[43] Kalinowsky was present at the earliest shock treatments and was responsible for doing neurological evaluations of the patients.

His initial reaction to the treatment was less than enthusiastic. "According to my wife—because I don't remember it exactly—she claims that when I came home I was very pale and said 'I saw something terrible today—I never want to see that again!'"[44] But somehow, that attitude soon changed to boundless zeal.

When the Axis pact between Germany and Italy required the return of German nationals to Germany, Kalinowsky fled to America. On the way he made stops in England, Holland, and France as a kind of shock evangelist, introducing the treatment to each country and finding time to publish on ECT as he went. But it was in America, where he landed in 1940, that he met his greatest success. He was immediately offered a position at the New York State Psychiatric Institute (P.I.) in upper Manhattan, a facility that was quite hospitable to German emigrés at that time.

On its Web site, P.I. takes full credit for "the introduction of electroconvulsive therapy to the U.S. by Lothar Kalinowsky."[45] But Kalinowsky said that the first shock in America was probably given by David Impastato at Columbus Hospital, a private hospital in New York City.[46] Others claim that it was given in Chicago a month earlier.[47]

Nevertheless, as we shall see, P.I. has played a larger role in the selling of electroshock than any institution in America. This is largely because it is a research facility that has aggressively and successfully sought state and federal funding. More funding equals more publications equals more influence. Although it is a state facility, P.I. has had, since 1925, a unique affiliation agreement with Columbia University's College of Physicians and Surgeons, which adds immeasurably to its perceived prestige.

Kalinowsky taught at P.I. for twenty years. In 1946, he authored a textbook on *Shock Treatments and Other Somatic Procedures in Psychiatry*, which influenced a generation of psychiatrists. In 1958, Kalinowsky helped found New York City's private Gracie Square Hospital, which was known then and to this day as a shock mill (a pejorative term long used for facilities that shock disproportionately large percentages of their patients).[48]

Kalinowsky trained many doctors to administer ECT at P.I. and later at New York Medical College in Manhattan. One of them was Richard Abrams. Abrams says that as a young medical student, he took to Kalinowsky like a lost duckling to its mother: "My synapses snapped shut like a steel trap; imprinting was instantaneous and complete."[49] With training from Kalinowsky and also from prominent ECT advocate Max Fink, Abrams, a former professor at the Chicago Medical School, has devoted his career to promoting shock.

Other German emigrés who played public roles in promoting shock were Zigmund Lebensohn of Washington, D.C.; Paul Hoch, who served as P.I.'s first chief of biological psychiatry and co-wrote the first shock textbook with Kalinowsky; and Leo Alexander, who served as an apologist for the Nazis at the Nuremberg trials and published extensively on ECT.[50]

These shock enthusiasts did far more to popularize the use of shock than its inventors, who abandoned the technique in favor of even more bizarre treatments. In March 1939, Ladislas Meduna entered the United States, ostensibly to give a lecture in Chicago; but he intended to stay and managed to do so, thanks to an appointment at Loyola University. After losing interest in metrazol, he told himself that "the next logical step, I think, will be the acceptance of carbon dioxide, and other gases yet to be discovered, as legitimate medicaments for treatment for suitable pathologic conditions." For the rest of his life his "treatment" consisted of inhalations of carbon dioxide mixed with nitrous oxide.[51]

Cerletti played no part in publicizing and promoting his invention. Until his death, he continued to believe neither the seizure nor the electricity caused the dramatic changes in mood and behavior, but some hormone secreted as a result of the shock. He electroshocked storks, hogs, sheep, and rabbits in an attempt to isolate this "defensive substance," which he named "acro-agonine" from the Greek for "supreme struggle for survival." He then tried to cure human patients by injecting them with extracts from the brains of electroshocked pigs. In the end he gave up, concluding that "the solution to these problems lies within the domain of the biochemists."[52]

The first electroshock patient was reported by his wife to have relapsed three months after his series of eleven shock treatments. Cerletti later found out that in fact, this man had received eight metrazol treatments in December 1937, less than four months prior to his being diagnosed as sufficiently ill to serve as the human guinea pig for the first electric shock. Apparently neither treatment had any lasting benefit.[53]

Acknowledging the Mental Patient Holocaust

It is only recently that mainstream psychiatry has acknowledged the mass killings of mental patients by their psychiatrists. In August 1999, the congress of the World Psychiatric Association in Munich, attended by 10,000 psychiatrists, featured an exhibition titled "In Memoriam," documenting German psychiatrists' extermination of their patients. They admitted to 180,000 killings. During the initial ceremony of the congress, the president of the German Society for Psychiatry, Psychotherapy, and Neurology publicly admitted that the killing of mental patients amounted to another holocaust.[54]

Some of those who killed their patients are likely alive as you read this book, and many of them lived well, rising to prestigious positions, without censure, shame, or guilt. For example, Austrian psychiatrist Heinrich Gross, accused of experimenting on thousands of children and killing many of them, died in December 2005 at age ninety. He was never tried for his crimes and died proclaiming his innocence.[55]

Though the massacre of mental patients took place on a smaller scale and was less well known than the massacre of the Jews, the larger holocaust could not have taken place without the earlier one. As one German physician said in 1947, "It is almost the same thing to see a human being as a 'case' or as a number tattooed on his arm. This is the double facelessness of a merciless epoch."[56]

Electroshock is the only one of the drastic somatic "treatments" developed in the eugenics era that is still in use today and the only one whose very name doesn't evoke derision or horror. The reasons for this are twofold.

First, the ECT industry was able to rebrand its product as "new and improved," a feat of pure public relations when it was nothing of the sort. Second, eugenic conceptions of persons with psychiatric labels have not gone away; they simply take different forms in an era, ostensibly, of informed consent and patient rights. When understood in their simplest form as *"They* are a threat to *us,"* they have not really changed at all. Without eugenic attitudes, no matter how brilliantly it was marketed, shock would have died off; countervailing forces would have been able to successfully unmask the marketing schemes. The genius of ECT's promoters and packagers has been to adapt, chameleon-like, to changing social attitudes, including evolving eugenic conceptions of mental patients, and to respond to challenges with unwavering and ever greater denial.

4   *A Little Brain Pathology*

If it were a drug or a medical device coming onto the market today, electroshock would have to be proven safe and effective in controlled trials, and would have to be cleared for use by the Food and Drug Administration (FDA). Because there were no such safeguards in effect in 1938, and because ECT's inventors and promoters had never thought it necessary to carefully study large numbers of patients before selling their treatment to the world, each patient became, in effect, a guinea pig.

This was a time before in vivo brain imaging was possible; the CAT scan, MRI, and PET scan were decades away. To study the effects of ECT, experimental animals had to be sacrificed and their brains examined under the microscope. Human brains could only be examined after death occurred, either naturally or as a direct result of electroshock. Both human and animal brain autopsy studies were common in the early years of ECT, and so many showed damage to the brain that, ever since, proponents of ECT have been obliged either to try to discredit their findings or pretend they didn't exist.

Animal Experiments

Lucio Bini, electroshock's co-inventor, first published a brief report of his and Cerletti's early dog experiments in the *American Journal of Psychiatry* in 1938. Though electroshock was already being used on humans by then, he described his use of shock on animals as "experimental researches." He reported that after shock "the alterations found by us in the nervous systems of these dogs were widespread and severe. Besides acute injury to the nerve cells, there was 'chronic cell disease.'" He concluded that with electroshock as with insulin, "these very alterations may be responsible for the favorable transformation of the morbid psychic picture of schizophrenia."[1]

In the 1940s and 1950s, studies were conducted on cats, rats, dogs, rabbits, guinea pigs, and monkeys. Virtually all of this evidence supports the position that ECT causes damage of various types to the brain. These include gliosis (a process in which glia, a type of central nervous system support cell, are overproduced and form scar tissue around a damaged area), pinpoint and large hemorrhages, and neuronal cell death.

In a 1946 review of the animal studies conducted to date, Dr. Bernard J. Alpers of Philadelphia—who'd done some of the earliest research himself—warned that "brain changes have been found even in those cases in which the experiments have been regarded as negative." In what could have been a response to Cerletti's mistaken conclusion that ECT was safe because the first patient survived, he wrote: "The problem is obviously not whether electrical shock is a cause of death, but whether it is associated with brain changes of any sort, and if so what those changes may signify." He warned against the danger of adding "injury to insult" in the life of the mental patient by the use of ECT and concluded, "Security in the application of shock treatments is ill-founded."[2]

Lothar Kalinowsky and his colleagues at the New York State Psychiatric Institute (P.I.) did their best to explain away findings of brain damage.

Even if we did find changes present, which we definitely believe to be pathological, what is their significance as far as the status of the patient or the status of the monkey is concerned? We merely have two coordinates here in our two sets of observations and they are manifestly insufficient to solve our question. If we subject an animal or a patient to electric shock and then find certain neurohistological or pathological conditions in the brain, and also find that the patient shows some peculiarity in behavior, are we justified in assuming that the changes in the brain and behavior are causally related? I don't think any of us would even seriously consider that as a compelling conclusion at all.[3]

In the mid-1940s, even animal research carried out at P.I. by stalwarts of ECT confirmed brain damage from the procedure. Two often-cited monkey studies were done by Armando Ferraro, a principal research scientist in neuropathology, and Leon Roizen, the chief of psychiatric research in neuropathology.[4] They found cell death and petechial (pinpoint) hemorrhages in monkeys given four to twelve shocks with low amounts of electricity, and had to attribute the findings to ECT. A second study in which monkeys received more shocks confirmed the findings of the earlier one.

The longest, most detailed, and most scientifically rigorous animal experiment to date is Hans Hartelius's 1952 cat study. Carried out at a prestigious medical university in Sweden, it took four years to complete, and was reported in a research paper that is the length of a book.[5] He shocked his forty-one animals with cat-sized electrodes and only enough electricity to elicit a seizure; that is, much less electricity, proportionately, than is now used on humans. The cats were pampered with fresh milk and Baltic herring. Within eight days of the last shock, their brains were removed for examination (under anesthesia while the cats were still alive, in order to rule out brain damage caused by the process of dying itself). Sixteen control cats were sacrificed in the same manner.

There were two parts to Hartelius's article: a review of the existing literature and the report of his experiments. In the review, he showed that the vast majority of studies on ECT showed brain abnormalities: vascular changes, changes in the glial cells essential to brain function, nerve cell changes, even "disappearance of nerve cells and areas of devastation." He critiqued the existing studies and gave reasons for some discrepancies in their findings (for instance, rabbit and rat brains are not similar enough to humans). Hartelius remarked that researchers who saw brain changes as "reversible" often made that claim when the damage had persisted for several months—in other words, they assumed that the damage would reverse itself at some point in the future. Other researchers claimed reversibility when they had killed the animals too soon after shock to know whether the damage repaired itself.

In examining the brains of the shocked cats and the control animals, Hartelius was "blind"—he didn't know, when he examined slides of brain tissue, which group they were taken from. But he had no trouble correctly identifying the shocked brains. He saw in them the types of damage that had been described in the earlier studies. And he statistically ruled out the possibility that any other factor besides shock could have caused the changes he saw in the brains. The most marked abnormalities, such as shadow cells (in which the material formerly housed in a cell nucleus has disappeared), were found in the cats who had had eleven to sixteen shocks, pointing to a direct correlation between the number of shocks and the degree of damage.

Hartelius concluded: "On the basis of the present results, the question of whether or not irreversible nerve cell changes may occur after ECT must be answered in the affirmative. . . . Either the actual electric current or the epileptic seizure may be the injurious factor."

In another cat study by Jules Masserman, a professor of psychiatry at Northwestern University in Chicago, animals deemed neurotic (purposely made so by maltreatment by their handlers) and normal cats were subjected to ten shocks in the same manner as humans.[6] They were given three shocks a week using the amount of electricity used on humans at that time, which is considerably less than is used today. All cats showed persistent deficits after shock: loss of spontaneity and initiative, disorientation for space and time, difficulty in shifting cognitive strategies to adapt to changing conditions, difficulties of retention, and "most evident of all, a marked impairment in the efficiency and facility with which the animal performed complex, recently-learned patterns such as operating the switch which opened its food box." It was also noted that six of the eight cats, "although ordinarily friendly," actively resisted being prepared for the treatment, and some showed anxiety and fear.

These effects of shock weren't specific to emotional disturbance; shock produced the same effects in normal and disturbed cats. In the case of the so-called neurotic animals, their induced abnormal behavior had been replaced by "simpler," more normal behavior—what in humans would be applauded as "recovery." But even in cats, it was clear to the researchers that "the price of recovery was a variable loss of certain higher adaptive capacities; e.g., even at the end of their post-shock testing period, four of the animals in this study had not re-acquired their normal facility and efficiency in complex skills of which they had formerly been capable."

The brains of the shocked cats, when examined under the microscope, showed slight but not gross changes. The researchers concluded that "the most likely inferences to be derived from the anatomical portions of our study were that the histologic and microscopic techniques employed were less adequate as an index of the molecular changes in brain structure or function produced by neurosis or electroshock than were the actual deviations of behavior observed in the living animals." The researchers noted that, similarly, in shocked humans, tests used on ECT patients are most likely not sensitive enough to disclose "subtle impairment of higher perceptive and integrative functions . . . similar to those that result from known organic lesions of the brain."

In 1974 neurobiologist James McGaugh reviewed the evidence on amnesia in shocked animals, mostly from studies conducted in the 1960s, and concluded that the memory loss was permanent: "Overall there is little evidence to support the view that ECS [the term used for ECT in animals] produces only temporary retrograde amnesia."[7] He hypothesized that ECS interferes with the memory storage process. But he did not go so far as to make the logical conclusion, that amnesia is permanent in humans as well.

Animal research on ECT slowed to a near-standstill in the 1960s and 1970s, with few studies reported in the English-language journals. A German study in 1966 found necrosis (neuronal death) and gliosis in shocked cats and concluded that "irreversible, intracellular dysfunction is unavoidable."[8] In 1971, Russian researchers documented brain damage in rats subjected to shock.[9] And in 1975, researchers looked at the brains of rats two months after electroshock and found "persistent decrease in neuronal volume." The authors concluded, "This constitutes a serious warning against the use of electroconvulsive therapy."[10]

Human Autopsy Studies

In 1942 the first published results of human autopsy studies began to appear, also documenting significant brain damage. One of the earliest cases was a forty-five-year-old woman who died after receiving sixty-two shocks. Bernard Alpers and Joseph Hughes wrote, "The importance of the case lies in that it offers a clear demonstration of the fact that electrical convulsion treatment is followed at times by structural damage of the brain."[11]

More than three dozen published human autopsy reports from 1942 to 1956 show brain abnormalities. Not all patients autopsied suffered cerebral complications, such as hemorrhage, severe enough to cause death—some died from other causes—but about 40 percent did. A review of these reports reveals that "by far the most frequent alterations reported were in the vascular system"—with twenty-three cases of hemorrhages large and small. Other brain changes symptomatic of damage included atrophy (shrinkage), edema (swelling in the acute period after ECT), necrosis (death of brain tissue), and "rents and slits similar to those reported in electrocution."[12]

One neuropathologist remarked, "What makes this picture, just like any other neuropathological picture a significant one, is the combination of changes; in all observations of sudden death after electric shock reported so far, petechial hemorrhages, cellular changes and some glial proliferation stand out prominently, as an almost constant whole."[13]

In 1957, ECT was found to have an overall mortality rate of one in one thousand, and one in two hundred in elderly patients. The rate was higher for those who had received what was beginning to be called modified shock, administered under anesthesia and using muscle-paralyzing drugs to prevent fractures of bones and teeth.[14] Autopsy reports of patients who died from ECT continued to be published into the 1960s.[15]

Doctors who observed large numbers of patients post-ECT warned that the patients were clearly suffering from an acute organic brain syndrome like that seen in other people with brain injuries. In 1942, Dr. Roy Grinker, the author of a neurology textbook, wrote: "There is not only an emotional but an intellectual change in the patients. Those who have seen fighters that have been in many battles know the 'punch-drunk' or 'slap-happy' conditions and may recognize a similar state in some patients after shock therapy . . . Careful studies by means of a battery of neurologic tests reveal a definite 'organic' change in memory which does not entirely clear up."[16] His contemporary, prominent Boston psychiatrist Abraham Myerson, observed that "the mechanism of improvement and recovery seems to be to knock out the brain and reduce the higher activities, to impair memory, and thus the newer acquisition of the mind, namely the pathological state, is forgotten."[17]

That these observations were consistent with the findings of brain damage in the histological studies was clear even to a proponent of ECT such as Max Fink, who wrote in 1958: "From the data available, it is probable that the biochemical basis of convulsive therapy is similar to that of craniocerebral trauma. . . . The electroencephalographic [EEG] effect of repeated induced convulsions is the development of . . . slow [brain] wave activity, occasionally with spike activity which is similar to that observed in severe head trauma."[18] (Today, Fink still tells his students that slow brain waves are therapeutic for mental patients, but no longer mentions that they are symptomatic of brain damage.)

There was no sense in which the doctors at the time who admitted ECT was brain damaging felt they were saying anything unacceptable to the profession or the public. In the 1940s, as we have seen, mental patients in Germany were being killed by their psychiatrists, without any outcry from the profession there or elsewhere. Portuguese neurologist Egas Moniz was awarded the Nobel Prize in 1949 for leucotomy—a type of psychosurgery that deliberately destroyed healthy tissue in the name of curing intractable mental illness. Psychiatrists in America, such as Walter Freeman, enthusiastically adopted the technique and renamed their version lobotomy. They used an ice pick or similar instrument and inserted it into the brain via the eye sockets to sever their patients' frontal lobes.

The widespread popularity of lobotomy in the 1940s and 1950s showed that mainstream psychiatry believed—as I hold it still does—that mental patients were less than full human beings. A little brain damage was thus of no consequence; in fact, it was therapeutic, as Abraham Myerson explained in 1942:

> I believe there have to be organic changes or organic disturbances in the physiology of the brain for the cure to take place. I think the disturbance in memory is probably an integral part of the recovery process. I think it may be true that these people have for the time being at any rate more intelligence than they can handle and that the reduction of intelligence is an important factor in the curative process. I say this without cynicism. The fact is that some of the very best cures that one gets are in those individuals whom one reduces almost to amentia [feeblemindedness]. It is impossible to conceive of that amentia without an organic base; there must be at least temporarily organic changes in the brain, and the cure is related to these organic alterations.[19]

Paul Hoch of the New York State Psychiatric Institute wrote in 1948: "This brings us for a moment to a discussion of the brain damage caused by electroshock. . . . Is a certain amount of brain damage not necessary in this type of treatment? Frontal lobotomy indicates that improvement takes place by a definite damage of certain parts of the brain."[20]

"Of course," opined Bernard Pacella (another colleague of Kalinowsky's at P.I.) in 1944, "one could always argue that a normal clinical status or at least a socially adaptable individual with a little brain pathology is preferable to a psychotic patient with no demonstrable brain changes."[21]

"Fueliginous Tenebrosity": Effects on Memory, Learning, Cognition

Today, nearly all articles on ECT appearing in medical journals begin, "ECT is a safe and effective treatment . . . ," thus precluding any investigation of shock's adverse effects.

But before the public relations era, when some doctors seemed genuinely interested in research whether or not the results were bad for business, there was a relative wealth of literature describing shock's effects not only on brain structure, but specifically on memory and cognition.

In 1942 not even the researchers at the Psychiatric Institute were convinced of shock's harmlessness to memory. As one colleague of Kalinowsky's put it: "I don't know how to account for the memory defect. I know that it occurs . . . even after two or perhaps three convulsions, these patients may appear to have a tremendous memory defect, and be greatly concerned over it; but I do not know the basis for this. I do not like to get entangled too much in what has been called 'fueliginous tenebrosity' on this particular matter."[22]

Leon Salzman, a professor of psychiatry in Washington, D.C., reviewed the literature up to 1947, and also studied patients who had had shock six months to three years previously, comparing them to patients who hadn't had shock: "The most persistent impression obtained is that the shock patients show a picture resembling the post-lobotomy syndrome. . . . In addition to their inattention and inability to concentrate there was some difficulty in carrying out tasks that they were well trained to do before their illness. One 55-year-old male who worked at the switch control tower in a railroad intersection found himself completely unable to handle the tasks he had previously done for 20 years. Even 6 months following shock therapy he found himself unable to return to his former employment."[23]

In a 1947 study done at P.I., Calvin Stone also recognized that it was not simply memory that was impaired by ECT: "Even the most cursory psychometric examination of patients who complain of memory losses will reveal a considerable degree of impairment in ability to comprehend what is heard or read, in simple arithmetical computations, in perception of relationships, in choice reactions, and in performance of tasks involving abstraction, classification, and arrangement of words or objects according to a specified plan. Therefore, it would seem to be not only more informative but more correct to speak of general impairment of the cognitive functions resulting from electro-convulsive shocks."[24]

British psychiatrist S. M. Cannicott, summarizing some of the work done in the 1940s and 1950s, wrote in 1962:

> ECT has proved the most widely used and successful of modern psychiatric treatments, but at a price. . . . Many patients . . . complain of memory difficulties associated with recent events; many show post-convulsive confusional states; and a minority complain of a feeling of blotting-out—"the agonizing experience of the shattered self" (Schildge, 1947; Stengel, 1951) whilst Anderson (1951 and 1953) quotes examples of poets who ceased creative work following electro-convulsive therapy and professors and students who forgot large parts of their knowledge. . . . Ritchie Russell (1959) says, "Intelligence seems to depend on the capacity to associate a vast number of memories with each other and one memory seems to be built on previous memories." . . . the impairment of memory involves a good deal more than a simple forgetting of recent events: *"if this memory disturbance is at all severe the intelligence will be, temporarily at least, affected."* The work of Cronholm and Molander (1957), applying a battery of tests to patients before and after ECT, tends to confirm these views . . . and Stone (1946) suggested a general impairment of cognitive function.[25]

Criticism from the Profession

In 1941, when ECT had been in use only three years, a standard psychiatric textbook called *Shock Treatment in Psychiatry* summarized the existing human and animal research as follows: "A great deal of evidence has been accumulated which indicates that brain damage is possible with this kind of therapy."[26]

As evidence continued to accumulate, organized psychiatry took the unprecedented step of issuing a warning to the field. In 1947, the Group for the Advancement of Psychiatry (GAP) reviewed the evidence and published a report called *Shock Therapy*.[27] GAP was organized in 1946 by Karl and William Menninger, two of the era's most respected psychiatrists and cofounders of the Menninger Clinic. GAP members held leadership positions in the American Psychiatric Association (APA) and at medical schools. In short, it was the very voice of mainstream psychiatry.

The report found that ECT was the most controversial treatment in psychiatry and was "dangerously" abused even by the lax standards of its advocates. It called for long-term follow-up studies as well as "definitive studies as to the possibility of irreversible brain damage," and in the interim, "instituting certain measures of control."

Shock practitioners immediately put pressure on the group to modify their statement. Two years later, having become president of the APA, William Menninger qualified some of the report's statements on ECT's efficacy and usefulness, though he stopped short of backing down on the safety issue. Although organized psychiatry would never again openly criticize ECT, individual psychiatrists, even very prominent clinicians, continued to publish on the dangers of shock in a manner that would be nearly impossible today. For example, Dr. Abraham Barhash wrote in *The American Journal of Psychiatry* in 1950: "From all over the country we get almost daily information about the indiscriminate use of shock therapy, not as an adjunct, but as the *only* approach to treatment. . . . We should at least ask ourselves whether it is true, as is often charged, that electroshock therapy is too profitable to be questioned or tampered with."[28]

Jules Masserman, author of the cat study cited above, reflected on the results of his work in 1950: "These experiments supported the growing conviction among psychiatrists that electroshock and other drastic procedures, though possibly useful in certain relatively recent and acute psychoses, produce cerebral damage which charges the indiscriminate use of such 'therapies' with potential tragedy."[29]

In his 1961 textbook he argued, without success, against the acceptability of brain damage for mental patients in special cases: "The damage produced [by electroshock] is permanent, with the result that the patient's higher intellectual functions may be irretrievably sacrificed. In less gifted patients, these finer capacities can be operationally spared with scarcely noticeable loss, but in patients with special intellectual abilities and highly developed talents and skills (e.g., scientists, artists, professional musicians) the permanent impairments produced by shock or cerebral surgery may be a tragic personal and social price to pay for the use of such drastic methods."[30]

Even Manfred Sakel, the originator of convulsive treatment, realized that electroshock was brain damaging and raised the seemingly obvious ethical question.

> If the amnesia is severe enough to dim out the outstanding psychotic ideas, the normal intellectual processes will suffer even more severe damage and impairment. This fact is still not generally recognized! In the amnesia caused by all electric shocks, the level of the whole intellect is lowered. . . . The stronger the amnesia, the more severe the underlying brain cell damage must be. To complete the clinical picture, it should be mentioned that the "slap-happiness" or "punch-drunkenness" combined with flatness, witnessed after too many "therapeutic" electroshocks remind one of the clinical pictures in cases of frontal lobe tumors, or in the small group of paretics, or again in lobotomics. . . . The question arises whether, in view of such experiences, this method of treatment should continue to be applied.[31]

The Failed Experiment with "Brief Pulse" ECT: 1941–1956

In the 1940s, when doctors openly admitted that ECT caused deleterious effects on cognition and memory, there was some hope that it might yet turn out to be possible to make the procedure less harmful. Beginning in 1941, they experimented with techniques to reduce the amount of electricity put out by the shock machines. If they could reduce it to the lowest possible amount necessary to cause a seizure, they reasoned, then perhaps they'd also minimize brain damage and memory loss.

The first simple attempts at this involved using direct current (DC) rather than alternating current (AC), thus reducing the power of the machines by half.[32] In 1945, W. T. Liberson built the first "brief pulse" (also known as square-wave) ECT device.[33] Basically, this meant altering the type, or wave form, of the electricity. ECT machines had been designed to use the form of electricity known as "sine wave," which is what comes out of wall sockets. With the brief pulse technique the standard wall current is systematically and continuously interrupted, and each "pulse" of electricity becomes briefer than it is with standard (sine wave) ECT. All other things being equal, this does, in fact, reduce the amount of electricity reaching the brain.

The September 1948 issue of the *Journal of Personality*, largely devoted to ECT, captured the mood of optimism at the time, and the industry's almost palpable sigh of relief. It stated that "progress in the application of electroshock has been made" with the use of brief-stimulus methods. "Comparative studies on the different techniques are coming to the fore, and we believe that it will soon be possible to decide whether the claims of the users of the brief-stimulus techniques are justified . . . memory impairment is much less conspicuous after convulsion than with the alternating-current method. . . . Brief-stimulus technique does not interfere with the function of the brain as much as the convulsions produced by alternating current. This lessening of the possibility of brain damage is naturally of real importance."[34]

There were claims that the lower-energy techniques reduced (but did not eliminate) memory loss, but the memory tests used in these studies were primitive.[35] Other studies found no advantage for the new techniques.[36]

However, although the lower-output machines could still induce seizures, psychiatrists complained that the treatment didn't work; it didn't produce the same "therapeutic" changes in patients as the sine wave version.[37] In an effort to compensate for the perceived lack of efficacy, Liberson recommended shocking patients for longer periods of time. To that end, he designed a machine that allowed AC current to flow through the brain for five seconds, or alternately, he recommended using many more treatments.[38]

The Liberson machines were not commercially successful. Psychiatrists preferred the high-output machines that had not only dramatically changed behavior but had predictable adverse effects on memory. They believed that the adverse effects were an essential part of the treatment without which it could not "work."[39] By the mid-1950s, Liberson's hypothesis that "the therapeutic effect of the treatment is due to repeated convulsions and not to the brain damage" had been deemed incorrect.[40] The idea and the manufacture of brief pulse machines were abandoned by the mid-1950s.

In the early 1960s, a couple of researchers experimented with machines said to use an even more benign "ultrabrief" stimulus, but this work went nowhere and was never commercially adopted. [41] Around 2000, some in the ECT industry began talking up ultrabrief shock again as a "new" technique, and they have recently begun using it as a marketing tool to sell shock to the media.[42] But in fact there have been no further experiments genuinely aimed at sparing cognition and memory since the 1960s.

Is "Modified" ECT Safer?

The term "modified ECT" is used to distinguish the type of shock given since the early 1950s—with anesthesia, muscle paralyzers, and, usually, oxygenation—from the shock of the 1930s and 1940s.

In its first decade, when ECT was given without anesthesia, the electricity knocked the patient unconscious. Patients almost never had any memory of receiving the electric shock afterwards, because ECT compromised their ability to recall the recent past, so they were spared the horror of experiencing the jolt. But patients' bodies would convulse so hard during the ensuing seizure that bones were frequently broken, a problem that could be only partly alleviated by their being held down by several attendants. The force of the seizure also caused broken teeth and bitten tongues. The broken bones and teeth cost hospitals many lawsuits in the early years of ECT.[43]

As early as 1938, curare—a drug originally used by Native Americans to make poison arrows—was used on ECT patients to paralyze their muscles during the seizures. Around 1952, it was found that the same effect could be achieved with a synthetic compound, succinylcholine, which has been routinely used ever since. Although the drug has made broken bones and teeth largely a thing of the past, it comes with its own cost: it paralyzes even the muscles used for breathing. Since patients can't breathe on their own right before or during ECT, beginning in the 1950s they were often ventilated with pure oxygen during the brief period of the treatment. However, the primary reason for this use was not to prevent adverse effects on the brain from lack of oxygen (hypoxia), but to make it easier to trigger seizures and to make the seizures longer.[44] In other words, oxygen actually fuels the seizure.

With the advent of the muscle-paralyzing drugs, it became necessary to anesthetize patients simply to spare them the terrifying feeling of being awake but unable to move or breathe. But again, the use of anesthesia comes at a cost. It raises the brain's seizure threshold, its natural defense mechanism against convulsions. The higher the seizure threshold, the more electricity must be used to overcome the brain's efforts to protect itself from harm.

Also, the use of anesthesia in and of itself is associated with a small risk of death; with ECT, since the anesthesia is repeated on a dozen or more occasions, this risk is additive. In short, far from making ECT safer, all of the modifications associated with so-called modern shock have increased its risks and therefore its mortality rate.[45] Doctors have known this since the 1950s.

The PR Line on the Early Research

By the 1980s, the shock industry had come up with a response to the over-whelming evidence of brain damage in the scientific literature. They'd ignore the best and most damning studies, while claiming that the early research was, without exception, so technically flawed as to be meaningless. Most readers wouldn't understand the discussion of the technicalities of preparing brains for examination under the microscope, but would take the word of the industry leaders that mistakes were made that skewed the results.

In fact, Hans Hartelius addressed and dismissed this straw man back in 1952. In part four of his elegant study, "Sources of Error and Interpretation of the Findings," he explains that there is no method that is without possible error. For instance, when the brain is removed from a living animal under anesthesia to lessen the impact of postmortem changes (the technique he used and which modern-day ECT apologists claim is superior), the anesthesia has its own effects on brain structure. Hartelius pointed out that even had his fixation method resulted in some slight artifactual changes, they would have been of one particular type only; they could not have resulted in the proliferation of many types of damage seen in his and a host of other studies.[46]

The other standard dismissal of the brain damage research is typified by a book about ECT written for the general public, published in 2006: "There were studies pointing to neurological changes in the beginning, when electroshock was given without oxygen to protect the brain, more treatments were given at a higher intensity, and damage was more likely and less of a concern to psychiatrists and patients desperate for an effective treatment."[47]

None of this is true, as we have seen. Oxygen wasn't given to protect the brain. Not only is today's shock more intense because of the use of anesthesia, but practices nearly unheard of in the early days of shock, like maintenance or lifelong ECT, mean today's patients are likely to receive many more treatments. For these reasons brain damage is more, not less, likely today than in the early days of shock. There is no evidence that patients' concerns about brain damage and memory loss, or the effects of these on their lives, are any less serious now than they were before modified ECT.

The Patients' Voices

Unlike animals and dead people, survivors of ECT can talk. Yet few researchers have allowed ex-patients themselves to describe the permanent effects of shock.

An exception was Dr. M. B. Brody, a British physician who interviewed five ECT survivors and published his findings in a 1944 article.[48] Besides noting, in a narrative fashion, what these women told him about their permanent amnesia and memory disability—such as losses of familiar skills and information—Brody let them speak in their own words about how the losses affected their everyday lives a year or more after shock. Each, independently of the others, described the same type, extent, and pattern of loss.

When I first discovered the article in 1991, I was profoundly moved to hear these women, probably all long dead, speaking the same words I, and so many other survivors, use so often to describe our permanent disabilities. Much has changed in the world in the sixty years since Brody's article was published. Two things have not changed at all: the human brain and electricity.

A thirty-two-year-old woman who had four shocks told the interviewer: "I want to go and do things and go to do it and find I have already done it. . . . I have to think what I am doing so that I know I have done it . . . it is uncanny when you do things and find you cannot remember it." She added, "I have met one or two people who seem to know all about me and I cannot remember anything about them."

Another woman who had fifteen shocks two years earlier reported: "It takes me a long time to remember. My memory seems 'slower.' It lets me down over small things I am doing, like posting a letter."

A forty-one-year-old described as a "much travelled woman" who once had an excellent memory for names and places wrote: "The following are some of the things I forget: the names of people and places. When the title of a book is mentioned I may have a vague idea I have read it, but cannot recall what it was about. The same applies to films. . . . I forget to post letters and to buy small things, like mending and toothpaste."

A woman in her mid-forties who had two courses of shock gave numerous examples of memory failure and embarrassment: "I originally had a very good memory for places and people. About two years ago we moved into this house. I have not the slightest recollection of taking it over, or of seeing it beforehand. Although detailed measurements in my own hand were produced, it awakened not the slightest chord of memory. Occasionally I concentrate in a determined manner, but so far can recall nothing more. . . . Three years ago I undertook a journey to enter hospital for an operation. . . . I have a great interest in travel, yet find I can remember nothing of the journey, the building, or the return home. . . . There are many faces I see that I know I *should* know a lot about, but only in a few cases can I recall incidents connected with them."

Brody could only add that these few women were representative of many more, and that all of them were completely free of mental illness, and too young to be experiencing age-related deficits. In short, there was no doubt their disabilities were caused by ECT. He concluded: "Even though the impairment of memory for the most part affects only trivialities and is one to which an otherwise well patient can adjust, it necessarily imposes a mental strain. It also contra-indicates electro-therapy in those, for example teachers and transport workers, in whom inability to remember names of persons and places may seriously impair working capacity. Finally, it implies permanent, or semi-permanent, damage to the brain."

Irving Janis, a psychologist at Yale, conducted a more rigorous scientific investigation of amnesia at New York State Psychiatric Institute.[49] He studied nineteen shock patients at great length in semistructured interviews before shock, four weeks afterwards, and in some cases again after some months had passed. The interviewer asked about the patients' entire lives. The same interviews were given to controls matched in all ways: age, sex, level of education, duration of hospitalization, and type and duration of mental disorder. In the first interview, the patients spoke at length and in great detail about their lives; after shock, every one of the shock patients and none of the controls had forgotten ten to twenty significant life experiences. They could not even recognize their past lives when the interviewer read back to them their pre-shock interviews.

Janis published excerpts from the interview transcripts, which illustrate in a way no one else ever has exactly how different ECT memory loss is from normal forgetting and how it has no parallel in ordinary human experience.

A thirty-eight-year-old woman, pre-shock, told Janis:

About four years ago, right after I lost my child . . . I took thyroid [medication] which caused palpitations. I didn't know, at that time, that that caused it. I felt terrified by them. It was a real panic, as if I were on the railroad tracks with a train coming. I was trying to be very brave about the death of my baby, going to work in the hospital where it died, collecting legal papers on it, and so forth, trying to be the super-woman. Then I had the palpitations; a friend told me I should get psychiatric help. I saw my family doctor and he sent for a neurologist. I spent the night at my doctor's office and then I went to the H Sanatorium for a week. I was hopeful of getting all better. They didn't feel I was really ill. After that, I began analysis.

After ten shocks she could not recall this information, even when prompted. In his paper, Janis reported the following series of questions and answers that took place after the treatment.

Q. Did you take some medication after the loss of your child?

A. I don't remember.

Q. Thyroid?

A. I think so.

Q. What reaction did you have to it?

A. I don't know.

Q. During that period did you have any special symptom which disturbed you?

A. I felt depressed.

Q. Anything else?

A. I don't recall.

Q. Did you have palpitations?

A. I vaguely remember palpitations now that you mention it.

Q. How did you feel about them at the time?

A. I don't recall how I felt.

Q. How did you feel at the moment you had the palpitations?

A. Probably not too well.

Q. Did you ever go to a sanatorium?

A. Yes, I remember going to one.

Q. What was the name of it?

A. I don't recall the name.

Q. What were the circumstances that led to your going there?

A. I don't recall why I went or what happened. I remember being there, though.

Q. How long were you there?

A. I don't remember. I don't think it was for very long. I really can't reconstruct that whole period.

In an interview with a thirty-four-year-old man, Janis uncovered a similar pattern of detailed autobiographical narrative before shock that was utterly diminished at the time of the post-shock interview.

I tried to commit suicide. I thought I was losing my mind because I had a funny feeling in my head. A dull feeling all through my head. It wasn't painful but I felt I didn't care about anything because of that feeling.

I tried to commit suicide because of that and because I thought I had syphilis. . . . I went to my room and got a scarf and put on a sweat shirt and blue work shirt. I had a few beers and at the bar I thought I heard a fellow say "That smell sure is syphilis." I got a pint of whiskey after leaving my room and then I took a train. I don't know where I got off the train but I had drunk a lot. Then I saw my brother at a bar in S— and I drank some beer there. Then I went to a private driveway to an old mansion up on a hill and I put the scarf over a stone and I stepped off the stone. I tried to hang myself. I don't know what happened but I came to down at a gas station about a quarter mile from that driveway. Maybe the scarf broke. I don't remember how I got to the gas station. I accused a fellow at the gas station of taking my coat and hat—but he was right. I must have left it back where I tried to commit suicide.

At one month after shock, his interview went like this:

Q. I believe you told me something about suicide several months ago when I talked with you.

A. About suicide? I don't remember anything about suicide. I can't recall ever thinking about suicide. . . .

Q. Can you remember ever going to the town S— once when you were drinking?

A. I don't remember.

A subsequent interview failed to elicit any further recall, underscoring that lost memories did not return over time.

Q. When I talked with you several months ago you told me something about suicide thoughts you had before coming to the hospital.

A. I've been trying to remember that, but I can't.

Q. Do you think you might ever have tried to commit suicide?

A. I don't think I ever did. Did I? At Staff one of the doctors said that I tried to commit suicide but I don't think that's true.

Q. I'd like you to take a look at this list and see if one of these things applies to you. [Reads a list of eight methods of committing suicide, including the one used by the patient.]

A. None of them means anything to me. Did I actually do one of these things?

Q. We'll talk about that later. Right now I want you to see if any of them seem familiar.

A. None of them do.

Q. Suppose that one of them did apply to you. Take a guess which one it might be.

A. I don't know. [Guesses wrong.]

Janis followed up as many of these people as he could, about half of them, one year after ECT, and memory had not returned to a single person.[50]

Most shock patients have stories just like those of the Janis patients. His patients were lucky; their pre-shock lives were preserved, at least on paper, and theoretically they could read about them. Without a pre-shock interview, we can never fully know what we don't know. My own list is long. I have a scar on my leg and don't know how I got it. I met a man who told me we had an intimate relationship, but I have no memory of it, and don't know if he's telling the truth. I forgot an operation I had on my teeth, another I had on my foot. I have records of bank withdrawals and no idea what happened to the money.

No one in the years since 1950 when the study was published has criticized Janis's methodology. When his work is not ignored or dismissed, there are calls for its replication. These calls have been made for over fifty years, but to date no scientists have heeded them.[51]

Research in the 1960s

In the 1960s, there were doctors more interested in investigating shock's effects on the brain than denying them or explaining them away. In 1966, a group led by Dr. Robert Morgan at Hawaii State Hospital proposed a research study to investigate the long-term effects of ECT, because "ECT and lobotomy never had to survive the rigorous checks most drugs pass before use. . . . A hospital staff using ECT in the absence of knowledge of its side effects is much in the position of those doctors who prescribed Thalidomide as a tranquilizer for pregnant women before the first malformed babies were born. A doctor now giving Thalidomide to a pregnant patient would be hard pressed to justify himself on the grounds that it's the most effective tranquilizer available and besides, she was keeping everyone up at night."[52]

In a very small sample (because it was difficult to find patients in the state hospital who hadn't been shocked), they observed and tested a group who hadn't had ECT and compared them with another group who had. The ECT patients did worse than the non-ECT patients on a simple memory subscale of an IQ test. Based on this, the researchers recommended a further study that would administer seven tests of intellect and memory likely to be relevant to ECT deficits, to be given at intervals over a one-year period. They concluded:

> Like lobotomy, ECT damage must be investigated and treated in its own right as an important mental impairment. To do this we must better define the consequences of X treatments on behavior as well as reliably sensitive measures for this behavior change. With enough data, it may some day be possible to deal therapeutically with ECT damaged patients, perhaps with some radically new approach to psychotherapy or direct re-education and modification of behavior. . . . Neurosurgery and neurological psychiatry may one day be able to restore the damaged sections of the limbic system and undo the pathological effects of the once well-intentioned electro-convulsive therapy.[53]

But that would have required that leaders in the psychiatric profession acknowledge the damaging effects of ECT. Perhaps, for a brief moment in the late 1960s, it was possible to imagine that this could happen. But the proposed study was never done. It was not funded. The circumstances that had made it imaginable were about to change, and would not recur.

"A Venal Spirit"

As the 1970s dawned, there could be no doubt that the shock industry was fully aware that ECT was brain damaging and disabling and of the precise nature of the damage, and knew its full impact on the lives of their patients, their families, and society. In legal parlance, if it did not know, it should have known.

Neurologist Robert Grimm summed up the industry's public relations crisis in one paragraph, with dead-on accuracy:

> There is sufficient information from both past studies and current electrophysiologic techniques to suggest that to one degree or another, organic damage to the brain occurs with ECT. I am keenly aware of the generally poor quality of clinical studies in ECT, as well as the fact that there have been no modern attempts (physiologic, histochemical or with Golgi or EM [electron microscope] techniques) to establish the nature of such defects in either humans or experimental animals. The argument over memory loss and intellectual decline remains intense; more, it seems a matter of preconceived notions and unscaled testing techniques than scientific agreement. As psychiatrists generally will not accept the statements of patients on these alleged losses, this issue continues to be a dangerous one and the source of considerable irritation. If it should turn out that ECT clearly does cause brain damage, then the public may well suspect that the protestations of psychiatrists to the contrary were an effort either to conceal an unacceptable (unpleasant) idea or, in some flagrant situations, a venal spirit. Arguments on practical grounds concerning the use of ECT are clear enough, but when made publicly, psychiatry becomes vulnerable to criticism as political and sociological aspects of the problem come into focus. Once in the public domain, professional control over the basic data asserting no or negligible brain damage is lost among these other questions or concerns.[54]

The solution, as the industry saw it, was to grab ironfisted control over both the data and the terms of the debate, using tried and true public relations tactics, and to stay its course, sticking to the script much like the Bush administration on the Iraq war no matter how many people were maimed or killed.

But it had other options. It might have chosen science over public relations, conducting the modern scientific investigation of ECT's effects on the brain called for by Grimm and others. Then, no matter what the studies showed, it could have fully disclosed the results to practitioners, the public, and potential patients. It might have addressed the needs and concerns of former patients who'd been harmed by ECT by, first of all, listening to them; second, by enlisting their expertise to design long-overdue scientific and epidemiological studies to assess the permanent impact of ECT on memory and cognition; and finally, by offering them neuropsychological testing and cognitive rehabilitation.

As we know, the industry did not make these choices. If it had, this history would have been very different. But there is no indication that the industry spokesmen ever questioned which course to take.

5 Informed Consent and the Dawn of the Public Relations Era

The ECT industry entered the public relations era in 1972. At that point the industry committed itself to a strategy to which it has held fast ever since. It made the decision to act *as if* ECT had been proven safe and effective. In effect, its power and credibility would serve as collateral against the fact that a thorough and unbiased scientific investigation had never taken place, and against the word of innumerable ECT patients. As its numbers and influence grew over the decades, its collateral would be more than sufficient.

The industry likes to point to the 1975 movie *One Flew Over the Cuckoo's Nest* as the source of its problems, as if they only began when large numbers of people saw electroshock used as punishment on the rebellious mental patient character Randle McMurphy, played by Jack Nicholson. However, the novel by Ken Kesey (which was far more critical of ECT) had been published in 1962, and not a peep was heard from psychiatry; the shock industry had no need or use for it back then. But beginning in the late 1970s, the movie served retroactively to justify the public relations strategy that was already well underway. *Cuckoo's Nest* is to this day a touchstone for the industry, a significant event in popular culture to which it can point and say with mock outrage, "Look how unfair!"

Cuckoo's Nest informed the strategy, to be sure, and put the meat on its bones. But it wasn't, could not have been, a Hollywood movie that precipitated what psychiatrists perceived as a crisis in ECT.

What fired up the industry, what precipitated the crisis? It was the idea that ECT patients have rights, including the right to informed consent and the right to refuse. In 1972, courts began to take this idea seriously and to rule in favor of patients.

There was another, equally compelling reason why the industry needed an aggressive public relations campaign in 1972, and that was the invention of the CAT scan, a method of three-dimensionally imaging the brain and the body (CAT is shorthand for computed axial tomography). The means for a scientific investigation of ECT's permanent effects on the brain was finally at hand. If ECT were to survive as a viable treatment, the industry had to make sure the new technology wasn't put to use to challenge its safety.

In the first three decades of ECT, patients were not required to give consent, and doctors thought nothing of shocking people who objected vigorously. Those who resisted were physically or chemically overpowered and dragged to the shock table. In fact, a leading shock doctor recommended that patients not even be told that they had been selected for shock, since in his opinion "such information could not possibly do the patient any good." Nor should they be asked for consent, lest they refuse; written consent should be obtained from relatives.[1]

Even less did the ECT industry concern itself with the idea of *informed* consent. This doctrine, which began to be put into practice in other fields of medicine in the late 1950s, holds that a consent is not valid unless a patient is fully informed about the risks and benefits of the proposed treatment, understands them, and agrees to them. Legally, informed consent is the difference between treatment and assault and battery.

In 1961, one doctor told a U.S. Senate subcommittee, "I think one should go to the extreme of always explaining to a patient if he is going to get electroshock why he is going to get it and what it is going to be like and so forth. But as far as getting permission from the patient is concerned, this is not necessary."[2]

The American Civil Liberties Union Handbook on *The Rights of Mental Patients*, published in 1973, stated that "generally speaking, mental patients do not have the right to refuse electroshock therapy."[3]

That began to change in the early 1970s.

The Pilot Project for "Trust Us, We're Doctors"

In 1972, *Boston Globe* reporter Jean Dietz began to write about ECT abuses in Massachusetts. She reported that in some cases patients had received over a hundred shocks. She also pointed out the money motive in ECT: it was being disproportionately used in the state's small, private, profit-making hospitals. Her conclusions were that both the science behind ECT and the laws governing its use were lacking.[4]

Other reporters picked up the story.[5] As usually happens when the media gets hold of something, legislators became seriously concerned, and legislative hearings were held. There was a real possibility that the Massachusetts legislature would enact laws to regulate ECT.

ECT practitioners rose to this first challenge (as they saw it) with a winning strategy that would be repeated over and over in the decades to come. They lobbied the state commissioner of mental health to convene a task force of psychiatrists to study the issues and report back to him. In this way they would have control over what the state did. If there had to be some regulation or legislation of ECT to assuage the public, as seemed inevitable, psychiatrists didn't want anyone from outside the industry shaping it. The damage from the bad public relations couldn't be undone overnight, but it could be controlled until the industry got its own sophisticated PR machine going.

The commissioner, a psychiatrist named Milton Greenblatt, was remarkably amenable to letting ECT practitioners tell him what should be done about ECT. He was an ECT practitioner himself. When the Massachusetts storm blew over, he soon became one of the principal mouthpieces for the American Psychiatric Association's new PR strategy.

So it was easy for shock doctors in Massachusetts to get official permission to effectively tell themselves what to do. Commissioner Greenblatt appointed the Task Force to Study and Recommend Standards for the Administration of Electro-Convulsive Therapy, made up of chairman Fred H. Frankel and ten other psychiatrists.

The first thing the task force did was officially agree with the journalists' conclusions: the science behind ECT was seriously lacking. It acknowledged this numerous times in its report. Scientific information on the treatment's risks, benefits, indications, and so on was "as yet insufficient"; the "relative merits and disadvantages" had not yet been thoroughly evaluated. "The weakness in the conclusions and recommendations of much clinical and research evidence stems from the scarcity of controlled and comparative studies of the long-term results. . . . Definite answers to some questions are still not available and the pressing need for extensive long-term comparative studies of the current treatment modes is clear." One of the questions that had not yet been answered was "whether brain damage results from the use of ECT."[6]

The task force planned to include a section in their report on "Follow-up Studies Concluded and the Findings." For lack of material, it ended up being the shortest section in the report, consisting of this single sentence: "The Task Force cannot emphasize sufficiently its conviction that only by means of adequate and unbiased follow-up studies will the true value of treatment methods be understood, and all who administer ECT are urged to familiarize themselves adequately with other treatment methods so that long-term comparative studies can be undertaken."

The dearth of facts didn't hinder the task force's work, since facts were largely irrelevant to its work. It is *the* basic principle of public relations that facts matter less than perceptions. Facts are at best irrelevant, at worst a hindrance to the PR man's craft. As articulated by the founder of modern public relations, Edward Bernays, in his 1947 essay "The Engineering of Consent," the first task of any public relations campaign is not to ask what the facts are but to conduct a survey of opinion.[7]

This is what—in fact it is all—the task force did. "In light of the great difficulty experienced in trying to clarify the main points of difference, the Task Force decided to add the opinions and practice of the psychiatrists in the State to its own general experience." It sent out questionnaires on ECT to 650 psychiatrists in Massachusetts. Only about 10 percent—sixty-six of them—responded. The task force's final report is a survey of these comments on selected aspects of ECT. Consistent with the manner in which the task force had defined its mandate, most were procedural questions about how to do it. Not all respondents answered all questions. But more than half of the respondents made comments in the section "Evidence of Adverse Effects of Shock Treatment."

The report noted that "the controversy regarding possible adverse effects of ECT, especially from large numbers of treatments, is captured by the nature of these comments. Ten respondents, in referring briefly to individual cases or in reporting generally, claimed that treatments leave unrecoverable gaps in memory and that large numbers of treatments cause intellectual deterioration, seizure, or personality blunting akin to the effects of lobotomy." In their recommendations section, the authors concluded that "the Task Force cannot accept the statements that adverse effects are never seen, or are transient should they occur."

They also concluded that there was no evidence supporting the use of ECT in children. Upon finding that the survey respondents generally gave no more than thirty ECTs in a course, they urged caution upon those who would administer more.

Commissioner Greenblatt followed their recommendations to the letter. In 1973, he issued regulations limiting the number of treatments any one patient could receive per year to thirty-five (but if a second psychiatrist not affiliated with the treating hospital approved, any number could be given). It provided that children under sixteen could not be shocked (unless an unaffiliated child psychiatrist gave his approval). Massachusetts became the first state to require reporting of basic statistics on ECT: the age and sex of patients, their diagnoses, number of shocks, and type of shock.

The state developed a consent procedure and required doctors to adhere to it, though it stated no penalties for those who did not. Voluntary patients had to give written informed consent. In the case of involuntary patients, a relative or guardian could give consent, even if the patient refused.

The data from the new reporting system were not compiled and publicly released until 1984. By that time, the industry's now well-oiled public relations machine, seasoned by campaigns in other states, claimed that the regulations had caused a drastic decline in ECT use.[8] They did this by misrepresenting the data; for instance, implying that it included reports from general hospitals, when in fact general hospitals were never included in the reporting requirements. The actual report published by the Department of Mental Health stated that, since not all hospitals which use ECT had to report to the state, there was not sufficient information to know whether the regulations had had any impact on ECT use.[9]

What was clear from the report was that a second opinion approving the use of more than thirty-five applications of ECT must not have been difficult to obtain. Under the new regulations, hundreds of patients got over thirty-five treatments a year, and some got an "inordinately large" number, just as Dietz had reported in 1972. It is impossible to know whether this was an increase or decrease from prior practice. Children under sixteen were still being shocked.

Dietz's original observation that ECT was used nearly exclusively in private profit-making hospitals as opposed to public hospitals was confirmed by a followup study. To be precise, private psychiatric hospitals administered twenty times as much shock as public hospitals.[10] This pattern took hold by the 1970s in other states as well, and remains true to this day. It is due to the growth in the number and proportion of psychiatric facilities that are private and for-profit, and psychiatry's shift to an insurance-based industry. Historically, state hospitals have provided long-term custodial care at public expense. But insurance companies won't pay for indefinite care for psychiatric conditions, which by their very nature don't resolve quickly. Drugs take several weeks to kick in, but ECT provides a dramatic appearance of improvement in a short period of time. Cheap to administer and unquestioningly reimbursed by insurance carriers, it is highly attractive to facilities seeking to maximize profits.

In Massachusetts, in part because a shock proponent held a key political position, the industry succeeded in its maiden attempt to essentially convince a state to allow it to regulate itself. Although some patients could now refuse shock, the status quo had, for the most part, been maintained. But there would be more "challenges" in other states.

States' Rights, Patients' Rights . . . Psychiatrists' Rights?

The state's ability to regulate ECT arises from its rational interest in protecting the health of its patients. The state has its own interest in medical care, too; it pays for it through Medicaid and Medicare, and it is interested in ensuring that its money is well spent and that the treatments it pays for are sound and helpful. For example, Medicaid and Medicare won't pay for what they deem to be experimental treatments.

ECT wasn't being unfairly singled out for scrutiny, as the industry strategists claimed; all types of medical procedures come under judicial and legislative scrutiny by their very nature. It was the historical lack of such scrutiny that characterized ECT, not an arbitrary excess.

There was nothing psychiatry could do to make the states' interests go away, or to claim they weren't legitimate. So the doctors downplayed or ignored them, while portraying any proposed legislation as a violation of their own fundamental rights: the "right to treat," the "right" to give as many shocks as they wanted to whomever they wanted, whether the patient consented or not, without government oversight or intervention. The shock doctors' rallying cry was "Let's keep the government out of the doctor-patient relationship!"[11]

As for patient's rights, they do not necessarily conflict with the rights and role of doctors. It was organized psychiatry's decision to act as if its financial stake in ECT equated legally and ethically with the right of patients to control their own minds and bodies, and as if one right impinged on the other. From this standpoint, their own patients were their adversaries. Rights long conceded to nonpsychiatric patients, such as the right to refuse treatment, were seen by psychiatrists as a threat against which they had to mobilize. The doctors' perceived financial interests (which they saw as entitlements) took precedence over patient rights.

Max Fink complained in 1974 that "the laws of the nation are being changed so that the rights and privileges claimed by physicians are eroding at a very rapid rate."[12] What was being eroded was the "right" to forcibly shock persons who didn't consent. There is no such right.

However, citizens do have rights under the law and the Constitution, including fundamental rights to privacy, free speech, free thought, bodily integrity, and freedom from unwanted medical treatment. These rights are not checked at the hospital door, even if it is a locked door. The rights of those of us considered mentally ill have historically been seen as less fundamental than the rights of others not so labeled; but still, when a state takes our rights away, it must justify its actions as an exercise of its *parens patriae* or police powers. In the former case it takes on the role of parent to one seen as unable to care for herself or himself; in the latter, it acts to prevent harm to others.

The state can intervene to make medical decisions for persons only when they are formally determined to be incompetent to make their own.

Competent persons have the right to refuse treatment even if their decision is seen as wrong or irrational. Persons labeled mentally ill, even those with acutely distressing emotions and behaviors, are not considered legally incompetent simply by virtue of their psychiatric label, nor is the ability to make medical decisions necessarily impaired by severe depression or other psychiatric conditions. The assumption that mental illness (the label and/or the condition of emotional distress) automatically renders people incompetent to make their own decisions is another widely accepted but false eugenic conception of our time.

The Right to Refuse

In one of the earliest lawsuits, *New York City Health and Hospitals Corporation v. Stein,* a judge interpreted a pending law mandating consent for ECT to mean consent was required from the patient herself.[13] A competent patient had a right to refuse ECT in New York State, "however unfortunate that decision may prove to be," even if the court disagreed with her choice. An adult woman's mother had sought to shock her, but the patient refused ECT and her wishes prevailed because, the court reasoned, she would bear "the greatest suffering from an incorrect decision." There was no state interest in forcing ECT on a competent patient, for there was no threat to public health or safety (as there might be in the case of a tuberculosis patient, for instance).

Besides New York, states that passed laws requiring consent for ECT in the 1970s included Delaware, Florida, Connecticut, and Michigan.[14]

Wyatt v. Stickney was a landmark case in Alabama that has shaped policy nationwide.[15] A multifaceted case that went on for over thirty years, it raised the issue, among others, of a patient's right to refuse both psychosurgery and ECT. In 1972, Alabama issued a court order establishing "Standard 9," stating that a patient could not be shocked without "express and informed consent." This amounted to an absolute right to refuse ECT, even for persons deemed incompetent. Even for a competent patient, ECT could be given only after indication from four psychiatrists, one neurologist, and two attorneys monitoring the proceedings.

Psychiatrists refused to comply with the new law. Three years later, patients who had been involuntarily shocked in Alabama sought remedy in

Wyatt v. Hardin.[16] A judge found that the patients had indeed been shocked against their will and that the defendant psychiatrists "resented" the new law, but declined to punish them under civil or criminal law. The state established a substitute consent mechanism whereby patients deemed incompetent could be shocked. Hospitals were to establish an Extraordinary Treatment Committee to make decisions for these patients. If the committee decided that shock was in the patient's best interest, it could consent for him or her. Patients had to be represented by counsel. All doubts about the wisdom of ECT were to be resolved against the procedure. Patients and relatives could appeal the decision of the committee. In the case of competent, consenting patients, ECT now required two recommendations from a qualified mental health professional and approval by the hospital director.

In Minnesota, a fourteen-year-old boy was shocked against his will and over his mother's objection, and his case went to court. In *Price v. Sheppard*, the Minnesota Supreme Court ruled that shock may be a violation of the constitutional right to privacy.[17] At the same time, the court allowed that, in some cases, the state's interest could supersede a patient's constitutional rights, and there must be a weighing of competing interests; therefore, patients who refused ECT were entitled to a court hearing as to whether treatment could proceed. While the judges expressed great concern over the intrusive nature of ECT, in the end competent patients were not granted the absolute right to refuse ECT in Minnesota; they could still be shocked against their will. The court spelled out the procedure to follow. It implied that the state's interest in shocking involuntarily committed patients would be greater than its interest in shocking voluntary patients. Unfortunately, it also made the unwarranted assumption that persons who were committed were incompetent, making it even easier to shock them. Other states do not allow that assumption to be made. In *Gundy v. Pauley*, the Kentucky appellate court ruled that state law gives a competent patient the absolute right to refuse ECT, even if she is involuntarily committed.[18]

Aden v. Younger, 1976: Patient Rights or an Attack on Psychiatry?

Of all the battles over basic rights for ECT patients in the early 1970s, California's was the most heated. That's probably because the nascent mental patients rights' movement was strongest and best organized in California—and conversely, the state had some of the most enthusiastic shock doctors.

In 1974 the Network Against Psychiatric Assault in San Francisco (an organization of psychiatric survivors, including shock survivors, founded to oppose all forms of psychiatric abuse) began documenting and publicizing the lack of informed consent to ECT at the University of California Medical Center's Langley Porter Neuropsychiatric Institute, as well as the general lack of studies on ECT's safety and efficacy. In April of that year, Assemblyman John Vasconcellos introduced a bill in the California Assembly (AB4481) which, in its original form, gave mental patients the absolute right to refuse ECT. It was subsequently modified so that persons considered incompetent could be shocked without their consent. But as passed on September 24, 1974, it provided new protections for patients. Competent patients could not be shocked without written informed consent. All the risks and possible side effects "thought to be associated with the treatment" had to be disclosed to a patient. The risks and side effects were also to be disclosed to a responsible relative. Three physicians would have to review a competent or incompetent patient's consent to shock. A statewide reporting system was required to be set up. And finally, ECT had to be shown to be "critically needed for the welfare of the patient."

As a reviewing justice later put it, the objective of the law was "to ensure certain medical procedures are not performed on unwilling patients." It didn't make ECT illegal. It made it illegal to force ECT on a competent patient who said no.

The industry concluded that if there were no unwilling ECT patients, there would be no patients at all. The Northern California Psychiatric Society wrote, "One of the most dangerous features of AB4481 is that it will serve to eliminate the use of ECT in California almost entirely, and it will do so for the voluntary patient who asks for it just as it will for the involuntary patient who objects to it."[19] Absolutely nothing in the bill supported such a statement.

Nevertheless, to defend against this perceived threat, a lawsuit was filed against the state's attorney general and its director of health, demanding that the law be repealed. The petitioner was psychiatrist Gary Carl Aden.

Between 1972 and 1980 (while he was passionately advocating for shock treatment), according to charges filed against him, Aden engaged in sadistic sexual abuse of at least three female former patients. He was charged with drugging them, beating them with a riding crop, using a hot iron to brand them with his initials, tying them up with hospital restraints, and forcing them to have sex with him. When the details became public in the 1980s, he gave up his medical license rather than have it taken away. The prosecution called Aden's "absolutely" the worst case of sexual abuse they'd ever seen.[20]

But in 1976, Aden made headlines only as the plaintiff in *Aden v. Younger*. His rather tenuous argument was that the law passed under AB4481 was unconstitutional. He said the informed consent provisions of the California law were unconstitutional because they violated a patient's right not to be informed; the reporting provisions violated patient confidentiality; and the requirement that consent be reviewed was an unconstitutional infringement on the doctor-patient relationship. Worst of all, Aden argued, if doctors would not order shock for unwilling patients for fear of the proposed $10,000 fine, those patients would die. A day before the law was to take effect, a restraining order was issued, staying its enforcement until an appellate court could review it.

The court decided that parts of the law were unconstitutional—but not the parts Aden claimed, and not for the reasons he claimed. Most of his arguments were dismissed as meritless and the decision came down firmly on the side of patient rights. ECT was not being unfairly singled out for unnecessary regulation; it needed oversight because it presented "a great danger of violating the patient's rights." The regulation of ECT was "a legitimate exercise of the state's police power." A reporting system was needed "to control possible violations of patients' rights" and was not a violation of confidentiality. Disclosure of ECT's risks was necessary because "the state's interest in protecting a patient's right to refuse treatment could not be accomplished by any measure short of such disclosure."[21]

But the wording of the law—the requirement that ECT be "critically necessary"—was unconstitutionally vague; the requirement that a competent patient's consent be reviewed by three doctors was unconstitutional; the provision that disclosure be made to a relative was an unconstitutional violation of the patient's right to privacy; and the protections for patients in danger of being ruled incompetent were inadequate. Rather than rewrite the entire law to remedy the defective sections, the appellate court ruled it unconstitutional in its entirety.

Gary Aden described the mood of the shock doctor brotherhood at that time as "ecstasy, as well as seasoned alarm." He and a few of the other doctors in attendance at the American Psychiatric Association annual convention that year came together to form an organization "to assert their right and to comfort them in their plight . . . supplying an effective voice in combating the emotional and unjustified attacks on ECT."[22]

No fiction writer could have made up a cast of characters like the members of the American Society for Electrotherapy (ASE; later renamed the International Psychiatric Association for the Advancement of Electrotherapy, or IPAAE). Its members had trouble staying out of the headlines for long. Besides Gary Aden, they included Shervert Frazier, one-time NIMH director, who plagiarized four major research papers between 1966 and 1975 and lost his professorship at Harvard as a result. He was the chair of the APA's public relations committee during the period in which the campaign to sell ECT was born.[23]

Then there was H. C. Tien, the first president of ASE, who devised his own bizarre synthesis of psychotherapy and ECT, which he called ElectroLoveTherapy. It involved intensive shocking of patients, mostly women, until the desired degree of "selective memory erasure" was achieved. Immediately after each shock they would be bottle fed like an infant by a spouse who would "reprogram" them. They would then take on new names to reflect their electrically altered personalities, and would be returned to their families as docile servants.

John Nardini, the first psychiatrist to be sued for lack of informed consent resulting in permanent memory loss and brain damage from ECT, was a founding member, as was Paul Blachly, the first American ECT psychiatrist to become a shock machine company entrepreneur. He began the tradition of ECT practitioners starting their own companies to sell the machines, a practice that significantly increased their incomes. Blachly died in 1977 but his company, Mecta, still makes half of the shock machines sold in the

United States. (It's now owned by husband-and-wife investors who hire shock proponents to design the machines.) Blachly advocated his own unconventional form of ECT in which several shocks were given and multiple seizures elicited at each session. He called it "multiple monitored ECT" (MMECT, the "monitored" part being a plug for his company's machine, which at the time was the only one that monitored the EEG and EKG).[24] MMECT could cause patients to regress to infancy. His machine, marketed as a "new" type although it had been invented in the 1940s, played a pivotal symbolic role in the public relations campaign to convince the public that ECT was safe.

Another board member was Milton Greenblatt, the psychiatrist who, in his position as commissioner of mental health in Massachusetts, had three years earlier steered the industry clear of legislative oversight.

An ad for the organization said it was formed "to ensure the sacred privilege of treating our patients according to recognized medical standards" as well as "to provide an effective voice in combating the emotional and unjustified attacks on ECT."[25]

Try as they might, they were never able to find a patients' auxiliary.[26] Today, the IPAAE survives as the Association for Convulsive Therapy, or ACT, and it has its own vanity publication, *The Journal of ECT*.

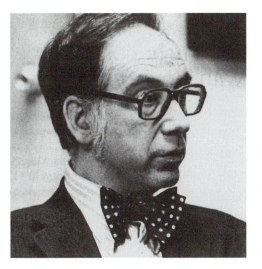

Figure 2. Psychiatrist/entrepreneur Paul Blachly, who sold "brief pulse" devices on the false premise that they were safer.
(Reproduced courtesy of Oregon Health and Science University).

California Passes Rights Protections

Although California's first law to protect ECT patients' rights was over-turned, another similar bill (AB1032) was introduced and passed in 1976.[27] It gave competent patients the right to refuse ECT. They had to be informed of the nature and risks of ECT, and had to give written informed consent.

The new law gave patients alleged to be incompetent the right to a court hearing on the issue of competency, after which, if adjudged incompetent, they could be shocked on consent of a relative or guardian. It went farther than AB4481 in another way: it outlawed ECT for children under the age of twelve.

The new law did not eliminate the use of ECT in California, as the shock lobby had predicted. If anything, it had the opposite effect. The use of ECT increased slightly in the year following the bill's passage, and then remained nearly steady with small fluctuations. However, from 1977 to 1978 there was a 50 percentage increase in the number of patients shocked against their will, suggesting that psychiatrists quickly found a way around any informed patients' refusals.[28]

Throughout its history the ECT industry has assumed, and acted as if, truly informed consent and the right to refuse ECT amounts to a total ban on its use. This speaks volumes about what the industry knows, but won't admit it knows, about the effects of shock. With each proposed law or regu-lation, it claimed—and still claims—that ECT was about to be outlawed, or "proscribed" to use the terminology of Max Fink. For instance, in flagrant disregard for facts that are a matter of public record, Fink claims that in the early 1970s there were attempts at "proscription of ECT in the Massachusetts, Michigan, and Alabama legislatures. . . . In 1974 in California, the legislature proscribed the use of ECT."[29] (In fact, ECT was outlawed in America exactly once, in one city, on the vote of the citizens of Berkeley, California; this ban lasted for forty-one days in 1982 until the law was overturned.) The industry continues to make these claims long after the evidence is in that the laws have not had the predicted effect. Yet in other contexts, such as promoting ECT to the media, it makes the opposite claim: that shock is being used now much more than it was before there was any regulation.

Bills to ban ECT never come disguised as informed consent or right to refuse bills, and there is no mistaking them for anything else. They say in plain English: ECT shall be prohibited. One can only conclude that the claim that regulations or laws result in a decline in ECT use, a kind of failed effort to ban ECT entirely, is so useful to the industry—enabling them to successfully defeat proposed reporting laws in state after state using the same argument—that it knowingly misrepresents the data.

In the early 1970s, the first attempt to ban ECT was a decade away, and came about at least partly *because* of the hard-line strategy the industry adopted at the outset of the 1970s. Had the industry been honest with its customers about the risks of brain damage and permanent memory loss, and allowed them to make informed choices about whether to take the risks, it is likely there never would have been any attempts to ban the procedure.

Instead, it acted as if it had a guilty conscience, as if it knew about the risks of its product. But like cigarettes, ECT machines had been in use for decades in which the end users of the product were not warned of its hazards. To disclose the risks now would invite scrutiny and legal liability: what had doctors known and when had they known it? Like the tobacco industry, the ECT industry was likely advised by lawyers to admit nothing, to take a strong and inviolable line of denial, forever, no matter what. Such a line didn't hold for the cigarette makers. But unlike smokers, former ECT patients, perceived as irrational and dishonest, cannot win damages lawsuits.

It is possible to imagine a different strategy. The shock industry might have welcomed in a new era of long-denied human rights for their patients, gaining in public opinion polls by seeming humane and progressive. Instead, the industry took an extreme stance in the other direction: it decided to act as if the very continued existence of ECT was incompatible with, and threatened by, any government regulation or legislation, no matter how innocuous. And it continues to act this way despite decades of evidence to the contrary.

PR Lessons Learned from the Early Legal Actions

Whether a state exercises its power to force treatment on a person depends largely on the perceived risks, benefits, and intrusiveness of the procedure. It also depends on the nature of the right potentially infringed by forced treatment. The more fundamental the right and/or the riskier the treatment, the stronger the state's interest needs to be. A mere rational interest could suffice to force a procedure of low risk and proven benefit, while only the most compelling interest can justify a very risky, unproven, or intrusive procedure—one which also by definition is more likely to infringe a fundamental right.

The courts in the earliest right-to-refuse ECT lawsuits made clear their concern over the intrusiveness and risks of shock. The judge in *Price v. Sheppard* called it "one of the most intrusive forms of treatment." The impact of ECT was "unquestionably great, for the result is the alteration of the patient's personality." The judge in *Aden v. Younger* concurred: "The legislature has determined ECT and psychosurgery are such intrusive and hazardous procedures that informed consent is a mandatory prerequisite to treatment. . . . The extent of memory loss and the risk of permanent memory loss are not fully known, but the fact of memory loss is not questioned. The risk of other adverse effects is possible, since the procedure is so little understood. Those possible risks include permanent brain damage in the local area of the electrodes, and a slowing of brain waves."

In both cases, the patient's right to refuse hinged on her right to privacy—privacy of her mind—a fundamental constitutional right that was compromised by ECT and which was balanced against the state's stake in forced treatment: "[The right of privacy] is not an absolute one and must give way to certain interests of the state, the balance turning on the impact of the decision on the life of the individual. As the impact increases, so must the importance of the state's interest. Some decisions, we assume, will be of little consequence to the individual and a showing of legitimate state interest will justify its intrusion; other decisions, on the other hand, will be of such major consequence that only the most compelling state interest will justify the intrusions."[30]

The more intrusive the treatment, the greater the threat to the person's privacy; but what was intrusiveness? It has been defined as follows:

1. the extent to which the effects of the therapy are reversible
2. the extent to which the resulting psychic state is "foreign," "abnormal," "unnatural" for the person in question, rather than simply a restoration of his prior psychic state
3. the rapidity with which the effects occur

4. the scope of the changes in the total "ecology" of the mind's functions

5. the extent to which one can resist acting in ways impelled by the psychic effects of the therapy

6. the duration of the change.[31]

In its 1976 ruling that courts would decide whether patients who did not want shock could be ordered to have it, Minnesota required the courts to consider, along with intrusiveness, the risk of adverse side effects and the extent and duration of changes in mental activity. Other states use similar criteria.

These were the factors that a competent patients would want to weigh in making their decision, perhaps the information that should be disclosed to them in obtaining informed consent. But courts were unwilling to be as specific in deciding what a competent, consenting patient should be told. For instance, New York State's consent form required only that patients indicate by their signature that "Dr. _____ has explained to me the reasons for the above-named treatment, its advantages and possible complications."

The court in *Aden* directed only that risks "thought to be associated with the procedure" need be disclosed. It didn't say *whose* thoughts counted.

The early shock lawsuits were a wake-up call to the industry, telling it exactly what it needed to do to survive and thrive into the next century. Arrogance and brute force wouldn't work in an era of patient rights; a gentler approach of persuasion and coercion was called for.

The key to shocking as freely as they had before rights protections was in the legal definition of competency. Psychiatrists had not lost their power to shock anyone who was deemed incompetent. In every state the definition of competency includes the patient's ability to understand the risks and adverse effects of the treatment. Organized psychiatry could define those risks as it pleased. If the APA said shock was harmless and could convince judges that it was, then any patient who disagreed with this assessment lacked an understanding of the risks of treatment, greatly increasing the chances that she or he would be ruled incompetent.

The industry couldn't make ECT safe. It couldn't prevent brain damage, permanent amnesia, and cognitive disability. But it didn't need to. It needed only to control public and professional *perception*: what people, including the rank-and-file doctors and the judges who would assess competency and grant permission for forced treatment, *believed* about shock, not what was actually true about it. The problem as reframed by the industry strategists was not a problem with ECT; it was a problem with the perception of ECT. Since it was a public relations problem and not a medical, scientific, or moral problem, its solution lay in public relations tactics. Bad PR simply needed to be replaced by good. As Milton Greenblatt, speaking for the APA, put it: "More and more time and resources will have to be committed to monitor and influence public opinion, legislative action, and judicial decisions."[32] For this, a CAT scan study of shocked brains was irrelevant and counterproductive.

Instead, the APA put its resources into ever more sophisticated public relations games—literally. For instance, its Division of Public Affairs developed a board game called "The Crisis Management Game," to train its local public relations officers to deal with perceived public relations crises. Moving pawns with the APA logo around the board, they'd land on squares such as: "A coalition of former psychiatric patients and their families has successfully petitioned for a referendum on the ballot in a city election. Passage will ban the use of ECT by physicians in that city. What will you do to try to defeat it?"[33]

The players then had to choose from a limited range of "solutions," including "contact the media," "utilize information and manpower resources," and "seek professional public relations assistance." There was no option for meeting with the hypothetical patients, for instance, or for defusing the situation by developing a truthful informed consent form. It was a given in this game that patients and doctors were enemies. The object of the game was to develop public relations strategies that would work in real life, such as cultivating a large group of media spokespersons.

The industry set out to shape public perception of ECT to such an extent that no one would be immune to its party line.

For this, it needed three things:

- A platform—an organization with power, numbers, money, and credibility; an official, quasi-governmental document.

- Control of the media—the ability to prevent, suppress, or defuse negative portrayals and to orchestrate good publicity through an aggressive PR campaign.
- Control of the literature—that is, the prestigious scientific journals that determine "truth"—by controlling access to funding and publication.

All were within its grasp; all would be achieved within ten years.

6   *The American Psychiatric Association Task Force*

In direct response to what it perceived as "challenges," including real and imaginary legislative initiatives, organized psychiatry took action. In the fall of 1974, just as California passed its first ECT patients' rights bill, the APA established the Task Force on ECT "to defend against the complaints that the treatments were dangerous and abused."[1] It was so pleased with the way the task force strategy worked to forestall legislation in Massachusetts that it appointed the chair of that group, Fred Frankel, to head the national effort.

The APA Board of Trustees selected the task force members. Five of the nine were ECT practitioners, and at least three belonged to the shock industry lobbying group, the International Psychiatric Association for the Advancement of Electrotherapy (IPAAE). Max Fink was the principal mover of the task force. The lone psychologist, Larry Squire, was a young researcher just beginning a long career in studying memory. His work would become central to the shock apologists' plan. The Task Force Report was funded by the IPAAE, who provided "important input," according to Gary Aden, as well as Fink's own private foundation, the International Association for Psychiatric Research (now Scion Natural Science Association). Larry Squire also paid part of the cost of the report from his federal grant money.[2]

In 1976, to kick off the task force's first public meeting, the APA declared a "crisis in ECT." The crisis, in the words of Fink, consisted of "public demands and legislative fiats to stop the use" of ECT.[3] The possibility of a problem with ECT itself was not on the table for consideration. Never did the industry stop and ask itself why patients didn't want ECT, or whether it really was dangerous. It defined its problem as a public relations problem only, and set out to polish the image of ECT.

The structure, tone, and content of the Task Force Report reflect that mission. From beginning to end it was a political, not scientific, document, written to achieve political goals. The authors relied on their M.D.s and

Ph.D.s to convince an uncritical public, including lawmakers, that whatever the task force produced would be upheld as sound science. That gave the authors the freedom to cut their public relations talking points from whole cloth: snipping with impunity, leaving out what didn't suit them, tailoring what was left to fit an agenda determined in advance.

A scientific investigation never begins with a public opinion poll, but a public relations campaign always does. Following the formula used in Massachusetts, the APA's first step was to poll a 20 percent sample of its members. They weren't going to investigate ECT; they were going to ask people's opinions of ECT. But of course the questions were worded carefully. There were few chances for participants to comment on the adverse effects of shock. Psychiatrists were asked whether it was likely that ECT causes slight or subtle brain damage, thus disallowing the possibility of more serious damage. Forty-one percent answered yes to this question, which must have alarmed the task force members. Organized psychiatry had reason to be concerned about winning over those doubters.

To give the illusion of openness, the task force held a so-called Open Forum paper presentation at the APA's 1976 convention in Miami Beach. But the panel was stacked with ECT advocates: Fink, Frankel, Salzman, Greenblatt. There was one exception: neurologist John Friedberg, author of *Shock Treatment Is Not Good for Your Brain,* presented a survey of the literature that the psychiatrists wanted swept under the rug. The APA newspaper, *Psychiatric News,* mused disingenuously, "It was unfortunate that Friedberg alone had to carry an entire side of the debate against five other speakers"— without revealing that in fact psychiatrists had been *forbidden* to speak critically of ECT, so that none of them dared step up to do so, even when Friedberg offered to cede his time to a psychiatrist.[4] The industry rag described Friedberg as "speaking more as if chanting a litany than reading a scientific paper."[5]

A second neurologist, Robert Grimm, urged caution on the task force in a written statement, pointing out that "the use of convulsions by one branch of medicine (psychiatry) to effect a therapeutic response while another branch (neurology) labors to prevent convulsions reveals a serious ethical problem which these generally collaborative branches of medicine should consider."[6]

For their part, the shock doctors made it clear that their mission was to improve the public image of ECT, not ECT itself, and that this was a direct response to criticisms from their former patients and new patients' rights laws. Fink called his paper "Myths of 'Shock Therapy.'" Since brain damage and permanent memory loss were myths, the task force could hardly take them seriously. He recommended "relinquishing our myths and changing our clinical attitudes towards ECT" in order to "improve the present unrest and common allegations of abuse," not conducting a scientific study of ECT's effects on the brain. Referring to the Massachusetts case, he said, "Medicine has failed to use its inherent powers of self-discipline, and the present malpractice crisis is the result."[7]

This, according to Psychiatric News, emerged as the major theme of the task force public hearings on ECT. Its July 2, 1976, front-page headline was: "MDs Protest ECT Regulation at APA Task Force Hearings." The story read: "Psychiatrists vigorously endorsed the therapy as a valuable component in the therapeutic armamentarium, and opposed efforts by legislatures, courts, or APA to regulate or provide guidelines for its use. The task force is not bound by the straw vote among the participants in the hearings in what it eventually recommends on APA's position (if any) on ECT regulation, but the message it received was unmistakable. Participants are generally angry that an effective, proven remedy for depression has been called into question by 'irrational' forces."

Three of the six who presented papers at the meeting (published in the September 1977 American Journal of Psychiatry) were task force members. Chairman Frankel announced that the purpose of the task force was "to weigh the evidence as carefully as possible and to assess realistically the cost/benefit ratio of ECT."

That this careful weighing of evidence never happened can be seen by comparing the papers prepared for the July 1976 meeting with the final Task Force Report of September 1978. Whole sections were simply copied virtually word for word from the authors' 1976 position papers. In other words, the Task Force Report was a foregone conclusion once shock proponents were chosen as its authors.

The Task Force on Amnesia, Memory Disability, and Brain Damage

Larry Squire's 1976 paper became the section titled "Memory and ECT." He cited largely his own work. Thirty-five years of literature on the deleterious effects of ECT on memory and cognition were simply ignored. Squire did cite three such studies, including what was then the longest-term follow-up study (ten to fifteen years), only to criticize their conclusions that ECT causes permanent memory loss and cognitive disability.[8] For example, even though the ten-year follow-up used a rigorous scientific method including matched control subjects and sophisticated neuropsychological testing, Squire concluded that there must have been something else besides ECT to account for the differences between those who had received shock and those who hadn't. However, the study results were replicated in a subsequent seven-year follow-up study that specifically addressed the issue Squire raised by controlling for psychopathology.[9]

Irving Janis's 1950 study was the only source for the section on "retrograde amnesia," but Squire distorted and discredited it, saying that Janis's patients only forgot experiences from the time period immediately preceding the shocks. But in fact Janis covered the patients' entire lives in his interviews and stated clearly that knowledge from all time periods was forgotten: "It should be mentioned that the amnesias are by no means limited to events of the recent past, although experiences during the six months prior to treatment are more likely to be forgotten than those which had occurred in earlier periods. Occasionally the amnesias involve events of early childhood that date back 20 to 40 years."[10]

In order to convince his readers that amnesia is temporary, Squire also had to omit Janis's conclusions, including his finding that memory loss remained stable one year after shock.

Squire's own work, done between 1974 and 1976, is far less rigorous than Janis's. It mostly involved using simple multiple-choice tests to assess the effects of ECT on memory during, or very shortly after, shock. These tests have not been validated (replicated and found to measure what they purport to measure) by other researchers. In his "TV test," he asked patients to recognize the name of a television program that was broadcast in a certain year. Patients have a one out of four chance of getting the right answer by guessing. If they answer correctly for whatever reason, it's assumed they remember everything that happened that year.

On the basis of these tests, Squire concluded that many years of memory can be lost to ECT—but not permanently. In the report he says variously that "memory loss largely recovered by one to two weeks" and "impairment in memory for remote events persisted for at least two weeks." It is important to understand that the task force's conclusions about the return of memory are based entirely on these multiple-choice, recognition-memory TV tests, on which patients can easily do well by sophisticated guessing on first testing, and even better when taking the test again within a short period of time. "Memory returns" would become a central tenet of the APA's public relations campaign, and remains so to this day. But there are no studies that show this.

Despite all his equivocation, Squire was forced to conclude that "ECT can affect memories acquired many years prior to treatment," and, as to amnesia for events one to two years prior, "A fully satisfactory study of this issue with maximally sensitive tests has not yet been accomplished."

The report tried to ignore the issue of ECT's long-term effects on memory ability. It cited only those studies of memory and learning ability that took place *during* ECT. It cited none of the studies in which memory ability of ECT patients was compared to that of normal controls. Nevertheless, Squire was left with the undeniable finding in his own studies that the majority of ECT survivors had "memory complaints" long afterwards.

The task force wouldn't own up to permanent memory disability, just the "complaints"—a not-so-subtle way of discrediting and trivializing survivor reports. Forced to acknowledge that such reports were "common," Squire seemed to be trying hard, at the end of the section, to explain them away. He allowed that his tests might be inadequate, but this caveat is all but lost to history. The sentence that lived on—the one that was seized on by the industry and repeated over and over—was this one: "ECT might lead many individuals (with or without psychiatric illness) to have persistent illusion of memory impairment."

The industry admitted no more than it was forced to. It was willing to acknowledge that memory for the "days" prior to treatment could be permanently lost. Even that concession was made to further a larger strategy of denial. The task force hypothesized that this short period of real amnesia could cause patients to be oversensitive to normal forgetting, and thus to think they had memory difficulties even though they did not. It cited no studies to support this theory. There were none.

The 1978 report omitted a critical sentence that appeared in Squire's 1976 presentation. The omission alters the meaning of the section in the direction of further denial of ECT's adverse effects. The omitted sentence was: "It is too early to accept or reject any of the hypotheses outlined here [as to causes of reports of impaired memory]; further work is needed before it will be possible to choose among them." Yet even though there had been no such studies between 1976 and 1978 to settle the question, the report led the reader to believe that there was evidence to show that patients were simply imagining permanent memory disability.

The report contained a section on "brain damage"—in quotes, to show it wasn't seriously considering the possibility that there was any. No longer was it politically acceptable, as it had been up until the 1960s, for psychiatrists to acknowledge that ECT caused brain damage, much less to openly condone brain damage for mental patients. None of the many authors who had done so were cited by the APA. The report dealt with the research showing brain damage in animals and humans dishonestly, either ignoring or distorting these studies. For instance, the literature on animals was dismissed in two paragraphs. Four of the many studies documenting brain damage were cited, only to have their findings characterized by the APA as "not extensive" and "reversible," conclusions at odds with those of the original researchers.

Four studies were cited in favor of the conclusion that ECT does not cause damage to animal brains. Each of the studies actually did find damage. S. Eugene Barrera (1942) found diffuse pathology; Joseph Globus (1943) found extreme, permanent pathological changes; William Lidbeck (1944) found permanent brain damage; and Karl Neuberger's 1942 studies of dogs showed widespread damage and severe pathology.[11]

None of the studies showing damage published after 1952 were cited.

The human autopsy literature was dismissed in similar fashion, with the task force speculating, for instance, that it must have been the "pain, fear, and panic" associated with ECT—not the ECT itself—that killed patients. The

APA said it couldn't find any studies showing brain damage with so-called modern ECT, implying that there are none when they do exist, as we saw in Chapter Four (note 16).

And yet, the task force's strangely worded conclusion was that "it seems proper to continue to investigate the question of whether ECT produces adverse morphological or metabolic effects in brain."

The Task Force Comes Down against
Regulation and Redefines Informed Consent

The large section of the report devoted to legislative issues consisted mostly of criticism of the Alabama and California laws. There was no equivocation about where the task force stood on the issue of regulation of ECT, or how it saw its own role in forestalling future regulations: "Our wish to avoid restrictions on clinical practice was more than balanced by our recognition of the fact that at this time in history where the profession fails to provide its own guidelines, they will be created by others who may be less well-equipped to do so."

Regulations, if any, should be "in the hands of psychiatrists" rather than legislators, and Massachusetts was held up as a successful example. Though the state had passed regulations, at least legislation had been averted and the industry had been able to control the outcome through its self-selected task force. The APA, expressing confidence in its ability to influence state commissioners of mental health (as opposed to legislators), said they could be allowed to regulate ECT in a "flexible" manner. This is exactly what would happen in state after state in the next decades.

In a defiant statement directed at future legislators, judges, or commissioners who might wish to regulate ECT, and using semijudicial language that would, in fact, be echoed by judges, the APA stated: "This Task Force finds that there is no division of *informed* opinion about the efficacy of the proposed treatment in appropriately selected cases and goes to great length in this report to indicate that when ECT is well administered, the risks and side effects can be minimized" (emphasis in the original). It added, as a further warning to meddlesome legislators, "We cannot accept that legislators are able to evaluate clinical data and believe that in California HB 1032 they reached decisions beyond their competence."

At the same time that it opposed all regulation of ECT, the APA had no choice but to appear to be in agreement with the idea of informed consent, in theory: "Patients must be provided with adequate information concerning the nature of the therapy, with its risks, discomforts and side-effects."

Yet it was defensive about the practice of giving ECT without consent, saying that "psychiatrists who have continued through the years to treat the mentally ill in the absence of fully informed consent have probably done so in good faith" and that such actions were justified by "the expressions of appreciation and gratitude of close relatives." It still believed, and continued to act as if, informed patients would not consent, but now it had a way around that problem. Through the Task Force Report and its subsequent editions, the APA itself would determine what informed consent was. It now had a vehicle to ensure that patients were told only what the industry wanted them to believe. The 1978 report offered practitioners an appendix with "Descriptions of ECT for Informed Consent," saying tentatively, "The following might be helpful to those interested in an example of how the information necessary for informed consent can be presented to patients, relatives, or guardians."

It became the most successful tool for selling ECT in its history. Today, virtually every facility in the United States offering ECT uses some version of the contemporary APA consent form. The form has changed over the years to reflect even greater denial of ECT's effects on memory and cognition than in 1978, but the essence of the industry's stance has not changed. The APA claimed then, and still does, that the majority of ECT patients do not experience permanent problems with memory. In its current incarnation, the 2001 APA Task Force Report consent form contends that "most patients report that their memory is actually improved by ECT."

Cuckoo's Nest Launches the PR Campaign

The ECT industry likes to say that *One Flew over the Cuckoo's Nest* caused its "crisis." In fact, as I have shown, the perceived crisis was well underway when the film came out in 1975. It could not have come at a better time for the shock industry. The film put shock in the national spotlight and gave the general public a way of talking about it—any publicist's dream, at no charge to the industry. Even better, *Cuckoo's Nest* handed the industry its public relations script, the one it has used successfully for over thirty years.

The book and film take place while the protagonist Randle McMurphy (the Jack Nicholson character) is confined to a mental hospital. Actually, shock plays a minor role in the story. McMurphy is not shocked until the very end, and it hardly seems to affect him at all. He comes out of each treatment feisty as ever, joking about having had his batteries charged. There is no mention of any memory loss or adverse cognitive effects. What finally reduces McMurphy to a vegetable is not shock, but a lobotomy.

What the movie does have is a graphic depiction, a minute or so long, of the shock treatment itself. Today most people know only this one scene from the movie and nothing else about it, since the clip has appeared on countless news programs.

Cuckoo's Nest allowed the industry to shift the focus of criticism away from the procedure's permanent effects on memory, cognition, and self—away from the mountains of evidence of harm, away from the decades of reports of real patients, away from the question of brain damage—to the few minutes of the administration of the treatment. The problem with the treatment in the movie was simply that it was given without anesthesia. That's why Jack Nicholson grimaced as the electricity hit him, why he appeared to be in pain. The treatment itself seemed so—to use a word repeated ad infinitum by the industry—barbaric.

At the same moment the industry was able to present this as the only problem with ECT, it was able to say loudly and clearly that the problem had been taken care of. *Cuckoo's Nest* took place in the 1950s. That would now be called the "old" shock. The industry would, cleverly, not attempt to deny the shortcomings of the treatment before the 1970s; it would instead use the free publicity provided by the movie as a springboard for marketing the "new and improved" shock.

The claim sounds good and resonates with a faith in the inevitability of progress so deeply rooted in the American character as to amount to a national religion. As the masters of public opinion knew, no public relations campaign succeeds unless it resonates with the preexisting beliefs, prejudices, and opinions of the public. The belief that things are always getting better as time goes on, due in large part to scientific and technological advances, has been called "escalator-faith." Ironically, the notion of upward linear motion doesn't come from science, but from philosophy. It's a spiritual belief, not a scientific fact.[12]

However, upon examination, every plank of the "new and improved ECT" platform turns out to be false. Each one was a lie back in 1978, when the APA first claimed that "ECT in the 1970s, administered by competent clinicians, is vastly different from the procedures used and described in the preceding 30 years. Problems and confusion result from a failure to make this distinction."[13] And, repeated twenty or thirty years later ("Electroshock . . . is no longer the bone-breaking, memory-modifying, fearsome treatment pictured in films. Anesthesia, controlled oxygenation, and muscle relaxation make the procedure so safe that the risks are less than those which accompany the use of several psychotropic drugs"), they are no less false.[14]

Shock is sold to the public the same way that laundry detergent and automobiles are sold: by exaggerating evidence or making up false claims about its benefits, and by omitting evidence as to its shortcomings or harms. Because nothing changes in the PR script, it's easy to detect the themes if you hear it enough times. Just as the founding father of public relations Edward Bernays prescribed, "These themes contain the ideas to be conveyed; they channel the lines of approach to the public; and they must be expressed through whatever media is used. The themes are ever present but intangible—comparable to what in fiction is called the story line. To be successful, these themes must appeal to the motives of the public."[15]

The ECT PR script, repeated over and over (by individual practitioners, by other health professionals, in journal articles, in the popular press, and on television) has been so successful that nearly every person I talk to about ECT will quote some version of it. It's as widely accepted as the "chemical imbalance" theory postulated by proponents of psychiatric drugs. In the useful language of discourse analysis (the practice of analyzing how the language we use not only reflects but shapes our reality), these systematic and stereotyped ways of talking about a subject are known as "interpretative repertoires."[16] They determine what it is—and isn't—possible to say about shock and therefore how we think about it.

"It Works"

A series of many electrically induced, closely spaced grand mal seizures, with the accompanying acute organic brain syndrome and cumulative amnesia, is guaranteed to temporarily change mood and behavior, no matter the condition that brought the person to ECT (and would do so in the same manner even if there were no psychiatric condition at all). It is a biological certainty that it is impossible to be depressed, or focus much on anything, while body and brain are struggling to recover from a grand mal seizure. This is ECT's biggest selling point, because patients come to ECT experiencing extreme distress and/or are extremely distressing to others. The claim that ECT works predates the public relations campaign, originating in an era in which virtually no other biological treatment existed to which ECT could be compared, but it has been subtly refined in an era of drug treatment and patients' rights.

With so many psychiatric drugs available today, why shock? Because there are many patients for whom the drugs fail, and they are in large part the market for shock treatment. An essential part of the interpretative repertoire on shock is the situation of ECT patients as, by definition, the most severely "ill." This has been called, by psychologists who analyzed the discourse of ECT practitioners, the "severe-end rhetorical device."[17] Read virtually anything on ECT, whether in a book, a medical journal, or the popular press, and you will see how this device is used at the beginning to set the terms of the discussion. In a journal article, it usually takes the form of a warning about the claimed severity of depression as an entity (such as a statistic on suicide that refers to 6 percent of patients who commit suicide rather than saying that 94 percent never do so). In another context such as a news program or article, it will be an anecdote about the dire circumstances of a particular patient. By the time you are finished hearing about the persons' troubles, you are willing to condone just about anything that might help them.

The effect of this rhetorical device is to downplay concerns about ECT's adverse effects. It works, doesn't it? What else matters? It is also used to justify involuntary shock. And it deflects questions about what the actual science says about ECT's effectiveness. For whom does it work, for how long, at what cost, and what other treatments might provide the same benefit without the risks? If some people for whom psychiatry had nothing else to offer, who had been dismissed as drug-resistant or treatment failures, are now getting out of bed, combing their hair, and playing Scrabble—is there any point in asking those questions? In the PR era, they are brushed aside.

Yet scientific evidence for ECT's efficacy is just not there. A commentator in the *New England Journal of Medicine* noted that between 1965 and 2008 there have been only two methodologically sound randomized controlled studies investigating whether ECT is more effective than drugs, and only five in its entire history.[18] And studies comparing ECT to nonbiological treatments are not done.

Studies comparing ECT to placebo (sham ECT, where matched controls are given anesthesia but no shock) are the best evidence available on efficacy. In 1992, British psychiatrist Graham Sheppard critically reviewed all the sham-versus-real ECT studies to that date. (There have been none since.) He concluded that real ECT was not more effective than fake ECT. Although he could not find a publisher for his article, his eighty-page paper was presented at a scientific conference.[19] In 2006, a review article which looked at patient outcomes one month after sham or real ECT also found no advantage for real ECT.[20]

A very large recent study found that nearly half of patients receive no benefit from ECT at all. One-hundred-thirty-one out of 290 patients (one of the largest groups of ECT patients ever studied) did not respond to a course of shock. Of the responding patients, 39 to 84 percent relapsed, most of them within a month, and at six months post-ECT, only twenty-eight, or 10 percent, of the patients had sustained any benefit from ECT.[21] It's important to note that the patients in this research study were treated by Mecta machines custom modified to put out twice the electricity of unmodified commercial devices, and that the efficacy rate with standard devices is even lower.

Rather than scientific evidence, the claim that ECT works is made by assertion and anecdote. There is no doubt that some patients are glad to have the short-term relief they obtain from ECT and willingly accept the trade-off of possible permanent impairment. Desperate relatives are grateful for short-term respite from the stress of caring for a family member. But there is no evidence that ECT has any long-term benefit.[22]

The claim that "ECT works" never includes the fine print that it doesn't work for a large percentage of patients, and that when it does it's a very temporary fix achieved only at the cost of unpredictable but possibly extensive permanent impairment. In fact, the word "works" itself in this context is a simplification at best, a faulty rhetorical device. We may be asking the wrong question. It is not whether ECT "works," but what we mean when we use that word. Psychiatrists find it useful and, indeed, could not get along without it, but is that the standard we should be using to evaluate a procedure that hasn't been scientifically studied and which has substantial risks to patients? Even the proponents of ECT don't have an answer for how it works. But others have a simple answer: both ECT's benefit and its adverse effects fit the clinical picture of brain damage.

"It Saves Lives"

The claim that ECT saves lives is the trump card in the PR deck, the one that shuts down discussion. To argue against this is to become the bad guy; would you take away their treatment and condemn these hypothetical people to death?

The belief that ECT prevents suicide has always been strongly held by psychiatrists. The function of such a belief is to dismiss concerns about safety and efficacy as relatively trivial, as in this statement: "So clear are the benefits of ECT for patients who might otherwise commit suicide . . . that there should be little controversy over whether it is safe or effective."[23] Yet prior to the PR era, there were extremely few studies which looked at the actual data on ECT and suicide. One such study in 1950 found that patients who had received ECT committed suicide at twice the rate of those who hadn't received it.[24]

The problem with this plank in the PR platform, like the others, is that it is not true. Although people have been killed by ECT and its complications and have killed themselves after ECT, there is no evidence, anywhere you look, that ECT has saved any lives or prevented suicides. In the PR era, many studies have been designed to investigate whether dogma on ECT and suicide is supported by evidence. Study after study from the 1970s to the present shows that if ECT indeed has any effect on suicide, it is that people who have had ECT may be more likely to die from suicide or other causes than persons who haven't had it.[25] Most recently, a 2007 study which reviewed the outcomes for all patients treated in a Danish hospital from 1976 to 2000 concluded that the ECT patients had a higher suicide rate.[26]

Even husband and wife psychiatrists Joyce and Iver Small (both of whom participated in the first two APA ECT task forces), who have been shock advocates for thirty years, could not design a study to show that ECT prevents suicide. They followed 1,494 patients for five to seven years (an eternity in shock follow-up research) and found that those who committed suicide were more likely to have received ECT. They were forced to conclude that "these findings combined with a close examination of the literature do not support the commonly held belief that ECT exerts long-range protective effects against suicide."[27]

Furthermore, even in the short term, the Smalls concede, "Factual data in support of this contention [that the immediate risk of suicide, when not manageable by other means, is a clear indication for ECT] are not readily obtainable."

ECT survivor and researcher Sue Kemsley, in a paper reviewing the literature on suicide and mortality, concluded succinctly: "ECT has built its reputation as a life-saving treatment not on the foundations of evidence, but on psychiatry's need to justify its use in an age when personal liberties count for more."[28]

"It's Not Like That Anymore": Oxygenation and Anesthesia

Ventilating a patient with pure oxygen while she can't breathe on her own has been done since the 1950s, as we saw in Chapter Four. Contemporary practitioners such as Max Fink claim that it "precludes ill effects on memory" and that research done in the 1950s proved this conclusively. But that can't explain why patients who've had ECT with oxygen experience the same amnesia and brain damage effects as patients treated in the 1940s without it.[29] They also claim that the human and animal autopsy reports showing brain damage don't implicate ECT because lack of oxygen, not the treatment itself, was the culprit.

But in clinical practice, as opposed to the PR statements, some doctors don't consider oxygenation a necessary part of the procedure.[30] Even today, at world-famous hospitals such as New York Hospital, patients are not routinely oxygenated, according to the industry's top spokesman and author of the current APA ECT practice guidelines. He says of oxygenation, "I don't think it's going to make a bit of difference . . . They [patients] don't turn blue."[31] As an ECT consultant to the hospital, he doesn't insist on oxygenation and doesn't believe it prevents memory loss.

Well into the twenty-first century, ECT is given without anesthesia to many patients in some countries; in Japan, for instance, two-thirds of hospitals use unmodified shock.[32] At least one contemporary shock practitioner in the U.K. recommends unmodified ECT as the treatment of choice in certain cases.[33] Even staunch ECT proponents acknowledge—when the media is not listening—that the use of anesthesia is for the benefit of doctors, not patients, because while lowering the risk of lawsuits against doctors over fractures and broken teeth, it increases the risk to patients of harm to the brain.[34] For instance, Dr. Jan-Otto Ottoson wrote in 1981, "The most decisive reason for the use of ECT with anesthesia are medico-legal reasons because of malpractice suits against psychiatrists."[35] Broken bones can and do recover, but brain damage and death are permanent.

However, the fact that limbs don't thrash and bones aren't broken has made ECT much more pleasing cosmetically, a huge advantage for the PR campaign. Virtually every television segment on ECT in the past thirty years has included a scene of an actual shock treatment being given. It looks like nothing is going on; after all, you can't see brain cells being destroyed or memories erased. To the uninformed viewer, ECT appears to be a benign process, and when the segment is juxtaposed with a clip of the shock treatment in *Cuckoo's Nest*, the viewer is completely sold on the "new and improved" claim. It's a cheap trick, one which always works.

"It's Not Like That Anymore": Less Electricity

Because of the now almost ubiquitous use of anesthesia in the United States, which raises the brain's seizure threshold, the "less electricity" plank of the PR platform is simply not true. However, there's another reason. The shock machine companies, like auto manufacturers, keep putting out new models, and each new generation has been designed with a greater electrical output than the last. This is at the request of the doctors themselves, who since the late 1970s have owned or consulted for the device manufacturers.[36] Thus the brief pulse machines of the 1980s, roughly when the claim of "less electricity" was locked into the industry PR template, were actually putting out much *more* electricity than those of the *Cuckoo's Nest* era. This is true as well for the sine wave machines that predominated until the mid-1980s and which are still used today, and it is true many times over for the newer generations of brief pulse models.

And the shock industry continues to clamor for still more powerful machines. Having reached the legal limit on the amount of electricity that the machines can put out, they are lobbying the Food and Drug Administration to allow them to make and sell machines like the ones used in research, which put out twice as much electricity as those in commercial use.[37] That's because they well know what the rest of us don't: that ECT is really not as effective as they have claimed. As we've just seen, it's not very effective even when researchers use custom-modified, amped-up devices. The high rate of relapse after ECT, no longer a secret, has become an embarrassment to the industry and a potential public relations disaster.

The shock doctors can't advocate for more electricity when the public is listening, because they must maintain the PR line that their machines use only a small amount of electricity. For example, Charles Kellner, a consultant to Mecta and Somatics, claimed on television in 1994 that contemporary ECT uses only "probably only one-fifth of the electricity that was used in the old days."[38]

There is little danger the media or the general public will read the medical journals or attend the professional meetings in which the shock industry spokesmen contradict their "less electricity" pronouncements. In these professional venues, the talk can be categorized as "turn up the juice." For example, at the APA annual meeting in 1996, shock machine company consultant Harold Sackeim told aspiring shock doctors that rather than administering the minimum amount of electricity to induce a seizure, as had been previously taught, they should make sure to multiply the amount of electricity

necessary for seizure induction by a factor of at least 2.5 so as to be sure the patient received enough voltage. It is the electricity, he said—not the seizure—that is the "therapeutic" ingredient in ECT.[39] The higher the electricity, the better the result, from the doctor's viewpoint.

That is the same conclusion reached by the shock doctors who first invented brief pulse ECT in the 1940s. Those first brief pulse experiments appear to have been, at least at first, an honest attempt to make ECT safer by administering the least amount of electricity possible. They failed because the lower amounts of electricity did not produce the desired "therapeutic" results. But they were what they claimed to be.

Around 1970, Paul Blachly of Oregon, the first American psychiatrist to start a shock machine company, had the idea to revive brief pulse, marketing it as a brand new treatment. The "crisis in ECT" was the incentive to package the old wine in new, souped-up bottles. This marketing strategy has been a success for Paul Blachly's company, and for the ECT practitioner entrepreneurs of rival Somatics (the company formed by Richard Abrams and Conrad Swartz in 1985).

However, in the 1970s as in the 1940s, there was no such thing as simply shortening the pulse width without compensating in other ways in order to disable the brain enough to cause dramatic changes in troubling behavior. The genius of the new shock machine company entrepreneurs was to find ways to compensate for the potentially lower (and ineffective) amount of electricity used in the earlier brief pulse machines. They built several design modifications into the machines, modifications that can't be undone or detected by the operator. These electrical compensations were first publicly unmasked by Douglas Cameron, himself a survivor of ECT.[40]

Cameron describes several ways the designers of the newer machines amp up overall output. The frequency of the electricity (that is, the number of pulses per second) is increased. The electrical current—electron flow per second—is increased. The amount of time the electricity flows though the

---

Figure 3. (*opposite*) A 1975 ad for the Mecta device.

brain is expanded as well—to up to six times the maximum duration of the old sine wave machines. Wave lengths can also be increased. And finally, all of today's ECT manufacturers have returned to alternating (AC) rather than direct (DC) current; ironically, this is exactly the opposite of the tactic the inventors of the original 1940s brief pulse devices utilized to try to reduce memory and cognitive impairment. If none of this is enough, the operator can augment the amount of electricity reaching the brain even further by holding down the shock button for as long as eight seconds.

By the 1990s, the so-called "new and improved" devices were more than *eight times* as powerful as the original machine invented in the 1930s. Cameron calls the vastly increased output of today's shock machines "a well-kept manufacturer's secret." Anyone can confirm his findings, using information from the manufacturers themselves and mathematical formulas. None of this is a matter of interpretation or opinion. Electricity can be measured and math doesn't lie. The sine wave shock devices of the 1940s–1950s were capable of lighting up a sixty-watt lightbulb for up to one second. Modern day sine wave machines can light up a hundred-watt lightbulb for up to one second. The brief pulse machines designed in the mid-1980s can light up a sixty-watt lightbulb for up to four seconds. Today's brief pulse shock machines are even more powerful.[41]

The sales hook for the brief pulse devices, of course, is the lie that they cause less memory loss than the "old" machines. For a time, shortly after I lost five years of my life to shock, Somatics' advertising materials proclaimed, in large type, "ECT Without Memory Loss." A generation of patients treated with brief pulse can tell you that this is not the case. Indeed, a systematic review by the United Kingdom's ECT Review Group in 2002 found "little evidence from randomized studies that sinewave causes more memory impairment than brief pulse."[42]

"It's Not Like That Anymore": Unilateral ECT

Another modification touted as a new and improved technique is unilateral ECT, or the practice of applying electrodes on only one side of the head. But again, this practice is nothing of the sort; it was invented in the 1940s. It was thought then that placing both electrodes on one temple, corresponding to the nondominant half of the brain, would reduce the overall amount of electricity used and thus minimize memory and cognitive effects. Some studies assert that it does minimize these effects and that this has been shown by formal testing. This claim comes with a catch: to assess amnesia and memory ability, researchers use verbal tests, such as learning a list of words.[43] However, the side of the brain not shocked, the dominant side (usually the left side for right-handed individuals) controls speech and verbal skills. The nondominant side of the brain is associated with visual memory and other nonverbal functions, such as musical and artistic ability. Thus, damage to the nondominant side of the brain is not detected when these abilities are not tested.

There's another catch: with unilateral ECT, much more electricity must be used in order to produce the same "therapeutic" effect as with bilateral. Any net cognitive savings are easily wiped out when the electricity is turned up to six or twelve or twenty times the amount necessary to induce a seizure. Shock machine magnate Richard Abrams quipped in the *Journal of ECT*, "As Sigmund Freud said to Wilhelm Fleiss when the latter informed him he had kissed a patient for therapeutic purposes: Why stop there?"[44] Some patients receive as much as *four thousand times* their threshold levels.[45] By 2000, industry leaders said that any type of unilateral besides "high dose" was ineffective and should not be used, once again shooting their "less electricity" PR script in the foot.

Whether unilateral ECT produces less damage or merely a different type of damage is a moot point now, anyway. Unilateral, even "high dose," is rarely used in clinical practice today.[46] Its main value is as a tool for selling shock to the public. (Sometimes, to induce them to consent, patients are told they'll be started out on the supposedly memory-sparing unilateral shock, but the doctor always reserves the right to switch to bilateral if it "doesn't work." By the time the switch is made, the patient has forgotten the original consent agreement.) Like the original brief pulse ECT, unilateral was just never popular with doctors. Fink has now assigned even the high-voltage version of unilateral to the garbage bin of history, saying "we have fiddled with this placement for more than 40 years, and no credible way has been found to make its application effective."[47]

The fact that *Cuckoo's Nest* was set in the 1950s was Hollywood's great gift to the shock industry. It inspired the industry's single most successful line of defense: "It's not like that any more!" and one of the most successful public relations campaigns ever (compare, for instance, the tobacco industry's lack of such a defense, and what happened to it). The shock industry was right, on the face of it. Shock wasn't like that; it was much more powerful, much more dangerous. The industry lie was that it was now *safer*.

But to cry "unfair!" and to keep crying it and endlessly referring to the movie was to cleverly replot the entire story. For instance, a now-typical reference to *Cuckoo's Nest* goes like this: "*One Flew over the Cuckoo's Nest* is an example of Hollywood doing a disservice to medicine. I wonder how many people were killed because of that movie—how many people did not get ECT treatment because of it?"[48]

The culprit wasn't shock, it was public misperception and the psychiatry-hating media. Now the shock industry could take on the sympathetic role of victim (of the cruel media) rather than the villainous role of disabler of innocent brains.

7 *The Making of an American Activist*

The American Psychiatric Association's PR script does not allow for any criticism of electroshock. It is so overbroad in its denial of harm from contemporary ECT, and so committed to its denial, that it must dismiss all its critics as irrational. It does this effectively, without ever addressing any of their claims, by maligning their character, sanity, or motivation. This is usually accomplished by using one-word epithets, whether they apply to any particular critic or not. For example, those who challenge the use of ECT are said to be "antipsychiatry." Scientologists. And in the case of former patients, crazy, hysterical, or some version thereof will suffice.

This cannot explain how the shock survivors' movement came to be founded by an ordinary, sweet, sane, middle-aged, middle-class woman named Marilyn Rice. In reality there is generally only one reason anyone becomes an activist critical of electroshock: bad luck. That is how ordinary people end up making history.

For nearly fifty years, Marilyn Rice led a conventional life. The most remarkable thing she did was to confound some contemporary notions about what a woman could do. Highly intelligent, she earned a college degree in the 1940s, then built a successful career as an economist for the federal government. As far as I know, she never expressed an opinion on any political issue of her day, whether it was race relations, women's rights, or the war in Vietnam. She was not the type. I only once heard her express an opinion on a politically contentious topic. It was smoking; as a veteran smoker, she was in favor of it.

She was a rule follower. A nine-to-fiver, a steady achiever, and the straightest of all arrows: a government bureaucrat. As she once quipped, "Russell Baker always uses the Gross National Product as the symbol of all that is stodgy and conservative and respectable, and it is the simple truth that I was the country's leading technical expert on that fat and ugly statistic."[1] She married late, by happenstance had no children, and supported herself

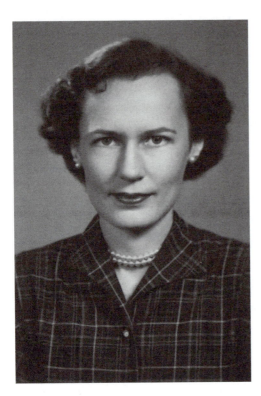

Figure 4. Marilyn Rice before her involvement with psychiatry.

and her husband while doing the cooking and housekeeping as well. In 1968, more or less for fun, she authored a thousand-page monograph on "The Anatomy of Federal Accounts." Study hard, work hard, get ahead, retire in comfort; that was the deal she'd signed up for. She saw no reason to complain.

Then she encountered electrical psychiatry.

How Marilyn Got Shocked

In the spring of 1972, when she was nearly fifty years old, her front teeth started to come loose, and she discovered she had serious gum problems. An orthodontist convinced her he could straighten her teeth while taking care of her gums, and she agreed, embarking on a series of periodontal treatments. But it quickly became apparent that this orthodontist was wreaking havoc on her mouth and her life. Each step in the process meant more misery. He pulled teeth and prodded others in such a way that her mouth became misshapen and she could hardly eat or speak, all the while assuring her it was for her own good. In constant pain, physically exhausted and emotionally depleted, she agreed to enter the Psychiatric Institute in Washington, D.C., in February 1973 for what she hoped would be some respite. She'd later call it "wall-to-wall carpeted Buchenwald."[2]

Her young psychiatrist, upon hearing that she was the sole support of her family, insisted on ECT, telling her it would get her back to work more quickly than psychotherapy. He didn't mention any permanent memory loss. ECT was presented as a harmless miracle. Rice was too worn down to resist what her doctor wanted. In March 1973 she had eight shock treatments.

She emerged in a kind of fog. She didn't know that she was in a psychiatric hospital, or why. She had no idea what was wrong with her mouth. When she returned home she didn't recognize her neighbors, and she didn't have enough short-term memory to read a book.

The fog lasted for weeks. Then she tried to go back to work. She realized that she had permanently lost years of her life, including the wealth of specialized knowledge she'd accumulated since college. Her psychiatrist, initially aghast at the realization that the procedure had ruined a fine brain, quickly became defensive. "Your work was too big a part of your life," he told her.[3]

Up to that point, Rice—like most people—trusted in doctors. But now, she slowly began to figure out what had happened to her, and it went against everything she thought she knew. Her doctors had lied to her.

She waited for her memory to return, as they had promised it would. It did not. Where there should have been memories was "an ocean of blankness . . . out of the ocean rolled great waves of horror: *Me! Brain damaged!*"[4]

She wrote, "All my beloved knowledge, everything I had learned in my field during twenty years or more, was gone. I'd lost the body of knowledge that constituted my professional skill. I'd lost everything that professionals take for granted. I'd lost my experience, my knowing. But it was worse than that. I felt that I'd lost my self."[5]

At first, she thought it would be possible to relearn what she'd lost, even if it took her another twenty years. What she found was that she wasn't able to hold on to new information. Her memory function was permanently impaired as well.

She assumed that her doctors hadn't known this could happen, and that they would want to know to ensure that it would never happen again. So she decided to tell them.

Marilyn Becomes a Brain Scientist

Beginning in July 1973, she began a two-pronged research project that would engage her for the rest of her days. She read everything that had been written about ECT by scientists and psychiatrists in the field, from journal articles to textbooks to its mention in the popular press. She made careful notes and summaries because she knew she couldn't trust her memory. She read all she could about memory, about brain science, and about brain damage as well. The work suited her lifelong love of learning and her addiction to research and scholarship as a way of life. Not even shock could change that. "I remain a scientist," she wrote in 1974, "although I have also become a guinea pig."[6]

She found the quality of the professional writings on ECT appalling. From the beginning of its use, it seemed, doctors had parroted the line that ECT cannot cause permanent amnesia or brain damage—based on research that actually showed the opposite (as we have seen in our survey of the early animal research), was too poorly designed to show anything, or on no basis at all.

On the other side of her exhaustive study, she questioned every person she could find who had experienced ECT. Since she was very open about her shock experience—it simply never occurred to her to be ashamed or to hide it—other shock patients had a way of finding her. These patients unanimously reported their memories had been permanently impaired by shock, in direct contradiction to the claims made by practitioners.

With great sincerity, Rice began mailing out educational materials on ECT's adverse effects to psychiatrists. She called it "shooting off my mouth and typewriter in all directions."[7] She shot off her first letter to one of the shock industry's biggest names, psychiatrist Max Fink, in August 1974, asking him whether he told patients they would get their memory back in three weeks. She got no answer from Fink, but wrote to others who had published books or articles on ECT. She wrote to the National Institute of Mental

Health (NIMH), the American Psychiatric Association, the American Medical Association, and various hospital directors. She suggested designs for research studies on memory loss. She even wrote a straight-faced spoof of the shock literature, poking fun at Fink in particular, and submitted it to psychiatric journals under the name M. Rice. She called it "The Delusion of Amnesia after Electric Shock Treatment." To her great amusement, she received equally straight-faced responses from the journal editors.

Retired now on a disability pension due to brain damage, Rice needed something to do with her boundless energy, intellectual curiosity, keen sense of injustice, and twenty years of free time. But even so, her educational campaign and her career as an accidental activist wouldn't have happened without two other key ingredients. First, she lacked an identity as a mental patient. If a devalued person internalizes the mental patient role, she can come to doubt her own ideas, experiences, and worth. Such a patient might be convinced by a doctor that her memory loss didn't happen, or that it happened only to her. Had Rice internalized an image of herself as crazy, she would have been too ashamed to tell the world about her psychiatric history. She was having none of that, because she never lost her class identity and privilege. The lifestyle and mindset of a middle-class professional was engrained in her. Losing her job couldn't change that. Many former ECT patients become poor very quickly after losing the ability to work, with only below-poverty disability payments to live on. But Rice had worked so long, at such a high level, that her disability pension was enough to sustain a middle-class lifestyle.

In short, she saw no reason why psychiatrists—with whom she shared this class identity—shouldn't listen to her: "I have always felt that the peculiar circumstances of my experience made me a first-rate laboratory animal for reporting what electric shock does to memory," she wrote in 1975. "Perhaps this is something that has only been done to really crazy people or not very bright people in the past, I innocently thought, and I can at least bring something good out of something bad by letting the psychiatric profession know of my important scientific discovery."[8]

As a professional, Rice expected high standards of other professionals. She assumed that psychiatrists at the National Institute of Mental Health were like the economists at the Department of Commerce. If the government said something, it had to have the facts and figures to back it up. No one at the Commerce Department would dream of printing an unsubstantiated statement.

Rice's job involved explaining how the government computes the gross national product. She was responsible for providing answers to the public to questions like, What do those big figures mean? Where do you get them? She expected NIMH to do the same. When they published a brochure for the public called *Facts about: Electroshock Therapy* claiming that "research now suggests" permanent amnesia does not occur, Rice contacted them, asking politely to be given the references for this research.[9] They referred her to two articles from the 1940s, three from the 1950s, and one from 1972. None of the research dealt with amnesia at all. None of the patients were followed up longer than six weeks.[10]

Some time afterwards, NIMH stopped distributing the brochure, saying "it would be appropriate to withdraw the pamphlet from circulation pending further evaluation of issues regarding the psychological and physiological impact of electroconvulsive therapy on the human organism."[11]

As Empty as Eve

Rice had friends who were, like herself, middle-class professionals, and one of them happened to write for that most middle-class of general interest magazines, the *New Yorker*. Through this friend, Berton Roueché, a journalist of impeccable credentials, came to be interested in her story, and she was glad to tell it. He changed her name (at his insistence, not hers) and added a fictitious upbeat ending, but otherwise got the details of her story right, thanks to many interviews and extensive written materials that Rice provided. His use of her letters to her family before and after shock especially spooked readers. In the most mundane prose, they reveal the full horror of suddenly, without warning, not knowing who or where you are or how you got there while at the same time *not knowing you don't know*.

Rice wrote shortly after shock, "Now I know how Eve must have felt, having been created full grown out of somebody's rib without any past history. I feel as empty as Eve."[12] The article, which appeared in the *New Yorker* on September 4, 1974, took this as its title. This was the first full-length, first-person description of extensive permanent ECT amnesia and disability to appear in the media.

The article took the APA by surprise. They weren't prepared to launch an all-out attack on the *New Yorker*. In the fall of 1974, the APA's public relations campaign was still to come. The task force had just been formed. Larry Squire, who—as we have seen—would contribute to the APA defense of shock in the Task Force Report, was still sitting on the fence between patients and doctors, maintaining a cordial and scholarly correspondence with Rice that had predated the article.

In just a couple of years, the industry would be fully prepared to launch an attack on any media coverage it deemed unacceptable. But in a note to Roueché, with whom she kept in touch, Rice noted that the response from the shock brigade was "a loud howl of silence."[13]

There were those, like Squire, who recognized Rice as the "Natalie Parker" of the article; and there were those who wrote to her care of the magazine and received a reply from Marilyn Rice. Either way, she heard from ex-patients and others from all over the country, and the lively correspondence she was already having with anyone interested in shock grew exponentially. Opportunities opened up for her; for instance, the chance to test-drive the early memory tests Squire was developing in order to measure ECT amnesia (her candid assessment was that they were either much too simple to assess ECT damage, or "phony"). She was able to have input into the Alabama shock legislation, and, perhaps most importantly, to network with others in the brand new ex-patients' movement.

The King and Queen of Shock

Leonard Roy Frank of San Francisco has been one of the key figures in the mental patients' movement since the 1970s. Frank's shock experience, sprinkled with quotes from his medical records, is told in John Friedberg's book *Shock Treatment Is Not Good for Your Brain.* He was locked up by his middle-class parents in the 1960s, largely because he had rejected their values. His "symptoms" included reading Ghandi, becoming a vegetarian, and growing a beard. Frank received fifty insulin shock treatments and thirty-five electroshocks, and lost years of his life. But even though his doctors shaved off his beard, the shocks didn't change his spiritual beliefs and countercultural lifestyle. He was part of the collective of former psychiatric inmates that put out the seminal texts of the movement, *Madness Network News* and *Madness Network News Reader*. He was Rice's introduction to, and connection with, sixties-style in-your-face activism: the protests, the civil disobedience, the guerrilla theater. The organization he co-founded, Network Against Psychiatric Assault, was instrumental in passing the California shock legislation.

There could hardly have been two people more different in style than the proud nonconformist with his long salt-and-pepper beard and the soft-spoken bureaucrat with her gray hair permanently styled in the 1950s manner. They were united only by their shock experiences and their desire to do something about it. After the *New Yorker* article, Rice wrote to Roueché, "I seem to have become the queen of the country's brain-damaged people. The Joan of Arc streak in me gets some satisfaction out of being the stronger nut standing up for the weaker ones."[14] If Marilyn Rice was the Queen of Shock, Leonard Roy Frank was the King.

Having lived by the rules her entire life, Rice was inclined to work through the proper channels—to ask politely and expect to be heard. "I don't call demonstrations 'action,'" she fumed in frustration over Frank's methods.[15] Frank had no illusions about the willingness of psychiatry, or the government, to yield anything on the basis of appeals to abstract principles like truth, law, and justice. Their relationship, originally warm and friendly, would eventually suffer as their philosophical and political differences became apparent.

By the time the *New Yorker* article came out, Rice was becoming disillusioned about her efforts to educate psychiatrists. She had honestly expected them to respond in the same good faith, and they had let her down. Her class had let her down, and she was never to get over it. "The profession didn't *want* to know about the effect of electric shock," she wrote to Frank. "Or," she continued darkly, "knowing, didn't want anyone making waves by telling."[16]

Her faith in truth, justice, and the American way shaken but not shattered, Rice, at her husband's urging, filed a lawsuit against her doctor. She even allowed herself the hope that it might succeed. As she later wrote,

"My purpose in pursuing the case was to try to establish the principle that shock doctors may no longer lie with impunity to patients about what will happen to their memories. I wanted something good to come out of something bad. And it was such an absolute beauty of a case."[17]

The Woman with the Ninety-Year-Old Brain

Previously, ECT patients had sued—and sometimes won—only when they suffered physical damage like broken teeth and cracked ribs, and only when they could prove the procedure wasn't done correctly. No one had ever brought a lawsuit for memory loss before. *Rice v. Nardini*, filed in Superior Court of the District of Columbia in February 1974, was the first to allege malpractice for lack of informed consent to ECT resulting in permanent amnesia.

> Defendant assured both the plaintiff and her husband that said electric shock treatments would impair her memory only slightly and for a period not to exceed three or four weeks. As a result of the electric shock treatments . . . the plaintiff has suffered what appears to be a permanent amnesia. The defendant, Dr. Nardini, did not . . . inform the plaintiff of the prospects of memory impairment resulting from the shock treatment; the plaintiff was prevented from exercising sound judgment before submitting to the treatment. . . . As a result of the defendant, Dr. Nardini's, failure to secure the informed consent of the plaintiff to the treatment given her, the plaintiff has suffered severe memory impairment and loss of ability to earn a living.[18]

The suit alarmed Rice's referring psychiatrist, Dr. Peter Mendelis. He had no reason to be afraid for himself, since he hadn't performed the shocks and wasn't named as a defendant. No, Mendelis frankly feared for the future of the shock industry. He thought he saw the handwriting on the wall bringing down the whole enterprise. So he wrote for help to the most senior shock proponent in America at the time, Lothar Kalinowsky.

Kalinowsky agreed with his assessment. There was good reason to fear both Mrs. Rice and a young psychiatrist named Peter Breggin, whom they suspected would be involved in the case. *Rice v. Nardini* could cause the industry irreparable harm; it might even force it into doing studies to prove that shock didn't cause brain damage. The case had to be defeated, but how to do that, they puzzled, when the plaintiff was a person of some stature, so talented and so obviously normal?[19]

Rice certainly was that person. But in a lawsuit, the truth often gets so twisted around that the plaintiff can no longer recognize herself or her life in the story told by the other side. That's just what happened in *Rice v. Nardini*.

Rice's lawyer, as well, had heard of Dr. Peter Breggin and his public criticism of ECT. The lawyer insisted that she needed a local physician as an expert witness and Breggin, like Rice, lived in the D.C. area. But she could tell that Breggin saw her first and foremost as a mental patient, and foresaw this as a deadly blow to her case. Indeed, he wanted to treat her by the hour for her "mental illness." She wasn't in need of any psychiatric treatment. Rice had lined up other experts and didn't want him, but Breggin sold himself to her lawyer.

In addition, she and her husband were repelled by Breggin's focus on money; he charged much more than any of the other proposed experts and insisted on being paid in advance. For all that, she couldn't get him to return her calls. She tried to get him off the case, but her lawyer would not hear of it. The lawyer, as well, treated her like an incompetent mental patient and shut her out of the case. She was stuck with a hostile expert witness.

Still, she hoped to put shock on trial. But the defense took the position that her amnesia was due to menopausal insanity. It might have seemed an easy task to discredit this position with logic and facts. But the defendant, John Nardini, was a trustee of the American Psychiatric Association. Breggin, in what Rice saw as a display of the medical profession's code of silence, caved in and sided with his peers. He wouldn't testify that her amnesia was due to ECT.

To her horror, the defense depicted her as a raving psychotic rather than an ordinary woman driven to despair by the stress and pain of botched orthodontic treatment. She couldn't even recognize herself or her treatment in the medical records that were presented to the jury; not only did they make her out to be a lunatic, but the doctor's and nurses' notes were almost comically inconsistent. For example, on the same day, the nurses called her pleasant, the doctor hostile. Another day she was "in good spirits" in one set of records, "profoundly depressed" in another. She could only conclude that the doctor's notes submitted by Mendelis had been forged for the trial. This would have been entirely consistent with his expressed desire to protect the practice of ECT as he knew it.

Rice would later ruefully call these the "crudest grossest *funniest* forgeries ever."[20] But they weren't funny at the time. She couldn't get her own lawyer to object to them; at the time, his daughter was in the process of having her teeth straightened by the same orthodontist who had ruined Rice's mouth.

Nor would Breggin believe that the medical records had been forged for the trial. "Doctors don't doctor records," he stated flatly, and he testified as if the records were authentic.[21] The defense tactic worked as intended to destroy all Rice's credibility with the jury.

"My lawsuit was an atomic bomb," she bitterly concluded later, "and Breggin worked to prevent me from detonating it. . . . Breggin stands firm protecting the American Psychiatric Association."[22]

To make matters even worse, her lawyer wouldn't let the jury hear three of her other medical experts, who were prepared to verify amnesia and brain damage due to ECT. Rice suspected it was because Breggin wanted the spotlight to himself.[23]

The defense had hired Lothar Kalinowsky as their expert. He testified that there had never been a case of permanent memory loss caused by the procedure.

The star witness was to have been Rice's brain scan. The computerized axial tomography (CAT) imaging technique had just become widely available. She believed, sensibly, that a brain scan would settle the question of whether or not the eight shocks had damaged her brain. So she had one. Even without a scan to show how her brain had looked before shock, a radiologist was able to compare her postshock brain with the norm for her age. Her brain had shrunk, or, in scientific terms, atrophied, so much that it looked like the brain of a typical ninety-year-old. Rice was fifty-three.

Had her case been tried on the merits, she would likely have won. But a jury is just a microcosm of society, with its hatred and dearly held stereotypes of mental patients. All a defendant need do is play to the jury's prejudices. The irony of Rice's case, of course, was that she was as far from the stereotype as could be. But with her own former psychiatrist testifying wholeheartedly against her, she was seen as nothing more than a crazed mental patient. "His unchallenged slanders about me had more influence on the jury than anything anybody said about electric shock," she concluded after the trial.[24] Compared to that, even the CAT scan was seen as irrelevant.

Breggin was, from her standpoint, quite simply a costly disaster, and one which didn't even end with the trial; he continued to demand money from her afterwards. She hadn't realized at first that his agenda did not correspond to hers: "Peter Breggin couldn't see our joining forces toward a common goal. . . . I think he did want to use the case to work against shock but in an indirect way, i.e., for getting financial support for the monograph he was writing and by promoting his own fame as a psychiatrist."[25] Indeed, his book (partially financed by the money she paid him) was published in 1979, and many other books followed. Breggin became famous and has had a long and lucrative career as an expert witness in ECT cases. But over the course of the next generation, not a single shock case in which Breggin appeared as an expert was won by a plaintiff. In January 1977, *Rice v. Nardini* was decided for the defendants.

She later pursued an action to have her shock case declared a mistrial, obtaining *amici curiae* briefs in support of her appeal to the court to reexamine the purported medical records.[26] That would be in the public interest, she argued, because of what was at stake in the case.

> It happened that plaintiff was not merely *a* patient suing *a* doctor. She was the typical shock patient of the new era, a middle-class middle-aged white woman who was a voluntary patient in a short-term hospital, was suffering from "depressive symptomatology," had 8 shocks, and had everything paid for by Blue Cross or other health insurance. Plaintiff fitted this description "to a T." She represented the *economic base* of present-day psychiatric hospitalization, and her informed consent lawsuit threatened it profoundly. . . . In summary, the issues and evils dealt with in the case of *Rice v. Nardini* were large social issues and evils. Plaintiff's injuries were the injuries of many, and her case represented a turning to

the courts for relief of large classes of persons from the ill effects of unbridled medical power. . . . It is perhaps not surprising that such "high" motives for denial of plaintiff's injuries should have worked themselves out through low motives on the part of the more immediate participants in the trial.[27]

Her pleas were not successful.

The whole experience left Rice with a distaste for the legal profession nearly equal to that she had for medicine. She found a little solace in designing a new letterhead for her correspondence, one which she used for a time after the trial. Under her name and address, it read: "Civilization in medicine and law is 500 years behind civilization in the rest of society."

The Truth in Psychiatry Letters: 1975–1983

Through all this, Rice had kept up her educational campaign. By 1975, she had developed an extensive list of correspondents and hit upon the idea of simply cc-ing each letter to multiple recipients. (This she did the old-fashioned way: with a typewriter and carbon paper. Ninety-year-old brain or not, Rice did not make typing errors.)

From 1975 to 1983 she sent out at least one mass mailing a week. These she called "Truth in Psychiatry" letters, because "it wasn't so much the *shocking* that was appalling about psychiatry, but the *lying*."[28] She wrote to psychiatrists, researchers, editors of medical journals, writers, television networks, the National Institute of Mental Health, the American Psychiatric Association, the American Medical Association, insurance companies, medical laboratories, drug companies, members of Congress, the Food and Drug Administration, shock machine manufacturers, former patients . . . and eventually to Jackie Kennedy Onassis, whom she'd heard had had shock, just in case the rumor was true. (Her secretary wrote back that it wasn't.) Each missive might be copied to ten to forty recipients besides its addressee.

The letters can be utterly disarming in their directness. Recipients must have been impressed by Rice's obvious wealth of knowledge and brutal honesty. Many did reply; for example, from France came a thoughtful response from a famous epilepsy researcher, and from Moscow, a letter from the world-renowned neuropsychologist A. R. Luria. Others didn't have the courage to place themselves under her scrutiny. One which surely must have gone unanswered by its primary recipient was addressed to the director of research at a state psychiatric institute and cc-ed to twenty-two others.

January 12, 1976

Dear Dr. Davis,

According to your article on electric shock in the October 27, 1975 issue of *Medical World News*, "memory loss . . . generally disappears within a month." According to the only study ever made of the state of memory after electric shock, no subject had a memory even remotely resembling normal. I enclose a protocol from that study in case you are not familiar with it.

What is the evidence that leads you to believe that memory is typically fine after shock?

Yours truly

Marilyn Rice

Others, like psychiatrist Lawrence Kolb, the author of a widely used textbook assuring doctors that "full return of memory finally occurs" and that shock "is not followed by any intellectual impairment," did respond, but only to insist that "there has been nothing in the scientific literature to show that good return and full intellectual functioning fails to take place in the vast majority of patients." Of course, there were two answers to that: the "scientific literature" had rarely chosen to study memory and intellectual functioning months after shock, and when it had, there was no such return to normal. Rice set the former APA president straight with her references, but all he could say was "I am grateful for your note and will continue to look into the matter further."[29]

The woman with the ninety-year-old brain also maintained a "sportsmanlike" correspondence with psychiatrist and shock machine entrepreneur Paul Blachly. Serious as she always was, she also had a droll side, which she'd use when she saw little hope of getting through by other means.

May 2, 1977

Dear Dr. Blachly,

Supplementing my letter of last week on psychiatrically-induced brain damage, I should like to call your attention to the phenomenon of accidental alleviation of nervous or mental disorders by brain-damaging experience. The phenomenon is often mentioned in the literature. [References follow, including one in which a doctor muses in print that "A doctor can't very well knock a patient over the head or fling him downstairs . . . but what about electric shock?"]

Dr. Blachly, I could easily set up a psychiatric hospital as good as yours. I would just put the patients down on the sidewalk and interfere with their cerebral function by dropping flower pots on their heads. I would put crash helmets on them to prevent external bleeding.

Yours very truly,

Marilyn Rice

References on request.

"One in 200"

As a statistician herself, Rice knew that statistics don't just appear all by themselves. Behind every statistic is a person. She herself had been such a person, and she expected no less of others who propagate statistics than the rigor and honesty of her own work.

Nothing disgusted her more than blatantly dishonest use of the tools of her former profession. In 1979, Rice worked closely with the New York State Assembly as it (unsuccessfully) attempted to pass legislation requiring reporting of ECT statistics. In this context, a Dr. Joseph P. Morrissey wrote a selective literature review that Rice read pre-publication.

Here, for the first time, was the claim that only one in two hundred ECT patients experiences serious adverse effects such as permanent memory loss. It was footnoted to an article by Max Fink. The trouble was there was no reference to any study or any data backing up the claim in the Fink article or anywhere else.

To her contact at the state assembly, Rice wrote, "No reference. No line of reasoning. No nothing. This happens all the time. A shock propagandist makes up a 'fact' out of his own head, publishes it, and then the rest of them start quoting it. Maybe you could prevail upon Dr. Morrissey in the name of honest scholarship to take that out of his paper before it gets published in the *International Journal of Law and Psychiatry*. I guess the statistician in me remains sensitive to crazy statistics."[30]

But of course it was published.[31] Rice didn't have the ability to prevail upon the doctor, and her correspondent, a junior aide to an assemblyman, didn't try. The one in two hundred "statistic," as she predicted it would be, has been repeated by industry spokesmen and irresponsible journalists for more than twenty-five years. It is stated as fact in the second Task Force Report of the APA, published in 1990. Because of this, it appears to this day in most hospital consent forms.

Marilyn and the Media

Nothing written or shown on television about shock or psychiatry got by Rice and little escaped comment. In a memorable letter to Arthur Ochs Sulzberger, publisher of the *New York Times*, in which she reprimanded him for a 1979 story that stated that a new version of ECT eliminated memory loss, she concluded: "With which news of fits, sir, you sank beneath what's fit to print."[32]

In 1976, television got interested in her, courtesy of Leonard Frank, who told her that ABC-TV was doing a documentary called *Madness and Medicine* on the burgeoning mental patients' rights movement. Rice put aside her concerns about her facial disfigurement to be interviewed on camera; she thought it was that important to tell her story. She was interviewed by what seemed like a sympathetic crew for three hours at her home.

When the show aired on May 26, 1977, she felt cheated. Only about a minute of the footage was used, and what was used seemed misleading and out of context. The viewer could easily have been left with the impression that dental troubles cause amnesia.

Still, the program packed a punch. Others appearing included Ted Chabasinski of the Network Against Psychiatric Assault in California, who had been electroshocked at the age of three, Peter Breggin, and Dr. Robert Grimm, who'd been one of Rice's expert witnesses. Electroshock wasn't the sole focus of the program; it was about abuses in psychiatry, but as the show's host pointed out, "More people get angry about electroshock than any other psychiatric procedure."

Shock machine entrepreneur Paul Blachly appeared for the industry, promoting his (now thoroughly discredited) brand of multiple ECT. Breggin pointed out, "If you look at the studies . . . that allegedly proved no damage, you actually find damage in them. It's a most amazing fact if you actually look up the studies." There wasn't much the then-president of the American Psychiatric Association, Robert Gibson, could say back to that. He admitted that ECT "has a certain hazard to it. . . . It can be felt as a kind of attack." The program ended with psychiatrist E. Fuller Torrey, before he did an about-face and became one of the nation's foremost proponents of forced psychiatric treatment, proposing that psychiatry be abolished. "Buried?" asked the interviewer. "Buried," said Torrey.

Madness and Medicine marked the first intersection of the mainstream media and the national mental patients' rights movement. It couldn't have come at a better time for the shock industry; at a time when its public relations strategy was at a critical stage of development, the show, like *Cuckoo's Nest*, gave them something to rally around.

8   *The ECT Industry Cows the Media*

Public opinions must be organized for the press if they are to be sound, not by the press.

—Walter Lippman

The campaign to sell psychiatry and its wares to the public began in earnest in August 1977, in specific response to the *Madness and Medicine* program. The newly elected president of the American Psychiatric Association, Jack Weinberg, sent out a letter to all its members that was also published in *Psychiatric News.*[1] It announced the beginning of the APA's campaign to win over the media in the classic public relations manner: each member was asked to donate at least ten dollars to conduct a survey of public attitudes toward psychiatry. "APA cannot launch a truly effective campaign to improve the accuracy of the public's perception of psychiatry," said Weinberg, "without a scientific analysis of what the misperceptions are, and why they exist." His choice of words defined the problem without seeming to: the public's attitudes were inaccurate, the public had misperceptions. Thus, the APA's problem could be solved without examining or changing anything about the practice of psychiatry itself. Framed that way, the problem could *only* be solved by public relations, and the Joint Commission on Public Affairs (the membership arm of its Public Affairs division) was assigned to do just that.

APA members gave more than $30,000 in just two months to the commission, chaired by Shervert Frazier of the International Psychiatric Association for the Advancement of ECT. The survey launched the APA's ambitious campaign for control of the media.

Beginning in 1977, the Joint Commission on Public Affairs developed and cultivated a "Roster of Media Contacts," a list of five hundred self-selected "experts" on various topics who signed on to do public relations for psychiatry. The commission provided training and guidance to these public relations spokespeople. Never again would a writer on ECT rely on dead doctors, dusty textbooks, and papers presented to strange-sounding medical societies at remote European conferences (to name three of the sources of information used by Berton Roueché in his 1974 *New Yorker* article).

Now, all she would need would be a single phone call to APA headquarters in Washington, where she'd connect with someone as much at ease in an interview or in front of a camera as in a hospital, maybe even someone whose name and face would be reassuringly familiar and instantly recognizable from previous articles and media appearances. The reporter would never be at a loss for the perfect quote of exactly the right length and tone, and no more digging up back issues of hard-to-find medical journals to corroborate those facts and figures; after all, she'd be talking with an expert.

Back in the pre–public relations days Roueché had cited eight experts of his own choosing. Only one of them made the cut to the PR team of the 1980s.

"Media psychiatrists," as they were called, were either recruited through ads in *Psychiatric News* or appointed, and were carefully trained. They were regularly supplied with "Public Affairs Guidelines" to hone their skills. "To ensure that a statement is used with a minimum of editing," coaches one such set of guidelines, "keep it under 45 seconds in length . . . listeners and viewers have a hard time absorbing facts and figures . . . on-camera impressions say more."[2]

None of this would have availed, of course, had the APA not been able to orchestrate consistent and unwavering consensus from the mouths of all media psychiatrists on a given topic. Task forces were formed within the APA to hammer out position papers. Since 1978, when the first Task Force Report on Electroconvulsive Therapy was published, to this day, the report has conveniently become the standard answer to any journalist asking about ECT. The task force strategy has been used to manage controversy and shape public opinion on other issues as well, such as tardive dyskinesia (permanent brain damage caused by antipsychotic drugs). The reports serve to legitimize psychiatric treatments in the eyes of the public and, just as importantly, become a de facto "standard of care" to protect the profession from malpractice lawsuits.

There remained the problem of how to train reporters and producers in this new way of conducting their business. Some of them, lamented the APA's marketing director, "prefer to ferret the news story out themselves."[3] The APA's solution made its debut in 1978, with the first APA-sponsored "National Symposium for Media Writers." Media people would be targeted, courted, and invited to this event, the first of many ostensibly designed to alert them to advances in the field. The 1978 event was held in the resort town of Snowmass, Colorado, during ski season. Those reporters who produced the stories the APA liked best were eligible for special awards for reporting excellence, to be presented at the APA's lavish annual conference.

Subjected to a steady diet of hand-fed stories, like squirrels in Central Park more than a few reporters in the intervening decades have lost their ferreting instincts, or failed to develop them at all. For instance, reporters who show up at the APA conference today are provided with free meals, phone lines, faxes, computers, and comfortable rooms for working on stories, as well as a stack of professionally written press releases—complete with quotes from "experts"—which they may submit as articles under their own byline, without bothering even to attend the conference sessions.

Even with all this damage control successfully underway, there was one more avenue to be pursued by the APA. This was a formal complaint made against ABC-TV to the Federal Communications Commission (FCC), under what was known as the Fairness Doctrine. The doctrine, adopted in 1949, was supposed to ensure that television news coverage was balanced and unbiased.

The APA's complaint read in part: "The *Madness and Medicine* program failed . . . to provide a fair or balanced basis on which the public could evaluate some of those patients who were specifically portrayed in the program." Marilyn Rice recognized herself as one of those whom the APA inferred were not necessarily credible. So she wrote to the FCC with so much more of her story of psychiatric mistreatment that it could reasonably have concluded that psychiatry had gotten off lightly in her case.[4] But it didn't offer to meet with her or any of the others interviewed for the program.

In response to the complaint, ABC agreed to broadcast an APA-scripted segment titled "A Consumer's Guide to Psychiatry" on the popular *Good*

Morning America program. The APA agreed to call this fair, commenting in *Psychiatric News* of June 16, 1978, "This ABC morning news program is typically seen by three to four times more viewers than are estimated to have seen *Madness and Medicine* in May of 1977."

The APA withdrew its Fairness Doctrine complaint. But a message had surely been sent to those journalists who would tread on psychiatry's turf as to what would happen if they got out of line again.

As part of the APA's new strategy to prevent such incidences before they occurred, it turned to public relations professionals. For instance, its largest branch, the New York State Psychiatric Association, hired a PR firm to fix psychiatry's "image problem." From then on, announced the chair of the public affairs committee, "Writers, programmers, and production staffers, and all other media people about to do something on psychiatry [will] learn to turn for help and information to the PR firm representing psychiatry. There has been no such service available to the media up to now." A spokesman for the PR firm said it had prepared a list of specialists to "guide the media" on a variety of topics, including electroshock.[5]

Media Falls in Line

Rice saw through the APA's public relations campaign from the beginning. She subscribed to the industry journals and kept track of everything about ECT in the media. She correctly dated the launch of the campaign to sell shock to 1978, based on the string of articles praising ECT that began to appear late that year. For her mailing-list audience, she kept up a running commentary on the APA's "all-out campaign to persuade the public that ECT is the best treatment for any emotional illness that is at all serious—much better than drugs—and that there are no risks in it."[6]

A *New York Times Magazine* piece on June 17, 1979, said that ECT was "like wizardry," and that a new "low energy" technique eliminated memory loss.[7] Ann Landers, the popular advice columnist, told her readers that ECT would make them feel "like a million dollars." Around the same time stories touting shock appeared on NBC's *Prime Time Sunday*, in *Reader's Digest*, and in *Parade* magazine. Fawning articles appeared in consecutive weeks in November 1979 in *Time* and *Newsweek*.[8]

The APA couldn't resist congratulating itself on how easily the media had been won. "In 1979," crowed the marketing director, "when NBC, *Time*, and *Newsweek* became interested in ECT, writers knew where to turn for official answers to their queries. . . . The fact that they knew whom to contact is no accident." He especially praised the *Time* article, which "follows the line of APA's Task Force Report, pointing out the importance of this life-saving treatment," and noted that "much of the material presented at APA's conference was contained in the *Newsweek* article." His prescient conclusion was: "Determination to articulate the profession's positions on patient care issues will determine what the public sees and hears about psychiatry in the future."[9]

But there was one last holdout, one final declaration of independence from the media for the APA to deal with, using the tactic that had worked so well with ABC.

"Electroshock: The Unkindest Therapy of All"

> For the most part, the press just meekly publishes the "party line" on medical matters—be it shock, dentistry, or anything else. If something critical happens to get published, the medics move in like the Nazi war machine to clobber the editor or publisher. The better (truer) it is, the more raucous are their shrieks of protest. . . . Actually the psychiatrists are the worst of the lot, probably because they are trying to maintain the widest discrepancy between truth and their propaganda, and nowhere is this wider than on the shock subject.
>
> —Letter from Marilyn Rice to Fred Hapgood, May 15, 1980

Out of nowhere, seemingly, considering the strength of what Rice called the pro-shock tide that was running in the press under the tutelage of the APA, came this article by science writer Fred Hapgood, published in the *Atlantic* in January 1980.

The focus of the article was the 1978 APA Task Force Report. Hapgood later said that his interest was sparked because "the tone of the APA's report was so patronizing. It radiated a smug arrogance that infuriated me."[10] As he put it in the article, "The reaction of the APA task force to fears about the use of electroshock is: first, they are completely unwarranted, mere 'imaginative beliefs'; second, it is no business of laymen to interfere with clinical practice. . . . It is somewhat alarming to see a group of physicians clinging to a standard of harm so high that the four horsemen of the Apocalypse could ride under it."

And as for what they tried to interpret as science, he wasn't buying it: "It is scandalous that each new version of ECT is not tested by first subjecting animals to experimental seizures and then examining them for signs of neurological damage."

Hapgood was able to see through the report's pseudoscience right to the public relations line. "A recurring pattern in the development of electroshock is for the profession to argue that while old versions of ECT might have had questionable aspects, the latest models have solved all those problems and are completely safe." His conclusion was: "The long, sad history of ECT should give caution to those who believe that when professional and popular opinions differ on medical issues, it is always the physician who is right."[11]

These insights, just as fresh and relevant today, explain why the article incurred the APA's wrath like no other before or since. Hapgood, a veteran writer, was shaken by the industry's response: "I had not anticipated such a furious, combative, uncompromising reaction."[12]

The New York chapter of the APA immediately complained to the National News Council, the counterpart to the FCC in broadcasting.[13] But its real coup was in getting a long letter from one Raymond Glasscote, said to be a happy shock patient, published in the *Atlantic* letters column. Glasscote denied any memory loss from his alleged treatment, in what seemed a too-calculated refutation of Hapgood's statements about negative public opinions on ECT. As Rice quickly discovered, Glasscote was no mere patient. He was in fact a psychiatrist, the editor of *Psychiatric News*, and a highly placed official within the APA's public relations office—his title being Director, Joint Information Service of the American Psychiatric Association and the National Institute of Mental Health. In her typical investigative reporter fashion, Rice contacted Glasscote and many collateral sources but failed to find any evidence that he was ever treated with electroshock. (He told her the hospital that had the records had burned down.) In disgust, she rallied other individuals and groups to try to get the *Atlantic* to publish Glasscote's affiliation. The legal reform organization HALT (Help Abolish Legal Tyranny) and the National Women's Health Network filed a complaint with the National News Council about the magazine's refusal to do so.[14] But nothing happened.

As the press continued to fall in line, the APA newspaper Glasscote edited reported glowingly on triumph after triumph, each "completely predictable."[15] All the favorable press was then interpreted by APA medical director Melvin Sabshin as a sign that green pastures lay ahead for psychiatry, the troubled times of the '70s being forgotten.[16]

Rice was having none of it. "The praise and optimism he refers to were put there by APA itself," she commented wryly. "Nevertheless, if the media continue to present evaluations of psychiatry ghosted by its trade association, his prediction could come true. . . . So unless we hear some sort of declaration of independence from the media, it appears that Dr. Sabshin is going to be right about the future of psychiatry. Its domination of everything should be complete by about 1984."[17]

As usual, she was right.

Unfortunately, my first contact with the media took place in 1985.

20/20

In early 1985, I was still suffering from acute organic brain syndrome due to the shocks three months earlier. I knew I had lost years of my life, including my college education, to amnesia, but I didn't yet know how many. I couldn't remember the work I had done before shock or understand my own writings. I was unaware that my brain had not yet recovered its ability to set down memories. Only once it recovered that ability, in 1986, did I realize I had no memory of 1985. My account of my experience with ABC's *20/20* comes from my writings made at that time.

"Balance" was the word that got me to open the door to my shabby apartment to a camera crew of several glossy people from ABC. I didn't want to be exploited, didn't want to be used, and I was, as anyone would be, nervous about appearing on national television. Appearing on national TV as an ex-mental patient was a hundred times scarier. My landlord, my neighbors, all kinds of people who hadn't known I was labeled would see it.

Don't worry, they said. Of course we want the show to be balanced. That line, plus the naive perception that the media has an interest in fairness as an ordinary person understands it, is their ticket to interview people who have good reasons to fear being interviewed.

We want to get *both sides*, they said as they set up their lights. We want to hear your story, they said, and I talked for three hours.

On May 23, 1985, I saw what a lie that had been.

The three-hour interview had been edited down to fifteen seconds. The audience simply heard me say that I didn't remember being in the hospital—as if that were all ECT had done to my memory and my life. Nothing about it having wiped out my college education or impaired my intellect. Following my segment, there was a big "but," and several minutes were allotted to three patients who were said to be happy with the results of shock and downplayed their memory loss.

Fifteen seconds later in the program were allotted to Peter Breggin, as the token professional critic of ECT. This was immediately followed by a disclaimer by the narrator that Breggin's position was based on "old" evidence. Then three APA-approved doctors were introduced as "cautious scientists" and allowed to say, without rebuttal from Breggin or anyone else, that ECT does not cause brain damage or significant mortality. Their financial interest in the treatment was not revealed. ECT practitioner Richard Weiner, M.D., who would become chairman of the second APA Task Force on ECT, was introduced as an "electrical engineer" without telling viewers that he put his talents to use designing shock machines for Mecta and Somatics Corporations. Nor were viewers told that psychologist Harold Sackeim did the same.

Larry Squire appeared in this context as an apologist for the APA, admitting that patients experience "rather severe loss initially" of up to several months, only to add that patients gradually recover memories and that six months post-ECT memory ability is "relatively normal." But that's not what his own research shows. By this time, he'd followed up his patients longer than the six-to-nine-month period he'd reported on in the APA Task Force Report, so he knew—and had published the finding—that not only was memory function impaired for the majority of patients at six months, it had not returned to normal three years postshock.[18]

The segment ran for fifteen minutes. Thirty seconds were allotted to critics, fourteen and a half minutes to proponents.

At the time, those of us outraged by the *20/20* piece focused on the imbalance of time allotted to the two sides in our letters to ABC, to the producer, to everyone we could think of. We thought we had a slam-dunk case—who could argue thirty seconds versus fourteen and a half minutes was fair? We also innocently believed, as most people probably do, that statements made by ABC and presented as fact, like "ECT may be making a comeback," had to be supported by data and would be retracted if we politely pointed out that these statements weren't factual.

As far as I know, I got no answer to my letter to Victor Neufeld, who produced the segment. But others got a short note saying simply, "We believe our report was fair and balanced."

In my two-page letter to Neufeld, I characterized the show as "a big commercial for ECT." I didn't mean it literally, but to my horror, it came true.

Somatics, the shock machine company founded by Richard Abrams, liked the *20/20* program so much they bought the rights to it. From 1985 until just recently, they have used the tape as a promotional tool to sell their shock machines. Yes, my image was used to sell the "treatment" that damaged my brain and ruined my life. I tried to stop Somatics from using me as a shock salesperson, and was told that the release form ABC made me sign before the taping gave them the legal right to do so.

Mecta consultant Richard Weiner was pleased with the show as well. Looking back at it in 1994, he said, "*20/20* was the first national portrayal of ECT that wasn't just an irrational diatribe against it."[19]

The *20/20* program set the template for the industry's public relations campaign that virtually every show for the next two decades followed. Of course, I didn't know there was a template then. It only became apparent over time, as show after show repeated the pattern. As the APA says, that's no accident.

The template requires that viewers be hooked in with the "new and improved" line. *20/20* promised "new findings" on shock therapy, and "new technologies." A person getting the "new" shock was shown, and this was contrasted with the old, "unpleasant" ECT. The *Cuckoo's Nest* shock scene was shown. Anesthesia and muscle relaxant, in use since the 1950s, were presented as "new," "improvements in administration." Brief pulse, forty years old, was also presented as a new technology. The APA's self-selected, carefully groomed media shrinks were presented as experts in medicine, not media. And at the end, no less an expert than Barbara Walters reinforced the central theme of the show by enthusing about how ECT is now "different from the way we used to see it."

ECT as Aging Rock Star

There was one more twist in the *20/20* show, which after all is supposed to be a news program. Pushing fifty, ECT got newsworthy the same way washed-up, middle-aged rock stars do: by making a comeback.

The "comeback" angle had been tried out by the industry some years earlier. The 1979 *Time* article had been titled "A Comeback for Electroshock?" It was posed as a question, not a statement. The article made clear that there were no data to support it.

But a national network news show like *20/20* doesn't need data; it makes its own evidence. If Hugh Downs or Barbara Walters or Tim Johnson says something, people believe it; and if people believe it, it's true enough. True enough, for instance, to be cited as truth endlessly by other journalists.

20/20's claim wasn't true, not by any measure. It couldn't be; there *are* no national statistics on the prevalence of ECT. There weren't then, and there aren't now. There are almost no statistics on the prevalence of ECT on the state level, either. In 1985, only three states (Colorado, California, and Massachusetts) required institutions to report how many people receive ECT. None of the state data supports a claim of a comeback. California has consistently reported that the use of ECT has remained steady; for instance, in 1986 and 1994 the number of Californians shocked was around 2,500, the same as in 1977. As we have seen, Massachusetts did not have sufficient data to tell whether the use of shock increased or decreased between 1974 and 1984, although some have interpreted what data there are as reflecting a decrease. Colorado reported an increase in the 1980s, but that state used negligible amounts of ECT, shocking fewer than three hundred people per year.

Speculations about the use of ECT on a national level are based on a sampling of selected hospitals, or on an extrapolation of one or two states' data to the whole country. Even these speculative "statistics" are few and uneven, and do not support a claim of an increase; if they can be said to show anything at all, they show decreased use of shock.

In 1973–74, Massachusetts' Department of Mental Health conducted a survey on the use of ECT in the state; based on that survey, it has been estimated that as many as 80,000 people in the United States may have received ECT in 1974.[20] The APA, in its 1978 Task Force Report, claimed there were 93,000 patients a year in the mid-'70s, but it had no actual data to back this up.

The results of a New York State survey on the use of ECT between 1972 and 1977, when extrapolated to the national level, yield a figure of only 32,000 people a year in 1977, and further reflect a 50 percent decline from 1972 to 1977.[21]

The National Institute of Mental Health, based on a sample survey of selected inpatient facilities, came up with a figure of 59,000 shock patients a year in 1975. It further estimated that use of shock declined to about 31,000 patients in 1980.[22] Using the same data, another group somehow came up with a slightly but not significantly different figure of 33,000 patients in 1980.[23] The former group, which included one of the ECT industry's foremost PR men, Richard Weiner, said that the use of ECT remained steady from 1980 to 1986.

A *Washington Post* reporter, assigned to a comeback story in late 1985, found herself confronted by data from insurers showing that the use of ECT was steadily declining in her city. With no evidence to support her claim, she simply quoted "top psychiatrists in the field" who assured her that the numbers didn't matter. One explained the data away by stating loftily that ECT was simply not the style of D.C. psychiatrists. Another said, "The data is hard to come by, but my impression is that ECT use has gone up."[24]

No matter where you look, there is simply no support for the claim that in 1985, ECT was making a comeback.

But that didn't matter. The American public could be counted on to believe it. As countless rock 'n' roll legends or washed-up movie stars can gratefully attest, Americans love an underdog, and the comeback story makes us feel good. It resonates at the deepest level with American optimism and the national belief in personal triumph over adversity.

Once *20/20* had broken this "news" story, ECT embarked on one of the longest comebacks ever. To date, there is still no end in sight.

The Media Come Full Circle

The APA must have taken particular satisfaction in one very significant measure of the success of its public relations campaign, and the way reporters swallowed up and regurgitated the party line whole. Jean Dietz—the same reporter who had helped to trigger the PR campaign in 1972 with her critical articles—published one of the earliest, most obsequious comeback articles thirteen years later.

The title alone—"Shock Therapy: Advocates Giving a Jolt to Villainous Hollywood Image"[25]—reflects the new style of shock journalism: no news here, just advertising. The article reads like an APA press release:

> *Electroconvulsive therapy is making a comeback.* [This in the first line, without attribution, without evidence; stated by the reporter in her own voice as fact.]
>
> *Hollywood's the villain, not ECT.* "Its poor image today is less a matter of bad practice than it is Hollywood stereotyping."
>
> *It's not like that anymore.* "Over the years, the technique has been refined."
>
> *Any memory loss is only temporary and trivial.* "Only some recent memories are lost; the brain's capacity for remembering is not permanently damaged."

With a wink and a nod to "balance," one token dissenting voice is allowed: "A few psychiatrists disagree . . ." (Only one is cited, Peter Breggin.) "Breggin's is a minority position." Four proponents expound on the virtues of ECT, including, ironically, Milton Greenblatt in a backhanded criticism of

Dietz's earlier efforts: "ECT is safe and has been needlessly overregulated."
The APA's "Fact Sheet" on ECT is cited verbatim.

At the end of the article, Dietz's former investigative bent surfaces, a
little: seeking support for that comeback claim early on, and finding none,
she turns to Max Fink. Fink has none, either: "In terms of statistics, there's
no real way of knowing" that shock is booming, he concedes. One of the
"subjective signs" of the boom, he admits frankly, is that he's making more
money; he's been hired as a consultant to two "venture capital companies"
wanting to start making shock machines. "Venture capital does not go where
the failures are," Fink says cannily.[26]

The American Psychiatric Association seems delighted by the success of
its public relations campaign in the media. It has opposed, and fought vigorously against, all proposed legislation requiring states to keep statistics on
the true number of persons shocked.

In retrospect, I should have given up on the media in 1985, but I naively
refused to accept that things could be as awful as they were, raised as I had
been to believe that in America journalists were held to high ideals such as
freedom of speech, objectivity, and balance. As the Dietz example shows, it
wasn't a matter so much of any individual journalist being biased; it was
more a matter of the ways in which it was possible or not possible at any
given time to practice journalism. Those who wanted to be published had to
write what they were allowed to write—or not at all.

In the coming decades, I would have dozens of contacts with print and
broadcast journalists from many venues, from small special-interest newsletters up to the *New York Times*; from low-budget cable talk shows to
Geraldo Rivera and *60 Minutes*. I would be forced to think deeply about who
journalists are, what they do, why they do it, and for whom. I would learn all
this the hard way, and my family and I would pay a very high personal price
for this knowledge.

At the same time as the industry had permanently tamed the media,
there was a new forum in which it would have to prove itself, a forum in
which facts and hard scientific data were supposed to prevail over PR. Here
was an arena with real danger for the APA, for unlike the media, the government had the ability to ban ECT.

The APA had to win over the Food and Drug Administration. And it would do this the same way it had won over the media: through sheer political pressure and expert public relations. The media coup was easy, the media eager to bend to the winds of money and power. The government was supposed to be different.

In the end, the government would not be won as easily as the media, but it would be won by the same strategy.

Long Strange Trip

ECT AT THE FOOD AND
DRUG ADMINISTRATION

In the 1980s the ECT industry convinced the federal government that ECT was safe *without ever doing a single safety study*. In place of clinical trials, it substituted a massive lobbying campaign to the Food and Drug Administration (FDA). The American Psychiatric Association, the National Institute of Mental Health, and doctors from the most prestigious hospitals and universities in America spoke as one to the agency, with a clear message: *Do not test the ECT device for safety*. And it worked. To this day, neither the FDA nor any manufacturer of an ECT device has ever conducted a study to determine the effects of the devices on patients.

The American public generally doesn't know this, and if it did, would have trouble believing it. After all, drugs have to go through clinical trials before being allowed to be used on humans. Don't devices also have to be tested and found safe? Wouldn't someone stop doctors from using a medical device that was dangerous?

The answers to the above questions are supposed to be yes. But the ECT machine has been treated differently from other medical devices. In the case of the ECT machine, the answers are no, and no.

The Medical Devices Amendment of 1976

Prior to 1976, there was no federal regulation of medical devices, even though Congress had originally intended that devices as well as drugs be regulated by the Food and Drug Administration. The call for regulation in the late 1960s was a result of medical horror stories told by patients who had been harmed by the Dalkon Shield intrauterine contraceptive device and other untested devices. These accounts were collected in a report commissioned by President Nixon in 1970.[1] As a result, Congress passed the Medical Devices Amendment to the federal Food, Drug and Cosmetic Act on May 28, 1976.

The law brought all medical devices—from tongue depressors to artificial hearts—under the jurisdiction of the FDA. It required that each medical device be classified on the basis of its safety and effectiveness. The FDA recognized that there are risks to all medical interventions, so it didn't set a standard of absolute safety, but reasonable safety, considered in light of the device's benefits. The law established three classes of medical devices. The classes have to do with the device's risk/benefit ratio, and in turn with the degree of oversight required.

Class I devices (like the tongue depressor) present little to no risk, so require only what are known as "general controls." This means that as long as they're manufactured with reasonable attention to quality control (in FDA-speak, using "good manufacturing practices"), they're safe to use without any more oversight. Many Class I devices are bought over the counter.

Class II devices are low-risk devices. Their safety is ensured by following instructions or protocols. Until 1990—that is, during the period when the critical battles over the ECT device took place—a Class II device was required to have a "performance standard" that set out the parameters for its use. An example of a Class II device is an MRI machine; a performance standard for this device might specify precautions to be taken to protect patients. The MRI could cause harm if not used according to the standard. (The oversight requirements for Class II devices changed in the 1990s and the current requirements will be discussed later.)

Class III is the high-risk classification for those devices for which general controls or performance standards are insufficient. The FDA defines Class III devices as those for which "benefits have not been shown to outweigh risks" and which present "a potential unreasonable risk of injury or illness" when used as directed by the manufacturer for their intended purpose. The degree of oversight necessary to ensure maximum safety was known as "premarket approval." The name reflected the fact that even though a device might have been on the market for many years, its status was similar to that of a new device. It hadn't proven itself to the FDA. Its manufacturers would, when called on by the agency, have to submit a premarket approval application (PMA) in which they would have to prove its safety and efficacy. Silicone breast implants were Class III devices before they were taken off the market.

Devices that had been on the market prior to 1976 could continue to be used and sold until the FDA called for PMAs. And there was a provision in the law that allowed new devices to be grandfathered in and sold without any scrutiny by the agency, as long as they claimed they were "substantially equivalent" to a pre-1976 device. Applications that claimed substantial equivalence, called 510(k)s, were routinely granted by the FDA with few questions asked. As a former FDA attorney said, "If you compared a device to a horse, you could get a substantial-equivalence decision."[2] This is how and why every ECT device since 1976 has been allowed to be sold. At the same time as the industry claims shock machines are so "new and improved" as to virtually constitute a new treatment, it must tell the FDA that they are just the same as the bad old devices.

Medical devices were to be classified by advisory panels made up of scientific, engineering, and medical experts. A consumer and an industry representative were to be included as nonvoting members. They were to review safety and effectiveness data, advise on any possible risks to health associated with the devices, and could warn that a device should be banned. They could also make recommendations on specific issues or problems concerning a device's safety and effectiveness.

Hundreds of medical devices were already on the market in 1976. For each one, the panels had to recommend a classification. Their decision would be published in the Federal Register for public comment before becoming final. Then each device in Class III would be investigated for safety. If it were not proven safe, it would be taken off the market.

At least, that was what was supposed to happen.

Here, apparently, was a golden opportunity for ex-patients. If there was anything Marilyn Rice knew, it was her way around a government agency. She knew how the government worked. She knew how bureaucrats thought. She spoke their language. Not many people know what the Federal Register is (it's the official daily record of all decisions made by agencies of the federal government) and fewer still get off the shock table knowing how to use it.

What she might not have known, at least at first, was that the FDA was notoriously ineffective at the job of regulating medical devices. The reasons for this were historical, financial, and political. Device law was largely written by the industry itself, and was focused on protecting trade secrets, not patients. From the beginning, FDA regulators were more interested in getting new devices onto the market than ensuring the safety of old ones. The medical device industry is a $34-billion-a-year industry, with all the lobbying power and political clout that implies. The regulators, on the other hand, were never given sufficient staff or funding to do their jobs. "Budget strictures" was the frank answer Rice would be given over and over, year after year, to questions about why the FDA hadn't done what the law said.

Looking back at the failure of the law from the perspective of the early nineties, one investigative reporter characterized the agency's approach as "regulatory minimalism" and said it had "disregarded entire sections of the law it was supposed to carry out." FDA regulators, including those who had been key players in the regulation of the ECT machine, agreed. "I was a pussycat," said John Villforth, director of the devices center during the 1980s. "I'm not an enforcement zealot," agreed James Benson, FDA commissioner during those years.[3]

The FDA Report on ECT

The ECT device was to be evaluated by the FDA's Neurological Devices panel. The FDA's first act was to commission a report on "Safety and Performance Requirements for Electroconvulsive Therapy Devices" from an outfit called Utah Biomedical Test Laboratory.[4] As the first and only supposedly independent investigation the FDA ever made of ECT, it was biased and deeply inadequate.

The Utah group was headed by psychiatrist Louis Moench of Salt Lake City, a proponent of ECT. After he worked on the FDA report, Moench would go on to serve on the APA's second ECT Task Force. Moench was the only doctor hired for the FDA report; the others were engineers.

The group did not, in fact, do any testing, of safety or anything else. It never came in contact with a shock machine or a patient. Its work consisted entirely of two things: a selective literature survey and a questionnaire survey of four ECT users—by which it meant doctors. It is important to understand how Moench's group understood safety and efficacy. Patient safety is hinted at in the report without further detail. Memory loss is also mentioned, but nowhere is safety connected with memory; "the only safety deficiency reported is the occasional production of minor burns underneath the ECT electrodes." The doctors surveyed interpreted safety to mean their own. One commented, "The principal safety problem is preventing an unintentional ground loop around the patient."

Efficacy for their purposes was interpreted as the ability of the machine to do what it is meant to do—put out a stated amount of electricity in a reliable manner—and had nothing to do with its effects on a patient. Indeed, the report is written from the perspective of an engineer, not a doctor, and certainly not a patient. The men who wrote it understood their task as akin to bench testing (that is, testing a machine by itself, to see if it works in the lab) and not clinical trials (testing patients to see what the machine has done to them). For instance, the report recommends using brief pulse rather than sine wave current, not because it is better for the patient, but because it is more "energy efficient."

The articles chosen for review were mostly those that focused on comparing different types of ECT machines with one another or on other technical questions. Many cited articles were themselves reviews or position papers (for instance, the 1974 NIMH brochure that Rice had successfully challenged as fraudulent). The Utah report does note, in passing, the need for "new neuropathological studies."

The report is important because it underscores that (contrary to what it consistently claimed in the case of the ECT device) the FDA can, if it so chooses, commission studies on matters of public health. Had it used this ability sensibly, the rest of this history might be very different. The agency could have, early on, commissioned a groundbreaking CAT scan study on the one essential question—does ECT cause brain damage?—a question that, from a logical and public health perspective, should be answered *before* asking how ECT should be given.

The story of the FDA and ECT is, from the outset, the story of basic scientific questions unasked and unanswered. It is the story of this scandalous lack of basic data smothered in endless literature reviews.

Class II or Class III?

In November 1976, the Neurological Devices Classification Panel met to discuss, among other things, the ECT device. Allen Grahn, Ph.D., represented the Utah group. He explained that the purpose of their study was not to determine the validity of ECT, but to evaluate the ability of the ECT device to safely produce a convulsion. He said that amnesia could be caused by mental illness, and that the only safety issue with ECT was electrode burns. No former ECT patients were in attendance.[5]

The level of scientific sophistication of the panel was reflected in the cavalier comments of the panel chairman, Harold Stevens: "Keep in mind that in this unique situation, it seems that the human brain can accommodate some massive doses of electricity without any consequence. We know from the Japanese, who took bare wires and plugged them in and gave shock treatments, that there are no ill effects. We are dealing, I think, with a unique situation, which means that the risk of over-regulation is much greater in this situation. There have been very few complications from shock treatment used in the most outrageous manner."[6]

After that meeting, the panel recommended that ECT devices be placed in Class II. The final version of the Utah report was delivered to the FDA on December 15, 1977.

By January 1978, Marilyn Rice had begun a correspondence with various FDA officials that would continue for the rest of her life. Some were interested in what she had to say, cordial, and courteous; others, aloof or simply puzzled as to why an ordinary citizen took such interest in, and knew so much about, their doings. But she always got the information she needed. Through her letters and phone calls, she developed a particularly productive relationship with James Veale, director of the Neurological Devices Division. She would frequently send him information about ECT he wouldn't otherwise have found. For instance, when a fellow survivor, urged by Rice to have the new CAT scan, sent her the results of the test (which showed cortical atrophy, as Rice's had), she sent the report on to Veale. And she encouraged others—ex-patients, concerned doctors, and organizations—to write to the FDA as well.

On November 28, 1978, the FDA took the first step toward placing the ECT device in Class II: it published a notice of its Proposed Rule in the Federal Register. However, the FDA was not convinced of the harmlessness of the treatment. It listed eight "risks to health" posed by ECT. Besides electrode burns, they included brain damage and memory loss.[7]

From Rice's point of view, the notice opened up an official window for patients to be heard. She knew that whenever something is published in the Federal Register, by law there is a designated period of three months for public comment. She asked survivors to write, as well as concerned professionals such as neurologist John Friedberg and neuroanatomist Peter Sterling.

There was also an open public hearing on the ECT device on May 29, 1979. Rice attended with her husband, Pierce. She focused the panel on the one clear, true point she always made: "Safety, in this context, means mainly safety to memory. It is the long-run effect upon memory that is causing so much worry about this treatment." There's no debate or honest disagreement over ECT, she reminded them, just one simple question: "Who is lying? Is it the doctors or the patients?" She urged the panel to place ECT in Class III, if only for its "educative effect."

Richard Weiner, M.D., Ph.D., spoke for the American Psychiatric Association. He was the chairperson of the APA's newly created Task Force on the Development of a Safety and Performance Standard for the ECT Device (which was separate from the ECT Task Force). He simply signaled to the literature review in the 1978 APA Task Force Report as proof that ECT was safe and should be in Class II.[8]

This was Weiner's public debut upon the FDA stage. He was, in a sense, Rice's archenemy at the FDA. He would spearhead the APA's twenty-five-year public relations campaign to persuade the FDA that ECT was safe *without* an investigation. What was not yet known, and would not become public for over a decade, was that Weiner was also an electrical engineer who was then designing shock machines for Mecta and would later work for Somatics.[9]

The strangest thing about the shock machine saga at the FDA, the thing that defies common sense, is why the manufacturers have never taken *any* part in the regulatory process. They never testified at hearings. Even though the records sometimes reflect the fact that they were present—for instance, a representative from the Medcraft Corporation attended the 1976 and 1979 hearings—they never said a word. They never filed any petitions. They never submitted any data on their own behalf, not even when the FDA warned that their machines would be taken off the market if they didn't.

The manufacturers, after all, not the doctors or their trade organization, are legally responsible for the safety of their machines. FDA approval, or a "license to market" a Class III device, can be granted only to manufacturers, not to doctors. There is no other medical device whose manufacturers have delegated responsibility for their product to a trade organization.

This can only be understood in the context of the financial ties of the self-chosen shock advocates (Richard Weiner, Max Fink, Richard Abrams, and later on Harold Sackeim and others). They represent the manufacturers because they *are* the manufacturers, or derive income from them in various ways.

But none of this has ever been revealed directly to the FDA. And in 1979, it wasn't as clear as it is today that individual psychiatrists as well as organized psychiatry could have financial conflicts of interest that might compromise their objectivity.

Despite Weiner's attempts to deflect the panel's attention to the topic of performance standards, thanks to Rice there was considerable concern about memory loss during the open committee discussion after all the speakers finished—whether it was unavoidable, whether there was enough information about it. The panel changed its mind and decided to recommend ECT devices for Class III.

On September 4, 1979, the FDA officially classified the ECT device in Class III, where it remains to this day.[10] Rice wrote to Veale: "As a long-time career Government employee, I was pleased to see that the FDA wasn't just the rubber stamp for the self-regulating medical profession that it is often accused of being. It would appear that there is opportunity for extra-professional involvement in policy-making and that it can be effective."[11]

Now the device was to be treated as if it were a new device coming onto the market. The manufacturers were required to submit premarket approval applications. A PMA has to contain evidence of the safety and efficacy of the device. It should include the results of tests on animals and humans and should show any side effects of the device. If the application is granted, it is a license to market the device. If not, the device can be taken off the market.

PMAs for the ECT device were due May 28, 1982.

Should ECT Be Investigated for Safety—or Not?

It's likely that the ECT industry believed in 1979 that it would face unfavorable consequences for ignoring federal medical device law. But it could not comply with the law. The companies who sold the machines had never done any animal studies, any human studies, any safety studies of any kind. They had no reason to believe that these studies, if done, would prove ECT safe, and a great deal to lose if the studies showed ECT to be damaging.

Ex-patients, potential patients, and the public in general could be expected to be on the side of the law, and for an investigation. Why *not* investigate ECT? If it were as safe as the industry claimed, the investigation would show that.

Once again—emboldened by their early success with the media—the industry chose a public relations solution to a problem that could only be solved by science. Instead of complying with the law and conducting a safety investigation of ECT, they set out to convince the FDA that no investigation should be done. Instead of testing, they would lobby.

Rice realized that the successful campaign to sell shock to the media in 1978–79 was going to be tied to the campaign to sell shock to the FDA. And she worried about the ability of patients—with no initials after their names, no public relations firm, no money—to counter the campaign. Her worries were justified; she was, in fact, once frankly told by an FDA official that "You can never outlobby the APA."[12] The simple fact that patients were only asking the FDA to do what its own regulations required it to do—its job—didn't seem to be enough. The stakes were high, the battle lines were drawn. Was ECT to be investigated like any other device or treatment, or was it to be given special exemption because of the political power of psychiatrists?

"An Exhibit of Patient Experience"

The APA, acting on behalf of the manufacturers, would have to file a petition with the FDA for reclassification of the ECT device; it was the only way to forestall the PMA process. It was also the key to getting around the manufacturers' unwillingness to take any part in the FDA proceedings; by law, any individual or organization can file a petition to the agency.

Rice began strategizing about ways to defeat the APA's petition before it was even written. She anticipated that the FDA would hold hearings on the petition; indeed, as early as the spring of 1980, she was seeking to make sure ex-patients would be involved. If patients could not have behind-the-scenes access to lobby FDA officials the way psychiatrists did, the public hearing requirement on most FDA actions was the way to go.

But there were both practical and political hurdles. On a practical level, patients whose livelihoods had been stolen by ECT had no way to pay travel costs to the Washington area. On the political level, even if patients could get there, how to make sure their voices would be heard and not dismissed, given their perceived lack of credibility?

In early 1980 Rice had conversations on this topic with Veale, who was at that time executive secretary of the Panel on Neurological Devices. She was sufficiently encouraged to broach the subject of the FDA's paying the expenses for patients to attend the anticipated hearings. In language a bureaucrat could love, she set out her argument:

> At first blush, one might conceive of patient participants as advocates of a particular point of view. It might follow that one patient spokesman might well be sufficient to represent that point of view, with two or more being duplicative. However, the logic that underlay my suggestion of patient participation in this proceeding was something else. Rather than appearing as advocates, they would constitute an exhibit of patient experience, from which the panel could draw its own conclusions. For this purpose a sample would be required, with each individual reporting factually on his own experience. The "interest" such patients would represent in terms of para. 10.220(c)(3)(i) and (ii) of the FDA Administrative Practices and Procedures (*Federal Register* of October 12, 1979, pages 59187/8) is that of future psychiatric patients. (They personally would have nothing to gain—economically, healthwise, or any other way. Sad to say, brain damage is irrevocable.)
>
> What they could contribute would be first-hand reports of experience with shock. In this sense they are "competent" (para. 10.220(c)(3)(iii)) to illuminate the panel about the permanent effects of shock, especially upon memory. From this voice of experience the panel could learn what have been the usual effects of shock, and be guided in deciding what future shock patients should be told, if their consent is to be considered informed consent.
>
> But no one shock patient could "adequately" (para. 10.220(c)(3)(ii)) represent this interest. . . .
>
> What is needed is a sample large enough to reveal consistency among diverse reports. The participating individuals would not give opinions or

summaries as to the shock experience of others, but each would report simply on his/her own experience—and answer questions about it. From perhaps ten or a dozen different reports, a consistent and typical pattern of shock effects in different circumstances might emerge.

In line with the intent of the reimbursement program, each participant would be making a "distinctive contribution that will improve the record for decision" (p. 59175, middle column), and FDA would be receiving "new and different information" (p. 59176, middle column). Certainly FDA would have succeeded in encouraging participation "of those who have traditionally not participated" (p. 59176, first column).

. . . I might add that, in staging a demonstration of this kind, the neurological panel would be conducting original scientific research.[13]

Meanwhile, the APA was preparing its petition. It was well aware of the urgency (though it miscalculated the date.) The chairperson of the APA's Council on Research wrote in the April 1981 *American Journal of Psychiatry*: "Unless a successful reclassification petition is filed, the manufacturers have until April 4, 1982, to prove safety and efficacy or discontinue production of their devices. There does not appear to be any great move on the part of the manufacturers to accomplish this. Thus, unless ECT devices are reclassified, the FDA ruling could potentially wipe out ECT as a viable treatment modality."[14]

No one counted on what happened next. The FDA underwent budget cuts in the spring of 1982. It said it couldn't afford the costs of taking the ECT machine off the market, even if it wanted to, even if its own regulations said it had to. The deadline for PMAs came and went, and nothing happened.

In August 1982, APA filed its petition to reclassify the ECT device to Class II. The petition was given the docket number 82P-0316. By section 513(e) of the medical devices law, a petition for reclassification has to be based on new evidence. But the APA kept citing studies done as far back as 1940. In an eighteen-page bibliography, only a handful of articles had been published since 1979.

The section on "The Safety of ECT" was just an appendix to the 366-page petition. It was very similar to the APA Task Force Report of four years earlier; not surprising, since its three authors were all task force members. Studies showing damage to brain and memory from ECT were either ignored, misquoted, or discredited, often by grasping at straws. For example, the Janis study showing extensive permanent memory loss months after ECT was discounted because, said the APA petition, the patients received large numbers of shocks (they didn't; they received an average number). Selected animal and human research of the 1940s to the 1970s was rehashed and said to yield "a confusing range of findings," and those studies showing brain damage were dismissed with tortured rationalizations.

The bulk of the petition consisted of the APA's proposed "performance standard." This set out guidelines for the ECT machine as if it were a toaster, as if it had nothing to do with patients. In fact, patients' heads only mattered for the standard as "load impedance"; because bone and skull slow down and diffuse (impede) the passage of electric current (load) to the brain.

How big should the electrodes be, how far should they be able to drop to an asphalt floor without damage, how long should a shock machine battery last? The petition was all about standardization, not safety. It was concerned with setting the parameters for the design of the machines and making sure they didn't malfunction. But these were nonissues. Of all the patients who had suffered harm from ECT, and in all the studies that showed harm, there was never a claim that any machine malfunctioned, was poorly designed, or did anything other than what it was designed to do.

Given that fact, why did it matter where the electrodes were on the head, whether the machine put out as much voltage as it was supposed to, or what type of electricity was used? The answer was between the lines: if we figure out how to do ECT right, the APA was saying, then maybe, *maybe* there won't be any memory loss—not that there is any memory loss anyway.

But the APA and the device manufacturers failed to conduct any safety tests to prove that claim.

As part of the proposed standard, the APA included an informed consent statement to be given to patients. It was a slightly altered version of the 1978 Task Force "Description of ECT for Informed Consent" and any changes were in the direction of less honesty. For instance, in 1978 the APA had acknowledged that amnesia could extend back for one or two years; that warning, or the word "years," did not appear in the 1982 version. The APA assured patients that any memory loss would be temporary, lasting only days or weeks, and that, anyway, the "majority" of shock patients don't mind these memory "changes."

The Public Hearing on the APA's Petition

On November 4, 1982, the public hearing on the APA's petition was held in Washington. Despite Rice's appeal to Veale on behalf of former patients, the FDA declined to pay the travel expenses for shock survivors. They showed up anyway, from as far away as California, sharing hotel rooms for $37 a night.

At the hearing, the agency acknowledged receiving sixty-five letters in support of a Class III designation, that the majority were from patients, and that they reported permanent amnesia or memory impairment. Thirteen people, ten of them survivors, spoke against the APA's petition for reclassification. The only one to speak in favor was Richard Weiner.

It wasn't easy for some who had lost years of life to ECT to be in the same room with him, to sit quietly all afternoon and listen to him after having been allotted only a few minutes of their own. Jeanne Lindsay, a survivor from Connecticut, experienced it this way:

> Dr. Weiner and his contingent of advisors sat in the row in front of me. I felt a chill of fear in being so close to this man. How many human brains had he personally damaged? How many lives had he fragmented by pressing that button? How many times had he thrown that switch which obliterated someone's memory and wiped out his identity at the same time? I felt like a Jew who had lost her family at Auschwitz, and now I had to sit politely in the same room with the Nazi Commander. Only it wasn't my family I lost but myself. . . .
>
> While people were testifying I had a chance to observe Dr. Weiner and his friends. They had a strange sense of humor. For example, one woman testified that her husband was so horrified by the deterioration of her personality after a series of electroshock treatments, he broke down and cried. Weiner and his lawyer snickered. Another woman—Joy Rose from Philadelphia—testified that although she has a degree in psychology, after her shock-induced brain damage the best she could manage was a job in a store; even then, she couldn't operate the cash register and so was forced to leave. Again Dr. Weiner and his cohorts snickered. The

examples are too numerous to mention, but the APA contingent displayed this sadistic sense of humor again and again throughout the morning. I guess to them we're not even human, so any pain we experience is funny? . . . That night I felt profoundly depressed on behalf of the human race. Is there anyone, anywhere, who can just listen to the facts and make a decision without regard to a person's title?[15]

Rice had filed a petition with the FDA asking that she be allowed to question Weiner.[16] In particular, she wished to tell the FDA panel about the history of failed experiments with brief pulse ECT, and to question him regarding the APA's claims that brief pulse ECT was a new technology that reduces memory loss. She would have enjoyed this immensely, but was turned down: only panel members were allowed to question petitioners. Weiner never had to face the type of hard questions Rice would have posed, because the FDA panel, under pressure from the agency to reclassify, was too tame to ask any.

Nevertheless, Rice was able to discredit Weiner in her testimony. She had read the studies he cited and knew they didn't show what he claimed they did. A listener who heard both Rice and Weiner speak and didn't know who had the medical degree might have concluded that she was the better scientist.

In the complete absence of any objective tests that have ever showed return of memory, the APA tries to invert the requirement. It devotes its discussion to finding fault with those studies that have seemed to indicate permanent impairment, and charges that this has not been demonstrated to its satisfaction. . . .

Can it point to histological studies of shocked brains showing no brain damage?

No, it cannot—neither in humans nor animals. . .

The APA has for several years had the instrument at hand to disprove patients' claims of permanent memory loss if it really did find them untrue. It could have made a CT scan study of persons who have had shock treatment and compared the results with what was normal for their age. Alternatively, it could have done a CT scan with shocked animals.

This is such an obvious line of investigation that the only reason for not proceeding along it would be to avoid facing expected results. And indeed, such unwillingness is revealed by the quality of the discussion of CT reports on page F-8.

Here the level of science and veracity in this report reaches an absolute nadir. . . .

In this situation I propose that the FDA not grant this petition at this time. Instead, it should cause a CT scan study of ECT effects to be made, and such study should be conducted by persons who do not administer shock treatment and are not cozy with those who do. Then, after considering the results of this study, it should again consider this petition.[17]

Arguably, patients won on the issue of safety. But Weiner was successful in deflecting the safety questions aimed at him to talk about standardization, as if this were the only relevant issue. He avoided a discussion of whether ECT causes brain damage by talking about which side of the head the electrodes should be on, implying that ECT could be made safe while not addressing the issue directly. It was a classic PR tactic: if you can't answer a question, pretend you were asked a different one.

ECT Survivors Change the World a Little

It has been said that it only takes a few people to change the world. Rice had understood this from the beginning. She had worked hard to get survivors to testify at the FDA because she knew that if they did not, the FDA would grant the APA's petition. She was right.

After the public hearing ended, when the panel met for closed discussion and to vote, it was clear that some of the panel members were deeply concerned about the testimony from former patients, and could not scientifically or in good conscience reconcile what they had heard with a vote for Class II. Among these were Susan Foote, a lawyer and professor from the University of California at Berkeley who served as the consumer representative on the panel; Ann Barnet, a pediatric neurologist; and Gyan Agarwal, a neurophysiologist.

On the other side was Michael Gluck, whom Jeanne Lindsay had observed sitting, talking, and joking with Weiner at the hearing. She had assumed he was a lawyer or an advisor to Weiner, and was stunned to learn later that he worked for the FDA. Gluck slipped and referred to Weiner as "Rich" in the closed session and quickly corrected himself. He also kept speaking for the manufacturers, saying he knew what they would or would not do, without revealing how he knew this—while at the same time Foote and others repeatedly asked about the manufacturers' absence from the regulatory process: where were they, why weren't they involved, didn't they have to be? As Foote pointed out in a letter expressing their concerns, "ECT devices present potential serious, long-term risks, and there is continuing scientific controversy about their safety and efficacy. The manufacturers of these devices have not been participants in the regulatory process. The petitioners are not the manufacturers, but the users, of the machines. Users are not liable for defects in design and therefore lack the incentive to demand high standards. The FDA has a responsibility in the absence of active manufacturers' participation to play a more active role in the standards process. . . . The regulation of ECT by the FDA is not just a technical question, it has become a public policy question as well."[18]

Some panel members were ordinary people—teachers, doctors—trying to do their best, struggling with a difficult decision that would affect people's lives for years to come. Others, like Gluck, seemed to have another agenda. It was clear that no one could reconcile Weiner's blandishments with the testimony of all the patients. Panel members had to choose sides.

As the discussion wore on, the FDA's general counsel was called on to answer questions about the legal ramifications of reclassification: could machines still be taken off the market if reclassified? Did Class III mean that a performance standard could never be developed? Panel members were split: convinced by patients that ECT was not safe, yet persuaded by Weiner that it could be made so. Thus, the discussion focused on which classification would best facilitate this theoretical making-safe process.

Survivors had shifted the terms of discussion. Instead of sailing toward reclassification, Weiner had to answer tough questions from the consumer representative, such as: If a performance standard could make ECT safe, why didn't the APA just come up with one? Why did it need the FDA's intervention or reclassification to do that?

Weiner flubbed around. He concealed his involvement with shock machine company Mecta, saying only, "We have talked to manufacturers," and they would not develop new machines (which he implied would be safer) if the panel voted for Class III. Twenty-five years later this bit of chicanery is obvious, but it wasn't so then. "I am told," he continued cagily, that if the devices remained in Class III and the FDA called for premarket approval applications, the manufacturers could not afford to submit them, and then, "there might not be any manufacturers."[19] Once again history has shown this argument to be a sham. There were two device manufacturers in 1982, whom Weiner and Gluck claimed weren't even making any money; by the end of the decade, there were four thriving shock machine companies.

Genuine concern for patients' welfare seemed to motivate most panel members, but they were deceived about what the problem was. Even Susan Foote, who was as sharp as a tack, was convinced that "some of the devices on the market are not properly designed," while at the same time unaware that the man responsible for those designs was sitting right in front of her, telling her what to do. Believing that a performance standard could solve the problem, she read out loud the section of the law that said a standard could be developed while a device was in Class III. Yet she and the others were swayed by Weiner's dire and deceitful pronouncements about how the manufacturers and APA just wouldn't do that unless the device was reclassified to Class II.

Several members expressed the viewpoint that they wanted to see some action on a device surrounded by so much controversy, and their concern that a vote for Class III would forestall this. They hoped to spur research and to see patient groups sitting down with doctors, motivating manufacturers to improve machines. In the end, the panel thought it reached a compromise between what survivors wanted and what the APA wanted. It voted unanimously to grant the APA's petition to reclassify the device to Class II, but to make the reclassification contingent on the development of a performance standard. The device would remain in Class III until that happened. They believed that the APA would come up with a standard that would make ECT safe in a short period of time and then patients like Marilyn, like Jeanne, like me, would not experience crippling amnesia and disability.

"I just don't want to see the state of limbo where nothing is happening two or three years down the line," said one panel member. No one seriously contemplated that their decision would mean more than twenty years of limbo.

In disgust, Rice fired off a letter to the *New York Times*, which was printed on November 25, 1982. She pointed out that the FDA had received hundreds of letters (not the claimed sixty-five) against reclassification, and none for it, except for those sent by organized psychiatry. Referring to the short-lived ban on shock in Berkeley, California, which had been voted on three weeks earlier, she wrote, "Here was a classic case of a regulatory agency being regulated by the industry it is supposed to regulate, and it illustrates why people are going to the ballot box over this treatment."[20]

When the FDA's Notice of Intent to Reclassify, the next step on the way to reclassification, was published in the Federal Register on April 8, 1983, there was a further twist.[21] The agency said it intended to place into Class II only those ECT devices intended to treat depression and schizophrenia. Those intended for mania would remain in Class III. The issue wasn't safety, exactly—obviously, the risks of the device are the same no matter whom it's treating. But the FDA said that the APA hadn't provided sufficient proof that ECT was *effective* for mania. In the FDA's risk/benefit equation, the less effective a device, the smaller the risks that are acceptable. The agency didn't believe ECT was effective enough for mania to outweigh its risks. It didn't say how it planned to differentiate those machines used to treat depression from those used to treat mania.

Now there was to be a public comment period on the Notice of Intent. Rice and her network of survivors and allies across the country got busy getting the word out.

10 The Committee for Truth in Psychiatry

Marilyn Rice had developed a core network of fellow survivors over the years, but she had never put together any kind of formal organization. "Organizing is definitely not my bag," she was known to say, but by 1984 people were interested and the time was right. The work they were already doing at the FDA begged for a formal structure.

Drawing on her own experience and that of so many others, Rice had already drafted a proposed informed consent statement for ECT, the first ever written by an ex-patient. The FDA had said back in 1979 that it could consider endorsing an informed consent statement. The APA had submitted its own "Statement of Patient Information" in its petition to the FDA. Rice wrote her version using the APA's as a starting point. A fair and generous negotiator, she was always willing to accommodate as much of what the other side brought to the table as she could. Where the two sides diverged irreconcilably, of course, was on memory loss and brain damage.

Everyone who has ECT experiences permanent memory loss, and no one is informed beforehand that this memory loss is certain to occur. This is what prospective patients most need to know, and this is what Rice's informed consent form tells them. It describes the loss, so different from normal forgetting because it is the most recent knowledge, not the oldest, that is hardest hit. It tells people that while some information may be regained, erased memory is gone forever and does not return. It warns that there may be a permanent effect on memory function as well as a time-limited amnesia, and cautions that this amnesia may involve years. What varies among patients, it says, is not *whether* permanent memory loss occurs, but the way this memory loss affects their lives and, in turn, how they feel about it: from not minding much to adjusting to disability to being unable to return to their previous way of life. In four paragraphs, it boils down what people considering ECT most need to know, and what we survivors wish we had known.

It is straightforward about the benefit that may be expected from ECT. Shock makes people feel better in the short run. It produces a powerful emotional relaxation. The same effect will happen with brain damage of any sort, whether inflicted by a blow on the head, a gunshot, or a doctor in a hospital. Most people don't realize, because it's counterintuitive, that brain damage can cause you to feel better than well, to the point of euphoria, temporarily. Rice had not only experienced this (and described it in the 1974 *New Yorker* article), but had a whole collection of references from neurological journals that corroborated it.

Rice saw her consent form as "an iron fist in a velvet glove."[1] While it acknowledged the temporary benefit of ECT, it had to be honest: the temporary benefit and permanent amnesia were two sides of the coin of permanent brain damage. Knowing this, a patient could make an informed decision about whether to trade a few weeks of relief from urgent distress for an unknowable extent of permanent amnesia and cognitive disability.

Organizing and Petitioning: The Committee for Truth in Psychiatry

Rice never wanted to ban shock. Here was the fundamental difference between the accidental activist and those like Leonard Frank who could not countenance the use of shock under any circumstances. To Frank and so many others, shock was first and foremost a human rights issue: a crime against humanity. Rice didn't see it in those terms. Maybe the difference had something to do with how each of them came to psychiatry. Frank had been forcibly locked up by his parents because they didn't like his behavior; Rice, on the other hand, had suffered a type of nervous breakdown and sought help voluntarily. She always maintained a healthy respect for the kind of emotional suffering that made people desperate for relief, no matter how fleeting. Some people would make the trade-off of amnesia for that relief, and she respected that choice. All she wanted was that it be an informed one. No one, not even those who would have given their consent had they been informed, liked being deceived into shock. All who had experienced consent-by-deception wished to protect others from that experience.

With that as the fundamental point of agreement, seventeen women came together in late 1984 to form the world's first organization of electroshock survivors. Its name was pretty much self-evident: Committee for Truth in Psychiatry (CTIP).[2] The name reflected both its history—it had grown out of Rice's "Truth in Psychiatry" letters of the late '70s and early '80s—and its mission. It was especially important to the founders to make the point that the organization stood *for* truthful informed consent, not *against* shock or psychiatry.

Rice was trying, quite reasonably, to set the terms of the discourse in a way that did not distort patients' position and did not shut down all discussion. For if you are simply totally "against" something, whether psychiatry or ECT or abortion, there is really no possibility of a dialogue. With nowhere else to go, the terms of public debate then invariably shift to maligning the motivations or character of individuals and organizations. This is why advocates of ECT perennially accuse CTIP of being out to destroy psychiatry—that is, of wanting to take treatment away from sick people—and of being Scientologists. It doesn't matter that the claims are false; just by being made, they cast doubt on whether we are what we say we are.

Whoever has more power controls the language, and thus the terms of debate. Consider how this plays out in the case of an equally controversial issue, abortion. There is no inherent imbalance in political or personal power between those who support legal abortion and those who oppose it. Thus, the terms of the debate evolved in a way that honestly reflected both sides' positions. Both chose to define themselves as *pro* (choice, life) rather than *anti*. For the most part, this is how people talk about abortion today. But former ECT patients have no political power, and so organized psychiatry controls the very words we use to say what patients want. Psychiatrists have redefined being *for* informed consent and choice as being *anti* ECT, and they've done so in such a way that the public doesn't notice or question it. This is exactly what Rice wanted to prevent.

The Committee for Truth in Psychiatry had no formal structure. There were no officers, no dues, and no funding. Rice paid any expenses out of her own disability pension, and others who were able to contribute and wanted to did so.

The informal structure might not have worked with other organizations, but it worked for CTIP because it stood for one issue and one issue only—truthful informed consent to ECT—and there was no disagreement among members on that issue. They were united to work for informed consent at the FDA and in any other venues that might present themselves.

Rice was aware that anyone could file a citizen petition with the FDA, asking it to do anything within its authority. She knew how to write such a petition. And she singlehandedly did so. CTIP's first official act was to file a petition asking the FDA to adopt its informed consent statement for ECT.[3]

The beauty of this strategy was that she could organize patients and petition the FDA at the same time. The patient-written consent form would serve in the future as the basis for membership. Each new member endorsed the form by signing a short statement: "I have undergone electroconvulsive therapy and I know or suspect that I was not truthfully informed of its nature or consequences. In the interests of the protection of future patients, I endorse the statement of *Patient Information about ECT* that has been proposed to the FDA by the Committee for Truth in Psychiatry (FDA Docket No. 84P-0430) and, in so doing, I become a member of the Committee."

In the organization's first year, with only no-budget, word-of-mouth organizing, membership grew to 120 people.

The Committee for Truth in Psychiatry's initial petition to the FDA was filed on December 20, 1984. The FDA turned it down almost a year later, on December 5, 1985, saying simply that it intended to reclassify the ECT device and adopt the APA's consent form. Rice rapidly wrote up an appeal, asking that the CTIP submission remain open "until FDA has determined whether ECT does or does not inevitably destroy brain tissue (or has, alternatively, without an investigation, taken a firm position on this fundamental scientific question.)"[4]

The FDA's denial of the reconsideration petition on June 3, 1986, said it all: "We believe it would be inappropriate for FDA to keep your petition in abeyance indefinitely."[5]

"Ordinary American Heroes": The Animal CAT Scan Petition

Undaunted, the group strategized its next step, with the same goal of prodding the FDA into investigating ECT's safety or disclosing why it wouldn't.

The APA petition rehashed selected animal autopsy studies from earlier decades, only to conclude that "virtually all reports of pathologic changes resulting from ECT are methodologically flawed."[6]

If so, then why not just conduct a clean study using modern technology? It was a simple, logical, scientific solution. But if it didn't occur to the APA or the FDA, then patients needed to propose it. In a second petition to the agency, filed August 29, 1985, and given Docket No. 85P-0422, CTIP asked the FDA to make a before-and-after controlled CAT scan study of shocked animals. The petition, written by Rice, was six pages long, including references. In it she clearly spelled out what was obvious to us but might not have been to the FDA: the public policy grounds for an unbiased investigation and the need for FDA intervention.

> The longstanding dispute is not between segments of the psychiatric profession but is, most pristinely, between psychiatrists and their patients. Any psychiatrist who administers shock treatment hears a constant stream of reports and complaints of permanent memory loss, and meets them with a stream of efforts at refutation—you are still depressed, you are getting older, you are overly sensitive, you are imagining things. Other doctors hear these same complaints and back their colleagues; while friends, relatives, newspapers, legislatures, etc., also hear them and sometimes back the patients. In this way the dispute has shaped up as between the public and organized medicine.

Letters poured into the FDA in favor of the petition. Organizations of ex-patients wrote, not just from the United States, but from Canada, England, the Netherlands, even Iceland. Senators wrote on behalf of concerned constituents. The general public wrote. Everyone was in favor of the investigation. No one opposed it except for Ted Hutchinson, a man whose adult son was shocked and who has subsequently made something of a career out of defending the treatment. (The son has never been heard from.)

This time, some media paid attention. It was certainly an unusual and dramatic story. *Dickinson's FDA*, an independent drug-and-device industry newsletter, wrote on September 15, 1985:

> "Truth in Psychiatry," a newly-formed national group of 120 patients (they would call themselves "victims") of electro-convulsive therapy (ECT) petitioned FDA 8/29 to require CAT scan controlled before-and-after

comparison studies of the technique in animals. . . . Arguing what organized medicine is increasingly realizing, that patients in chronic therapy can come to know as much, or more, about their illness as the treating physician, "Truth in Psychiatry" says contrary clinical findings of no brain damage predate modern methodology, such as CAT scans.[7]

On March 1, 1986, it followed up with the headline "CT-Scan ECT Pressure on FDA Grows."

It may become a classic litmus test of the Reagan Administration's mettle in balancing the interests of "ordinary American heroes" against those of the medico-business complex. In this case, the "heroes" are psychotherapy survivors who still have enough coherency to mount an impressive FDA petition campaign, without lawyers, for CT-scan animal testing of electroconvulsive shock therapy (ECT). Their file is nearly an inch-and-a-half high, laced with persuasively pathetic hand-written pleas for FDA intervention. Their latest co-fighters are the National Committee on Preventing Psychotherapy Abuse, which in a 2/11 filing challenged FDA that "if the study is refused, what is it that is being hidden?" Permanent brain damage, that's what—and FDA's embarrassment over a long-stalled attempt at rulemaking that's in the "too hard" basket.[8]

To all this, the FDA had no response at all. It never granted the petition. It never denied it. Instead, it decided to treat it and all the comments submitted to it as just one big "comment" on the APA's reclassification petition. Comments, unlike petitions, don't require acknowledgment or response. Rice called this "the ultimate mark of contempt for patients."[9]

The Consensus Development Conference

In early 1985, Rice's sources at the FDA told her the proposal to grant the APA's petition would be published right after the National Institute of Mental Health's Consensus Conference on ECT. This was the perfect opportunity—orchestrated by the APA—to give the industry what it wanted in a face-saving way. A "Consensus Development Conference" is a type of conference held periodically on different topics by different branches of the National Institutes of Health; the aim is to bring together experts and come up with a position paper on which all can agree. One and only one such conference has been held on ECT, in June 1985. Under the political circumstances, since the FDA's proposal to reclassify was already written, there was only one possible outcome of the conference: an endorsement of ECT sufficient to justify reclassification.

Though the National Institute of Mental Health is a public agency and the American Psychiatric Association a private trade association, for all practical purposes the two are coterminous; with the same men (rarely, women) holding leadership positions in both organizations as in a game of musical chairs. Though not every APA member is associated with NIMH, every psychiatrist at NIMH is a member of the APA. Those who seek positions at NIMH are those who are most motivated, for whatever reason, to set the nation's mental health agenda. NIMH controls a $28 billion-plus research budget; it decides what is researched, what is not, and who gets the money.

The director of NIMH at the time was Shervert Frazier, a founding member of the International Psychiatric Association for the Advancement of Electrotherapy (IPAAE). Not surprisingly, the June conference was stacked with industry representatives. The planning committee included psychiatrist Richard Abrams, who, despite the proclamations that the FDA's Class III ruling was a deterrent to business, had just started up his own shock machine company, Somatics. It also included Richard Weiner, who not only was in charge of the APA's lobbying campaign at the FDA, but had a long-standing relationship with Mecta Corporation and would consult for Somatics as well. Psychologist Harold Sackeim, who consulted for both Somatics and Mecta, was also on the committee. Of course, all three presented themselves as scientists, and no one at the conference or in the media was told that all had financial conflicts. The committee also included Michael Gluck, Weiner's associate from the FDA, and psychiatrist William Z. Potter, a public promoter of ECT.

Some of the conference planners, such as Abrams, Fink, Sackeim, and Weiner, were featured speakers as well. Other speakers were selected from those who already had reputations as shock advocates, such as Joyce Small and, from the U.K., Chris Freeman.

Nevertheless, one vocal critic, Dr. Peter Breggin, managed to get himself onto the program as a speaker, the only psychiatrist who didn't toe the party line. His topic was "Neuropathology and Cognitive Dysfunction from ECT." While other speakers would go on at length about how to place the rubber bit in the patient's mouth so she didn't bite her tongue off, or what type of electricity to use, Breggin was succinct: "ECT can never be made harmless . . . the potential patient has the right to know about the controversial and dangerous nature of ECT."[10]

Not a single survivor of ECT served on the planning committee or the consensus panel, or was invited to speak. But activists from the mental patients' rights movement got wind of the conference in its planning stages and began pressuring the organizers to include ECT survivors.

As a result, an hour at the end of the first day which had been set aside for "public and organizational issues" was reframed as "patient issues" (as if these were separate matters from those the panel had already placed on its agenda, such as, "What are the risks and adverse effects of ECT?"). Shock survivors and authors Leonard Frank and Janet Gotkin were allotted ten minutes each. It was only enough for Gotkin to point out how the conference was stacked in favor of ECT, and it was so little that Frank had to leave out his prepared remarks about the FDA. A prominent mental patients' rights activist got ten minutes to suggest "alternatives," and two professional critics of shock, psychiatrist Lee Coleman and psychologist Edward Opton, spoke for fifteen minutes each.

The next morning, as if the patient issues panel hadn't happened, attendees heard psychiatrist Chris Freeman claim that half of ECT patients find the procedure less distressing than going to the dentist.[11]

In the end, the Consensus Conference came out with a statement that was in no way the same one it would have written if ex-patients hadn't put pressure on NIMH to include their perspective and that of nonindustry professionals.[12] Peter Breggin had challenged the attendees to come up with a single study showing ECT had any effect on mood that lasted longer than four weeks, and when they couldn't, the final statement reflected that ECT had only that very short-term benefit. Despite his denials of memory dysfunction made to the media less than a month earlier, Larry Squire now had to admit that his own studies conducted since the Task Force Report showed that permanent memory loss could be extensive. In 1983, he had published the results of his study following up ECT patients for three years. The conference statement adopted the findings of that study that ECT patients lost an average of eight months of their lives, six months prior to shock and two months after.[13] Without conceding that Squire measured amnesia accurately, this means that half of ECT patients lose more than eight months. The conference statement also included Squire's finding that for "many" (a majority of 58 percent in the actual study) ex-patients, memory function remained impaired three years after ECT.

The conference report further stated: "There are other possible adverse effects from ECT. Some patients perceive ECT as a terrifying experience; some regard it as an abusive invasion of personal autonomy; some experience a sense of shame because of the social stigma they associate with ECT; and some report extreme distress from persistent memory deficits. The panel heard eloquent testimony of these attitudes from former patients who had been treated with ECT. The panel also heard moving testimony from former patients who regarded ECT as a wholly beneficial and life-saving experience."

In fact, there was one patient who spoke of the benefit of ECT, Pat Wheaton from Illinois. What the final report didn't mention is that she also experienced permanent memory loss. She speaks of her amnesia quite frankly, but laughs about it, a response not typical of most former patients.

Thirteen members of CTIP and an equal number of local and national ex-patient activists attended the conference. We paid our own way and stayed in cheap motels. We quickly put together a press release, calling ourselves the Ad-Hoc Committee for a Moratorium on Electroshock. We made the following points:

1. Electroshock *always* causes permanent brain damage.
2. Electroshock *always* causes permanent memory loss.
3. Patients' reports of memory loss and other severe adverse effects, including loss of creativity and the inability to learn new material, are systematically ignored or denied.
4. The "improvement" described by the shock doctors—confusion, apathy, and euphoria—is actually the result of the organic brain syndrome caused by electroshock.

5. Electroshock causes more suicides than it prevents. Ernest Hemingway is only the most famous example.

6. Electroshock causes a small but significant number of deaths.

7. Electroshock has never been proven to have any long-term "therapeutic" effects. In fact, no study shows that these effects persist more than thirty days following the last shock.

8. Informed consent to electroshock does *not* exist because shock doctors deny the procedure's harmful effects, and because psychiatric institutions are inherently coercive.

9. None of these statements has been disproved by the American Psychiatric Association or the Consensus Development Conference.

10. The burden of proof must be on the shock advocates to scientifically and conclusively demonstrate the safety and efficacy of electroshock.

The Food and Drug Administration should not grant the APA's petition to reclassify ECT devices from its current high-risk class to a lower-risk class without conducting a full-scale public investigation.

For these reasons, we call for an immediate moratorium on electroshock.[14]

I said "we." I've heard stories about my own participation in this conference. That's all they are, just stories; I have no memory of any of it. Seven months post-ECT, my brain had not yet recovered its ability to hold onto the events of my life. Yet sometime in those seven months, I'd faced the same moral choice that Rice had twelve years earlier. What do I do with this horrible knowledge? Should I try to put it behind me—and how would that be possible? If it were, did I even want to? What responsibility did I have to those who came after me, those being deceived into signing up for brain damage? Was I the kind of person who could walk away from that responsibility, or was I not? If I knew of such injustice and did nothing, how would I live with myself? Somehow, even hollowed out by shock, I figured out what I was made of. Another accidental activist was born.

It's amazing what you can do while you don't have any memory. You're not aware, at the time, that your memory of each day is rapidly disappearing, and that in the end you will have no memory of what happened to you. I was on a television news show. I've also been told that I stood up at some point and talked about how I would have preferred to die rather than be subjected to ECT, had I been given a choice. One of the persons who heard me say that was the nurse who had attended my ECT treatments. It wasn't surprising that she would be there, considering that the director of the clinic where I had ECT was on the consensus panel. The story is that she came up to me—she remembered me, I had no memory of her—and said, "But you never used to brush your hair in the hospital. You *look* so *good!*" This inane comment inspired jokes about how there ought to have been a panel about the cosmetic benefits of ECT.

Besides myself, three other CTIP members were on television. Janet Gotkin took on panel chairman Robert Rose on the *Today* show.[15] "She slew him," Rice noted with satisfaction, "by asking why, if shock is so safe, the FDA has been calling it dangerous for the past six years."[16]

And we were successful in getting questions about brain damage into reporters' mouths when they interviewed psychiatrists. Rose answered these questions with stock phrases: "No brain damage." "No actual nerve cell death." "The vast majority of the studies which showed brain damage had methodological flaws." To which Rice pointed out that he was, of course, referring to studies made forty years ago, without the slightest suggestion that they should be replaced by up-to-date studies without flaws.

Survivors Offer Our Brains to Science

If neither NIMH nor the FDA would make such a study, who would?

There was only one answer to that question. We would.

No, we didn't have brain scanners. But we petitioned the FDA again, this time asking that a brain scan study be made on humans. For subjects, we'd volunteer our own brains.

I was designated the first guinea pig. Rice drafted the initial petition. As a twenty-six-year-old woman who had never suffered any other form of trauma to the brain and was not taking any drugs, I was an ideal subject. It would be difficult to argue that my brain damage was due to menopause or aging.

The one-page petition was succinct:

> I am aware that FDA is contemplating reclassifying the ECT device from
> Class III to Class II upon the assurance of the American Psychiatric
> Association, backed by the National Institute of Mental Health, that
> ECT is a safe treatment. I am also aware that no examination of ECT
> patients' brains has ever been made by the APA, the NIMH, or the FDA,
> neither by autopsy nor by CT scan.
>
> Although I recognize that CT scan findings in any one human brain
> could be the resultant of many influences and would have to be inter-
> preted in the light of that patient's history, I nevertheless believe that
> research on even one shocked brain would be preferable to research on
> none.[17]

I have no memory of filing my petition on December 28, 1985, but sometime in the next few months, my ability to form memories recovered, and I
remember receiving a denial letter the following May.

The petition was turned down by the FDA on technical grounds.

> FDA is denying your petition because, contrary to your contention, the
> results of a CT scan of the head of one patient could not alter the
> agency's position on ECT. . . .
>
> The principles of valid scientific evidence are discussed in section
> 860.7(c)(2) of Part 860, Title 21, Code of Federal Regulations. This para-
> graph states, in part, that isolated case reports are not regarded as valid
> scientific evidence to show safety or effectiveness of devices. The prin-
> ciples of well controlled clinical investigations are discussed in Section
> 860.7(f). . . .
>
> FDA concludes that the results of a CT scan of your brain would not
> constitute valid scientific evidence. Therefore, the results would not bear
> on the agency's proposal to reclassify ECT devices intended for certain
> uses. Thus, FDA denies your petition.[18]

In my petition for reconsideration on June 12, 1986, I cited chapter and
verse of the Code of Federal Regulations, under which one case study could
indeed fit the description of valid scientific evidence. But if they wanted

more, I asked that the FDA keep my petition open until it had received enough similar petitions for a respectable study.

Rice and I then got to work organizing other survivors to send in CAT scan petitions. One hundred twenty-three people did so. She was so tickled with my work she wrote a laudatory column in her newsletter about me: "From Art Critic to Brain Scientist." I thought that was a bit much. Besides, it was still much too painful to think about what I had lost.

My petition for reconsideration was denied, not on the merits, but on administrative grounds. The agency said I had to prove that they hadn't adequately considered the information in my petition, and claimed I hadn't done that. It also said that "regardless of the number of similar petitions that are received and filed, FDA does not intend to initiate any studies of the type you are requesting."[19]

Each of the other one hundred twenty-three petitioners was eventually sent an identical denial letter, ending with: "At the present time, there are no funds available to the agency to conduct the requested study, and it is not anticipated that the necessary funds will become available in the near future."[20]

Rice saw this nonsense as "a devastatingly good opportunity to arouse Congressional interest in what is going on at the FDA." She urged everyone to write their congressperson with a simple question: "Is it true they don't have money to find out what shock treatment does to brains?"[21]

Through the rest of the 1980s and 1990s, survivors and shock doctors continued to lobby the FDA, eventually building up Docket #82P-0316 into a stack of more than forty volumes that would reach from floor to ceiling. Survivors claimed the voice of truth; doctors, the voice of science. But survivors would not cede science to the doctors. The two groups would clash over the very definition of science: who got to define it, who had access to its tools and methods, who decided which questions it could ask and which it would not.

In these same years the controversy over silicone breast implants highlighted the fault lines of the ECT debate. The women who'd experienced toxic implants could not be dismissed as "mentally ill" and incredible; they were able, therefore, to bring and win lawsuits, something ECT survivors, by definition, could not do. The silicone breast implant, as a Class III pre-Amendments device, came under the scrutiny that should have been brought to bear on the ECT device. Its users and manufacturers were not able to prevent a call for PMAs, and when they could not prove their devices safe they were effectively taken off the market. In other words, the law was followed and it worked, however belatedly, to protect patients. This happened even though, in great contrast to the ECT device, few former implant patients who wrote to the FDA reported adverse effects and the vast majority reported good outcomes. In an unsuccessful effort to divert some of the publicity over breast implants to ECT devices, CTIP members wrote to the FDA and the media with the provocative question: "Are breasts more important than brains?"

In the next four chapters we will examine the two rival discourses on ECT, as patients attempted to shape federal policy and public opinion through direct appeals to the FDA, while shock proponents did so through control of the scientific literature and the media.

11   *Anecdote or Evidence?*

The APA was convinced that it needed to bolster its position with letters to the FDA from former patients who were satisfied with their treatment. It was aware of the letters pouring in from ex-patients reporting permanent memory loss and cognitive disability. In an effort to neutralize the effect of these reports, Richard Weiner begged for letters in support of ECT from ex-patients in the APA newspaper *Psychiatric News* (April 4, 1984), publicly admitting that the majority of letters received by the FDA were anti-reclassification.

Many years later, as the battle between doctors and patients dragged on, he tried again. He drafted a form letter to be sent to the APA members, who numbered around 30,000 at the time. He asked psychiatrists to write to the FDA in favor of reclassification, but it was just as important, he stressed, that they get their patients to write. He even sent guidelines to be used in drafting patient letters and a sample form letter, with instructions, for doctors to send. ("Do not mail this form letter" was one of the instructions—but someone sent it in anyway.)[1]

Similarly, as early as 1981, Gary Aden of the International Psychiatric Association for the Advancement of Electrotherapy (IPAAE) had attempted to establish a patients' auxiliary for the purpose of influencing the proceedings at the FDA. He failed to talk any of his patients into becoming public spokespersons for ECT, then felt obliged to write a long-winded letter to the FDA rationalizing his failure.[2] The shock advocates were so desperate for evidence from patients to back up their claims of ECT's safety that one of them, Dr. Lester Margolis, copied either medical records or other documents pertaining to his patients and sent them to the FDA docket. (He also sent a note boasting about giving ECT to patients in his office without anesthesia.) But because the docket is a public record, it cannot accept confidential medical information. The FDA clerk, in the absence of any evidence that the patients had known about or consented to the release of any of their records, properly withheld them from public view, placing them in their own separate volume and sealing them.[3] Only the cover letter from the doctor, identifying himself and saying that he wrote at the suggestion of IPAAE, is viewable by the public.

Later on, when IPAAE was succeeded by the Association for Convulsive Therapy, that organization's president, Conrad Swartz—while not revealing to the members or the FDA that he was co-owner of the ECT device manufacturer Somatics, Inc.—tried, also without success, to get patients to write to the FDA praising ECT.[4]

Meanwhile, Marilyn Rice, in a one-page monthly message sent to Committee for Truth in Psychiatry members, kept up the call for patients to write to the FDA. The message went out to the same one hundred people each month, year after year, from 1984 until she died in 1992.

The 1982 FDA docket, designated No. 82P-0316, was not designed to be a representative or randomized sample of ECT patients. Nevertheless, some conclusions can be drawn from the data that came in to the docket over the next two decades.

It would be expected that patient letters in favor of reclassification would far outnumber those against. The APA, an organization of 30,000 with vast resources and paid staff, should be able to mobilize hundreds of patients for each one who heard about the FDA proceedings by word of mouth from another ex-patient. This is what would be expected *if* it were true, as the APA claimed, that the vast majority of ECT patients experience no long-term adverse effects. On the other hand, if the vast majority of patients experience permanent amnesia and other disabling outcomes, then no matter how many people are looking for satisfied patients, it will be hard to find them.

In fact, 93 percent of the letters from those who identify themselves as former ECT patients are against reclassification. A small representative sample of the hundreds of letters from ex-patients can be found in the appendix to this book. In twenty-one years, only fourteen of these ex-patients made positive comments about ECT. But even these are not very positive. Many of those writing in favor of ECT don't indicate that they know to whom they are writing or why—for instance, they are addressed "To Whom It May Concern." In several cases, the letters were sent in by their psychiatrists. Some of these are actually scrawled on hospital stationery, suggesting that APA Task Force member Iver Small, who sent them in, approached his patients while they were undergoing treatment, when the confused patient could not very well refuse a request from his or her psychiatrist. And in fact, in his cover letter Small says the patient letters were written "during or after their course of ECT."[5] Of those sent in directly by patients, most say they were asked to write by their doctors. Even so, four of the fourteen specifically mention experiencing memory loss. None of these letters inspire much confidence in ECT.

> I have been asked to put down my feelings pertaining to having had shock treatments. I am sure only the doctor knows if they helped me or not. Being depressed you forget many things. I am sure they did not do any damage to my brain, at least not any more than the illness has already. I don't want any more. But I have every confidence in Dr. Kellams, and if he were to say they would be necessary again I am sure I would trust him and have them.
>
> —Mary Whitenack, C109, May 15, 1984

> I am a former patient of Dr. Louis A. Moench. It was his recommendation that the ECT psychotherapy be tried. The treatments were successful and were given me periodically though July of this year. It is now November and the Drs. as well as my family consider me a happy, well, normal functioning person.
>
> —Claudia Warner, C674, November 5, 1990

> I didn't consider the immediate loss of memory a hardship, a handicap, or destructive nor an inconvenience.
>
> —Pat Wheaton, C640, November 11, 1990

> I have become more confident, with a personility easily acceptable and more likeable than before. Also my outlook on life is positive and affirmative. Shock treatments, the eight that I had, gave me the will to continue my life with my family and friends unafraided of the future. Willing to change my personality, and thinking according to the situations developed.
>
> —W. Golbreath, C112, May 15, 1984

It is possible that only a fraction of a percent of patients are permanently damaged by ECT and that *all* such patients just happened to write in to the FDA. It is also possible that patients who did not know one an other just happened to describe the exact same effects by chance. But how likely is this?

At least a fourth of the FDA letters don't give any clues about the letter writer's affiliation. These are, presumably, letters from the general public. These letters highlight the enormity of the public relations problem still facing the industry a decade after the launch of the PR campaign: much of the public, if it thinks of shock treatment at all, is genuinely alarmed. All but one of the letters that appear to be from the general public are against reclassification and in favor of a safety investigation. There are hundreds of these. Some are form letters, originally designed by Marilyn Rice and used by other individuals and organizations, which simply ask that the FDA not grant the APA's petition without an investigation. Rice was right, as always, when she said, "The general public, if it hears of the issue, can be expected to be in favor of an investigation."

In 1986, every state established an agency under the new federal law (PL 99–319) known as Protection and Advocacy for Mentally Ill Individuals. These state agencies are charged by the federal government with protecting, and investigating possible violations of, the legal rights of persons with psychiatric labels. In 1987, Rice had a brainstorm: she'd explain the FDA situation to the director of each state agency and ask them to write a letter opposing reclassification from Class III to Class II. She put it to them reasonably; they need not take any position for or against ECT, only on whether the FDA should investigate to find out if it is brain damaging. Once she had the idea, it took off, and others did much of the work. The campaign was 100 percent successful; every single state went on the record opposing reclassification from Class III to Class II, calling on the FDA to investigate the safety of ECT. Rice's only miscalculation was in supposing that this would have any tempering effect on the FDA's determination to reclassify.

Survivors of ECT also contacted their congresspeople with a simple request: see to it that the FDA investigates the safety of ECT like they're supposed to. Tell them not to reclassify the device unless they do. Those federal and state senators and representatives who queried the FDA were sent an obfuscating response meant to deflect any criticism of the agency. Still, not every elected official was hopelessly befuddled by this tactic. Every single elected official who took any position on the ECT device—and there were many—opposed reclassification.

The letter sent to FDA commissioner Frank Young by the longtime representative from New York, Charles Rangel, was typical.

> Dear Dr. Young,
>
> Thank you for your last letter on electroconvulsive therapy (ECT). I found your letter very informative.
>
> However, I have one question. Does the FDA believe that ECT causes brain damage or not? If the FDA does not believe ECT causes brain damage, I would like a copy of any before-and-after anatomical medical diagnostic ionization studies (CAT-scans, MRIs etc.) that have been conducted on this issue that helped the FDA reach its conclusion.
>
> I would really like a response. It will help me make up my mind on this issue.[6]

If former patients, the general public, the Protection and Advocacy agencies, and elected officials were all against reclassification, then who was for it?

The ECT Industry Opposes an Investigation

Not surprisingly, the people opposed to a scientific investigation of ECT's effects on the brain were the doctors who use it and the shock machine manufacturers (though they were careful not to reveal to the FDA that they were the same people).

Officially, the shock machine companies made only a brief, one-letter appearance on the FDA stage during each comment period. Their letters are remarkable for their passive tone—let the psychiatrists take care of everything—as if the manufacturers had no conception that they, not the users, are legally responsible for the safety of their devices. For example, Mecta's then-owner, Rex Hiatt, wrote, "From our reading of the literature and meetings with individual psychiatrists, it would appear that ECT is a valid treatment for certain psychiatric illnesses."[7] Mecta's current president, Robin

Nicol, argued that manufacturers should not have to prove their devices safe because safety studies cost too much money.[8]

A representative for the Medcraft company had simply this to say: "We understand that the APA has petitioned the FDA to reclassify ECT devices to Class II and has provided, in support of its petition, significant information to establish the proposition that a generic safety and performance standard for such devices can be developed. We support that position with the *belief* [emphasis added] that ECT remains a valuable therapeutic device in the medical armamentarium."[9]

From Somatics, the company that started up after the ECT device was placed in Class III, the FDA heard nothing—officially. The company's owners did not write on Somatics letterhead, but Richard Abrams and Conrad Swartz wrote to the FDA on many occasions. They wrote before and they wrote after they began manufacturing the devices at issue, claiming all the while that if the FDA did not reclassify, the use of ECT would somehow be restricted. But they never told the FDA that they gone into the business of making shock machines. Twelve letters were sent to the FDA from Abrams, Swartz, or their co-workers at the Chicago Medical School, constituting the single largest bloc of letters from one institution.[10]

One hundred thirty-three letters, about 5 percent of the total, were sent to the FDA by psychiatrists. A small number of these opposed reclassification, but the vast majority were in favor. The opposite was true of the rest of the docket: the vast majority of writers were against reclassification. It is impossible to avoid the conclusion that the doctor letters carried vastly more weight with the FDA than the other 95 percent.

All of the heavy hitters of the industry were represented: officials from the APA and NIMH, Task Force members, prominent doctors from every one of the major universities that were heavily invested in ECT (Duke, Columbia, University of Iowa, Stony Brook, and others). Instead of making their case against an investigation of ECT on the evidence, the psychiatrists made themselves the evidence: their books, articles, research grants, professorships, directorships, and so on. For the most part, their statements that ECT is safe were made without citation or proof; the credibility of the author was seen as proof enough. For example, Herbert Pardes, at the time the director of both NIMH and the New York State Psychiatric Institute, wrote: "Studies which meet contemporary scientific standards are available on the safety and effectiveness of ECT."[11] But no studies were cited. By virtue of his positions, Pardes's statements were unassailable.

Not only did they not have to provide studies, but the psychiatrists even enjoyed the luxury of stating their personal experience or opinion in a way that would be dismissed as anecdotal or unscientific were a patient to do the same.

> A scientific fact can sometimes be established as a matter of common and frequent observation. I doubt that a systematic study has ever been published concluding that human beings have single noses with two nostrils at the bottom, and yet this is a genuine fact established by common and frequent observation. Let us not throw out the baby with the bath water as we pursue true facts about ECT and its effectiveness. In my clinical experience I have used ECT to treat patients with both typical and atypical presentations of mania—six different patients during the past nine months and dozens of other patients over the past seven years. It has worked rapidly and safely in all these patients, and has been most humane. I have personally seen that ECT has been much more effective for mania than for schizophrenia. My medical colleagues have had identical observations.[12]

The shock issue is not unique in being a social problem in which the one party who controls the technology to resolve the issue scientifically refuses to do so, apparently because to do so would jeopardize its own interests and the validity of the position it has already taken. How, then, is the issue ever to be resolved?

Consider the example of an oil spill, such as the one which occurred in California in 1969.[13] Citizens concerned about the extent and environmental impact of the spill were called on to back up their position with data. Clearly, they lacked the equipment and technology to get out on the ocean and measure the spill, so they turned to the universities. But they found that no oil experts were willing to help them because the experts were funded by the oil industry. The very process of becoming recognized as experts had created in them a conflict of interest.

In the case of ECT, the technology needed to resolve the scientific issues includes Ph.D.s and M.D.s, laboratories, brain scanners, human or animal subjects, access to neuropsychological tests and the expertise to read and evaluate the results, the financial backing and credibility of institutional affiliation, and more—none of which would mean anything without the ability to win over the editorial boards of the medical journals. Lacking these resources, ordinary citizens must find "experts" who have them, but discover that the so-called experts, without exception, are already invested in shock and unwilling to investigate it.

What cannot be resolved on the facts ends up being resolved politically, more like an election than a scientific debate. But by simple majority, those forces opposing reclassification had the edge by far. Legally, logically, morally, they carried the day as well.

Instead of conducting studies to prove ECT safe, proponents of ECT were able to argue, successfully, that no studies needed to be done because the FDA had their word that it was already safe. Put more cynically, their argument was, "Trust us, we're doctors."

How did they get away with this?

On Gender, Knowledge, and Science

The letters at the FDA reflect the gender demographics of ECT: 75 percent of those who identify as ex-patients are female, 25 percent are male, a figure that has been cited consistently over the years by various sources.[14] Ninety percent of doctors who give ECT are male, and females who have invested enough in shock to become known for it can be counted on one's fingers.[15] Only five of the 133 doctor letters are from women.

The survivors report their firsthand experience with ECT. They believe that they are the experts on their own experience, and this motivates them to write. They do not consider that it is possible for someone who hasn't lived their experience to doubt or discount it. Personal experience is highly valued and held to have an authority that is beyond question. The writers have a remarkably high level of confidence, or at least hope, that the FDA will recognize and value this authority.

The male doctors, on the other hand, do not recognize it. Personal experience (of persons who aren't doctors) is unreliable, suspect; simply, not a valid way of knowing. It is automatically doubted and interrogated, and is guilty until proven innocent. It does not lend authority; to the contrary, it is dismissible as anecdote. Its opposite, science, is the only way of knowing the truth. This is the way the doctors have been trained to think; this is, they have been told, the only way to think.

It seems to me that the perspectives of the mostly female survivors and the male doctors correspond with two distinct, differently valued ways of knowing which some believe are gender-related. Feminist scholars call these two ways of viewing oneself and the world separate and connected knowing.[16]

Separate knowers, more likely to be men, see themselves as autonomous. Truth, for them, emerges from impersonal, external methods such as reason and science. They recognize as authorities only those who have been formally designated as such, by virtue of degrees, publications, or appointments. Truth is what these authorities say.

The survivors insist that authority can come from personal experience and is not necessarily what the "experts" say. Connected knowing arises from a perception of oneself in relationship to others, and it emphasizes the need to understand others' viewpoints and to respect differences. It values empathy over autonomy.

Connected knowers realize that there are many ways of knowing. The survivors don't say experience is the only way of knowing. Far from it; we are eager to collaborate with doctors and to use the scientific method to get to the truth. We are confident that brain scans and our own observations will validate each other, and we recognize the need for validation. Let's get together, we say, and share what we know for greater understanding.

The doctors are not interested in what the patients have to say, and don't feel any need to acknowledge, understand, or address our claims. They have no compunction about dismissing us as crazy or liars. Separate knowers don't hesitate to judge without understanding, whereas connected knowers are hesitant to judge a viewpoint wrong until they understand it. Nor will they dismiss another's viewpoint out of hand based on some prior belief or principle.

At the heart of separate knowing is "the doubting game," described as "putting something on trial to see whether it is wanting or not."[17]

The presumption is that there is some flaw or defect in your opponent's thinking; the object of the game is to find it, and the game is over once it's found.

This is exactly what the shock industry lobby does—to the extent that they acknowledge the patients' claims at all, which most do not deign to do. However, shock advocates don't need logic or reason—the traditional weapons of separate knowers—or even evidence to discount mental patients. The patients, they say, are imagining deficits because they are mentally ill. Or else they must be Scientologists. Or else they had the "old" shock so their experience is no longer relevant.

The doubting game is the key to keep from "knowing" ECT causes permanent amnesia and cognitive disability. You start out from the assumption that it cannot, then dare your opponent to prove you wrong. The amnesia and disability are ascribed to some other cause, any cause, no matter how improbable, even if it does not apply to the person in question. This puts the burden on the patient to rule out all other possible causes, even pink elephants and cell phones, which is impossible to do.

Consider, for instance, how this game played out in the cases of two women who were treated, respectively, by Drs. Fink and Sackeim of the APA Task Force in the mid-'90s. They were brave enough to return to these doctors to tell them that decades of their lives had been erased by shock. In neither case, the doctors said, could ECT be the culprit. Had either of them by any chance had a head injury or a case of meningitis? No, and no. Nor had they been diagnosed with Alzheimer's. The doctors then told each woman that she must have had a stroke without knowing it. Since the women could not prove that they hadn't had a stroke, the game was over. The doctors won. They did not examine the women to see if there was any evidence of a stroke.[18]

The doctors believe that to raise any doubt (no matter how far-fetched) about permanent memory loss and disability from ECT is to discredit it. Once they have done so, their job as "scientists" is done. Separate knowers are "like doormen at exclusive clubs. They do not want to let anything in unless they are pretty sure it is good."[19]

Doubting is the name of the game in what passes for scientific literature on ECT. By the rules of the doubting game, you can prove ECT doesn't cause brain damage by poking holes (real or made-up) in the studies showing brain damage, as the APA does in its petition. Thus, there is no need to do new studies.

Men tend to find the adversarial doubting game easy and natural, while women typically find it difficult. They are much more comfortable with "the believing game." The believing game is all about trying to understand others and how they came to their beliefs. For believers, truth is grounded in firsthand experience. They may be hurt and angry when their own experience is doubted. They focus on the preventable harm that was done, even if only to one person. Because of this chance of harm, it is not acceptable to give ECT the benefit of the doubt. Doctors should have to prove the treatment safe, rather than patients having to prove harm—a rigged game when the technology to prove either claim is in the hands of the doctors.

Patients Become Scientists: The Neuropsychological Reports

Is it ever possible for patients to take the tools of science into their own hands—and what happens when they do?

The obstacles are overwhelming, but some of us tried.

No one who experiences memory and cognitive problems after shock is offered followup. No one is told that there are tests that can diagnose these problems, let alone what they are or how to get them. If former patients have the courage to tell the doctors who hurt them about their deficits, they're simply told that any memory loss is only temporary. And when it doesn't resolve, they're on their own, months or years later, trying to figure out what happened to them and what to do about it. My own doctor hung up the phone on me when I called, six weeks after shock, to say my memory hadn't come back as she promised.

Shock survivors have to be able to think outside of what they've been told. What worked for me was to ask myself, "If I had these problems from any other cause besides shock, what would the doctors do?" This is how I learned about brain injury and neuropsychological testing. Then I told others who'd had shock and urged them to get tested.

We faced formidable obstacles, like doctors who refused to even consider that ECT could be damaging and insurance companies who wouldn't pay unless a doctor said brain injury was suspected. Nevertheless, in the late '80s and early '90s at least six other survivors who had insurance or could pay out of pocket had the testing done, and we informally compared the results. The similarities were striking. We did poorly on the same tests and shared common deficits. Those of us who had prior IQ test scores for before and after comparison found we'd lost roughly the same number of IQ points—thirty to forty. In all our cases, the results indicated acquired brain injury.

The evidence that has come in since then has only strengthened the case for significant permanent intellectual disability caused by ECT. More survivors have now shared their test results with me, and they are like the others. The only study ever to ask if shock had caused loss of intelligence found that about 40 percent of former patients said it had.[20] Survivors who have had neuropsychological testing have written and spoken publicly about their cognitive deficits—for instance, Anne Donahue to the Vermont legislature in 1999; Jonathan Cott in his book, *On the Sea of Memory*, published in 2005 by Random House.[21] How significant is a loss of thirty-some IQ points? Quite simply, it is the loss of much of your ability to understand, interpret, and enjoy the world.

The tests we had were far more extensive than any tests that have been given to ECT patients in any experiment or study that has ever been published. We had batteries of tests that take days to administer. There simply isn't the time or the money to do this in a research setting, even if there were an incentive. Our more thorough testing makes mockeries of published studies that claim to have done neuropsychological evaluations (and found no deficits) using a couple of carefully selected, very simple, and often inappropriate tests.

We sent our results to the FDA. *Here,* we said, in effect: it's not just us saying this now, it's our doctors. Here is your scientific evidence, in the language you accept.

But it didn't make any difference. Technically, the FDA had no responsibility to consider all the evidence in the ECT docket. It was supposed to acknowledge the comments made in the official comment period, but even so it could pick and choose which to respond to. And as far as scientific evidence, it decided to accept only articles published in medical journals and proclamations by perceived authorities. A point-blank question by Marilyn Rice to the chairman of the FDA group that was surveying the literature on ECT—Had they reviewed the contents of their own files?—elicited a clear response: No.[22]

In the late 1980s, the APA's slightly reconfigured Task Force on ECT had begun putting together a second report, one designed to press the FDA into action at last.[23] The group was made up entirely of proponents of ECT: Fink, Weiner, Sackeim, Moench, and Small. Its conclusions were no surprise. When the new report, *The Practice of Electroconvulsive Therapy: Recommendations for Treatment, Training, and Privileging*, was issued, the APA used it as a public relations and lobbying tool. An item in the January 5, 1990, issue of *Psychiatric News* spoke to the success of the organization's renewed push to sell shock.

Press Conference on New ECT Report Nets Wide Coverage

Representatives from *United Press International*, the *Associated Press*, *Clinical Psychiatric News*, *Psychiatric News*, and *The Journal of Hospital and Clinical Psychiatry* met with APA President Herbert Pardes, M.D., and Richard Weiner, M.D., Chairman of APA's Task Force on Electro-convulsive Therapy (ECT) on December 21 at APA Headquarters for a briefing on APA's new Task Force Report on Electroconvulsive Therapy. In addition, the Division of Public Affairs responded with ECT information to inquiries from *The Wall Street Journal*, *The Los Angeles Times*, *The Boston Globe*, *The Washington Post*, *USA Today*, *The Chicago Tribune*, *Science News*, and the *CBS National Radio Network*. The result: items on the front page of *USA Today's* "Life" section, and in the *Los Angeles Times*, and stories on both the AP and UPI wires, which should result in many more articles among the wire services' customers. In his opening remarks, Pardes voiced unequivocal support for ECT, saying: "I would like to state, clearly, at the outset: ECT is a safe and very effective treatment for certain severe mental illnesses."[24]

With all that media coverage, could the FDA have missed the message?

The 1990 Decision

On September 5, 1990, the FDA finally published its Proposed Rule to Reclassify the ECT device.[25] Ex-patients, the public, the Protection and Advocacy agencies, the legislators: all had, in the end, only delayed but not deterred the FDA from the position it had taken seven years earlier in its Notice of Intent. The agency proposed reclassification to Class III for all devices intended to treat severe depression, while devices used for other indications would remain in Class II. The reclassification would not take effect immediately, but only upon the development of a performance standard.

For a document seven years in the making, the proposed rule was a shoddy piece of work by any standards. The FDA's pro-industry bias was apparent throughout.

By federal law the reclassification of a device must be based on "new information," that is, information not available at the time of the original classification. But there was precious little new information in the proposal. The reclassification was said to be based entirely on a "literature review" that included not only articles from medical journals, but selected pronouncements of doctors and organizations using ECT. Of the proposal's 125 references, only 26 had been published since the original classification in 1979. Some dated from the 1940s. The FDA rationalized a proposed reclassification based on old information by saying that new information could include reevaluation of old information, "where the re-evaluation is made in light of changes in 'medical science.'" It didn't say what those alleged changes were.

Many of the articles the FDA cited were not scientific studies at all, but were actually policy statements or review articles with their own slant. The result was far from real science: a literature review of literature reviews. Marilyn Rice made fun of some of this purported valid scientific evidence in her scathing critique of the proposal. "Here is an example of what the FDA means by 'new information' and 'valid scientific evidence': 'The Royal College of Psychiatrists, the American Psychiatric Association, and the Canadian Psychiatric Association have . . . reviewed the use of ECT in recent years and concluded that, given contemporary refinements in technique, ECT is a safe and effective treatment for major depression.'" The references supporting this statement are the APA Task Force Report, a quote from some unnamed person from the Canadian Psychiatric Association that appeared in the APA's newspaper, and a memorandum on ECT from the Royal College of Psychiatrists (the British equivalent of the APA).[26]

The FDA simply left out the literature which didn't support its position that ECT was safe. By this time two CAT scan studies had been done on people with labels of depression or schizophrenia, showing that those who had received ECT had more brain atrophy and other abnormalities than those who hadn't. A third article reviewed the CAT scan records of people labeled depressed in order to compare the results in shocked vs. unshocked patients, with the same results.[27] Although these were not before-and-after studies specifically designed to isolate the effects of ECT, they were the best evidence that existed regarding its structural effects on the brain. But the FDA ignored them.

They also ignored Larry Squire's 1983 study in which he found that the majority of ECT patients hadn't regained normal memory functioning three years after shock.[28] And they did not include his 1988 study showing that amnesia in ECT survivors is caused by ECT and can be distinguished from any temporary cognitive problems associated with depression.[29] Even his work that was cited was not represented accurately. For example, the findings of his 1981 study, which found that "for information 1 to 2 years prior to treatment, some memory problems might persist," were inverted by FDA as "[information] acquired 1 week to 2 years prior to treatment may be recovered." [30]

To the extent that the FDA acknowledged what it called memory "complaints" and a number of studies showing memory deficits, it was to dismiss them as invalid with a string of discreditors: inconclusive, anecdotal, suggestive, poorly designed, not adequate, beset with numerous sources of error, seriously methodologically flawed. A long-term study by Donald Templer et al., that looked at nonmemory cognitive functioning in ECT patients—and found ECT had permanent adverse effects on cognition—was misrepresented as an investigation of memory loss and criticized as beset by error because it didn't find any such loss.[31] The FDA complained that eight studies that showed ECT causes memory deficits were not valid because they were uncontrolled. It then cited uncontrolled studies approvingly as proof that "memory is regained." But there are no studies showing return of preshock memories.

For the most part, it seemed that no one at the FDA had read the literature it was citing. The agency flatly denied that ECT ever caused permanent damage to nonmemory cognitive functioning; the proof that it cited on this point was a review article on "Acute Memory Impairment Following Electroconvulsive Therapy." Another study that tested patients ten to fifteen years after ECT on nonverbal measures of cognitive function (the Benton and Bender-Gestalt tests) and concluded that "ECT causes irreversible brain damage" was dismissed by the FDA as irrelevant because the results "were unrelated to memory loss."[32] The FDA made a big deal of claiming that ECT prevents suicide and "personal injury"; this benefit was said to outweigh the risk of possible "brain changes." But the single study it cited in support of this "benefit" actually found that ECT had no effect on the frequency of suicide.[33]

The FDA's review was so careless that it even used the same 1973 study in support of two contradictory claims. When cited to show that memory was regained, it passed methodological muster; when cited to suggest that "ECT causes memory deficits," it was said to be poorly designed. But the study doesn't show that memory is regained; it found that one year after ECT, ex-patients still had retrograde amnesia when asked to recall fifty items from their pre-ECT history.[34]

Long-term (six months or more) studies are the only way to determine whether ECT's effects on memory are temporary, as the FDA clearly wanted patients to believe, or permanent. In the PR era, long-term research came to a halt. The last study to follow up patients as long as six months was done in 1986 by Richard Weiner. Even using a questionnaire he designed in collaboration with his fellow shock machine company consultant Harold Sackeim—which, not surprisingly, is extremely biased toward asking about the types of information shock patients do not forget—he found that after six months, people could not recall 30 to 40 percent of the information known prior to shock.[35] The authors themselves admit that their results are "provocative evidence for autobiographical memory loss lasting at least six months."[36] The FDA was aware of this study, because it listed it in its references, but in its discussion of adverse effects it never mentioned the study's primary finding that ECT causes permanent amnesia.

There remained one study documenting permanent amnesia and cognitive disability that even the FDA couldn't dismiss. This was a 1982 retrospective study done by C. P. L. Freeman, D. Weeks, and R. E. Kendell.[37] It assessed ex-patients in the very long term, longer than any other study: nine months to thirty years postshock, with a mean of ten years. All of them described memory and cognitive difficulties that had begun with the shocks and never remitted. The authors (one of whom, Freeman, is an ECT advocate) tested the patients on a wider range of neuropsychological tests than has been used anywhere else, and found their reports of memory and cognitive dysfunction to be substantiated by formal testing. When compared to matched control subjects, the former ECT patients were significantly impaired. The authors then tried to attribute all of the ECT patients' permanent deficits to drugs or depression, but could not do so. They were forced to conclude that their results were compatible with the possibility that ECT causes permanent memory impairment. And so did the FDA, which cited the study in support of "the possibility that some individuals may have a persistent organic deficit."

In the end, the best the FDA could say about memory loss was, "Permanent effects on memory *should not* occur and cognitive functioning *appears to be* unaffected by ECT" (emphasis added).

The unavoidable conclusion is that the FDA bought the APA public relations line and tailored its proposal to that theme. It even quotes the claim that "risks associated with ECT are primarily related to the technique of administration, which has been significantly modified over the past 40 years" without attribution, as self-evident truth.

The FDA proposal noted that in contrast to the literature on adverse effects, "the clinical literature is consistent" on ECT's efficacy. And although this meant it had to devote three times as much space to discussion of risks as to discussion of benefits, it was said to justify its decision that "the risk/benefit assessment of ECT intended for severe depression is favorable." However, its own small ECT Task Force (an internal ad hoc group put together to look over the articles published in the 1980s so that the proposal wouldn't appear to be based entirely on old literature) was not so sanguine. Its conclusion, as reported in the proposal, was as follows: "The questions of possible damage caused by ECT, the damage thresholds, and margin of safety for each treatment modality and various intensity levels remain unanswered." Left out of the proposal to reclassify, though, was a finding that could have skewed the risk/benefit analysis: "For severe depression an apparently effective use of ECT may cause irreversible brain changes of unknown magnitude."[38]

The FDA's Treatment of the Letters

In the end, the FDA dealt with the hundreds of letters in a fashion both dishonest and bureaucratic. It acted as if the only letters that counted were those received within the official ninety-day comment period, but then it lied about the number and nature of letters received in that ninety-day window. In reality, it combed through all the letters to find those that supported the position it had decided to take, and if those hadn't been received in the official comment period, it pretended they had.

For example, in its proposal the FDA claimed "about a hundred" letters were received in the 1983 comment period. In fact, it received exactly forty-two letters. Thirty-one were opposed to reclassification, five were fence-sitting, having bought into the belief that shock could be made safe by a performance standard, and six—all from psychiatrists—were in favor of reclassification.[39]

Of the letters from patients, it wanted to highlight letters from former patients who, it claimed, supported the use of ECT. None were received during the official comment period, so someone at the FDA picked out eight letters received later and claimed they were happy patient (or spouse) letters. In fact, three were not from patients at all but from ECT practitioners.[40]

The rest of the patient letters had been summarily dismissed by the FDA. According to its assistant commissioner for legislative affairs, "FDA has received hundreds of letters from individuals, including many former ECT patients, and groups opposing both the reclassification and the use, in general, of ECT devices. These letters did not contain any new information to assist the Agency in reaching its decision concerning reclassification."[41]

He did not explain why the letters construed as favorable to ECT counted as new information.

The Letters as Science

According to its own law (21 CFR Ch 1 860.7 (c)(2)), the FDA recognizes "reports of significant human experience with a marketed device" as a form of valid scientific evidence. The law does exclude "anecdotal" evidence. The word has a specific meaning in this context: "isolated case reports, random experience, reports lacking significant details to permit scientific evaluation, and unsubstantiated opinions."

The question of whether the FDA could give weight to our reports as "valid scientific evidence" hinged on whether our experience was "random" or "significant." The FDA doesn't define these terms, but by dictionary definition random means "by chance" and significant means "having meaning." Was it really possible that hundreds of patients who did not know each other and who had ECT at different times and places with different doctors would describe the same adverse effects of ECT by chance? Or, did the fact that so many survivors said the same thing have meaning?

Whether patients' experiences could be taken seriously as science was a value judgment. In ignoring the letters, the FDA seemed to be weighing the value, or lack thereof, of not just shock patients' words but their lives. It was also making a different, even more businesslike, calculation about the costs and risks to itself, if any, of negating those words and lives. We have seen how, historically, these kinds of calculations have come out.

In the end, the FDA totally rejected one form of discourse—patient reports—and unqualifiedly embraced another, "the literature," on the grounds that only the latter was science and thus the only valid form of knowledge. It could not admit that there are good reasons to distrust what passes for science in the field of ECT.

12   *Shaming Science*

The main prerequisites which served man in the achievement of high goals in science are not available in psychiatry. It is therefore small wonder that in the field where no defined borders can be established and fixed, there was and is an enormous place for anyone who wants to postulate theories. He cannot experience the inhibitions or limitations which might arise from the need for proof or disproof. His conviction is sufficient. The only quality which seems to be required, and which indeed is attractive, is brilliancy of presentation. This is, of course, human, and human beings, not having concrete scientific tools to handle, naturally resort to this method in their frustration.

—Manfred Sakel

Medical science today is a practice far removed from the idealistic notions of helping patients or advancing scientific knowledge. Scientific research now requires institutional support and competitive funding. It's a high-stakes, profit-driven enterprise where stakeholders with conflicting interests compete to influence and spin the results. Billions of dollars in industry profits, billions of dollars in future grant funding, and careers are riding on those results. Research findings showing no or negative effects of treatment serve none of these interests.

Like the tobacco companies who promoted cigarettes despite mounting evidence that their product killed people, the ECT industry is in a position to suppress evidence of permanent harm from the treatment, or to define the research agenda in such a way that experiments that might lead to such findings are never done. The gap between science for the sake of science and science in the service of profit is as egregious for the shock industry as it was for the tobacco industry.

This is no less so because the vast majority of ECT research in this country is funded by the federal government through the National Institute of Mental Health (NIMH). Some money comes from private foundations; Max Fink and his children have their own foundation, called Scion, that supports research favorable to ECT and recently funded a book on the history of shock that takes a decidedly pro-ECT position.[1] But researchers who ask for money from the government have to put together a research proposal that will compete with other research proposals. The process involves review by a panel of perceived experts.

On a superficial level, this system seems to build in protections against bad science and bad medicine. But in practice, expert reviewers are those who themselves have a history of winning research grants; they aren't likely to award funding to those who ask inconvenient questions that might challenge their findings. Those who know or are known to the reviewers have an advantage. Once selected for funding, those most motivated to set the research agenda can themselves become reviewers, and then reviewers of reviewers, and then reviewers of the entire national research agenda. In this way the system creates an insular, self-serving body of expertise, whereby the cycle of bad science (and risks to public health due to shoddy or biased research) perpetuates itself. Financial conflict of interest plays an absolutely central role in this story.

Conflict of Interest in Research

In 1999, Jesse Gelsinger, a teenager who had volunteered as a subject in a federally funded research project, died after an experimental gene therapy procedure caused his organs to fail. It was soon discovered that the scientist who ran the experiment had a financial interest in a related biotechnology company.[2] Gelsinger's death touched off a long and heated national discussion about ethics in research—in particular, about the prevalence of researchers' financial conflicts of interest and the ways in which they corrupt the entire medical research enterprise. The story had legs; it ran for years, and it's still running. After so many reports in mainstream media outlets such as the *Los Angeles Times* and the *Wall Street Journal*, the issue of conflict of interest in medicine is now widely recognized by the general public. A survey of the headlines tells the tale:

Study Shows Journals Report Few Conflicts of Interest
Can Medical Research Findings Be Trusted?

Almost Half of All Faculty on Institutional Review Boards Have Ties to Industry

Clinical Guides Often Hide Ties of Doctors

Cash Gifts from Grantees Prompt Congressional Investigation of NIH Officials

Stealth Merger: Drug Companies and Government Medical Research

NIH Scientists Broke Rules, Deals with Companies Went Unreported[3]

And, in that most august of medical journals, *The New England Journal of Medicine*: "Is Academic Medicine for Sale?"

According to editor Marcia Angell, the answer was clearly yes. "The ties between clinical researchers and industry include not only grant support, but also a host of other financial arrangements. Researchers also serve as consultants to companies whose products they are studying, join advisory boards and speakers' bureaus, enter into patent and royalty arrangements, agree to be the listed authors of articles ghostwritten by interested companies, promote drugs and devices at company-sponsored symposiums, and allow themselves to be plied with expensive gifts and trips to luxurious settings. Many also have equity interest in the companies."[4] Psychiatry was at the epicenter of the scandal, Angell said: "You are seeing played out in psychiatry the extremes of what is happening elsewhere in medicine."[5]

By the time the spotlight shone on the corruption of academic research, a small group of ECT users had already taken full advantage of the darkness to build their names, fortunes, and fiefdoms. To this day, the ECT industry has largely escaped scrutiny because the sales of any one shock machine company pale in comparison to the profits of any pharmaceutical company, because those who own or consult for shock machine companies receive their research funding from the federal government rather than directly from the companies, and because journalists and lawmakers believe the researchers' denials.

By 2004 the story of academic and government-funded psychiatric research tainted by financial conflict was huge. It's best summed up in a five-word headline from September 2004: "Eli Lilly's Bitch: The NIMH."[6] Still, no one but survivors of ECT made the connection between what was happening with drug research and what had been happening for the past twenty years with shock. NIMH had become Mecta's bitch.

ECT Research Enters the PR Era

Very little ECT research had been funded by NIMH prior to 1980. The 1977 ECT Task Force Report says that in 1972 and 1973, less than $5,000 was provided for the study of ECT. Of all the research dollars allocated to somatic therapy research between 1968 and 1973, less than one percent went toward ECT research.[7] Larry Squire had a long-standing grant, but it was to study memory, not specifically ECT. At the dawn of the public relations era, ECT research was up for grabs. What questions would be asked, which would not be allowed? Who would set the research agenda? Who'd get to decide who else got funded?

The first Task Force Report contained three pages of sample research questions that it considered important to answer. They included these: How long after ECT do memory complaints persist? Is there any permanent loss of memories acquired during the period of one month to three years prior to ECT? How important to the patient is memory loss? How do patients view the ECT experience six months or more after treatment? Whether the questions would ever be officially answered would depend on who beat out everyone else for NIMH funding.

Harold Sackeim staked his claim. Prior to 1981, he had landed a total of $5,000 in grant money. That year, he got around half a million; when that money ran out his funding was doubled. He has been continuously funded to the tune of millions ever since.[8]

It is impossible to understand what qualified Sackeim, an inexperienced psychologist fresh out of school, for a $500,000 grant. He holds a Ph.D., not an M.D., and has had no formal medical training. He had no experience giving ECT and, in fact, could not and cannot legally administer it since he is only a psychologist. He had published very little by 1981, and nothing on ECT or any medical topic. He wrote his master's thesis on "the psychology of self-deception." His Ph.D. dissertation in 1977 reached the conclusion that "selective nonawareness of cognition, at times, is motivated." In other words, people believe what they want to believe. Turning the study of self-deception into a specialty, Sackeim published several journal articles with titles like "Self-Deception: A Concept in Search of a Phenomenon."[9]

In 1979, the newly minted psychologist came to New York and became the director of the ECT research program at Columbia University. Columbia is affiliated with the New York State Psychiatric Institute (P.I.), and Sackeim had the luck to arrive there just as it was renewing its strong interest in biological psychiatry, an effort begun by Dr. Sidney Malitz. Malitz, the director of P.I. from 1981 to 1984, took Sackeim under his wing; they were co-principal investigators on the ECT research grant for the first years, until Malitz dropped out of ECT research in 1986.

Sackeim lacked any scientific or medical credentials as an ECT expert. But the industry didn't need a scientist. In the PR era, it needed a PR person, "an applied social scientist who advises a client or employer on the social attitudes and actions to take to win the support of the publics upon whom his or her viability depends."[10] Sackeim was qualified for that.

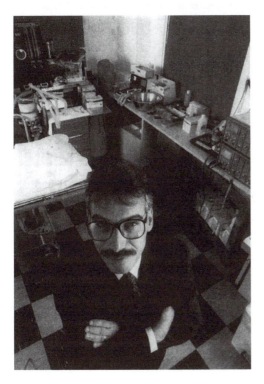

Figure 5. Psychologist Harold Sackeim.

The key to building a career and a reputation as a researcher, and therefore becoming a recognized expert, is to ensure that your grants are renewed over and over. At NIMH, funding is generally granted for three or four years at a time, no more than five (although a special award can extend that time). It is in a researcher's interest to pose questions in an open-ended way and to continually redefine them so that there need be no endpoint. In the case of ECT, "How should the treatment be administered?" is the question without end, never answered because it is always contingent on further research. What matters more than a clear answer is that the grant result in a number of publications in medical journals. As long as that happens, grants may be renewed indefinitely. This is exactly what's happened with the NIMH ECT grants; they've remained in the hands of the same men for decades. In addition, there are no constraints on how many concurrent grants a researcher may hold or how much money he or she may be awarded.

Max Fink calls Harold Sackeim a "research study entrepreneur."[11] I think this statement is meant as a compliment to Sackeim's ability to multiply federal research money by corporate money. Once he landed the research grant, he signed on with the Mecta Corporation as a consultant, and has worked for them since at least 1984. He has also worked for Somatics, their rival.[12] Since the death of Paul Blachly, the psychiatrist who founded it, Mecta has been owned by investors with no medical or engineering expertise. They've consistently hired the most prominent shock doctors to advise them. As Gorham Nicol, Mecta's co-owner, put it, "The doctors in research centers provide the medical requirements and information we need to build the equipment because our function is strictly as a manufacturer."[13] But when researchers tailor their research to the needs of industry rather than those of patients, science gets lost.

It is because of this inherent conflict of interest that the federal government adopted the Objectivity in Research rule when it reauthorized funding for NIH (and NIMH) in 1995. The law made it illegal for federally funded researchers to accept funding from the corporations whose products they are testing without disclosing it.[14] Disclosure is now also mandatory when presenting at medical conferences and publishing in some medical journals. But public records show that prominent shock doctors haven't disclosed that they receive money from the shock machine companies.[15]

Tools of Bias #1: Redefine the Questions
to Get the Answers You Want

The official title of NIMH Grant No. MH35636 is "Affective and Cognitive Consequences of ECT." It is one of the only NIMH grants that could have been applied to basic research into the effects of ECT on the brain, memory, and cognition. That is precisely what the grant was initially intended to accomplish, according to the original proposal submitted to NIMH by psychiatrist Sidney Malitz and psychologist Sackeim:

> The major objective of the proposed research is to examine the effects of bilateral and right unilateral electroconvulsive therapy on affective and cognitive functioning. The consequences of the two treatment modes will be studied in regard to neuropsychological functions that previously have not been investigated. . . . Drug-free inpatients presenting major, unipolar depressive disorder will be tested before, during, and after treatment, and a matched normal control group will be tested at comparably spaced times. . . . Posttreatment assessments include a two-month followup and retesting a sample of relapsed and nonrelapsed patients.[16]

However, in the mid-1980s, when he took over the grant reins as principal investigator and simultaneously began taking money from device manufacturers, Sackeim redefined the grant agenda. In each subsequent successful bid for renewal of federal funding, he has continued to direct it farther and farther away from the basic unanswered research question: What does ECT do to the brain? The initial stated goal of the grant, isolating the effects of ECT by comparing ECT patients to matched controls who haven't had ECT, or to themselves before treatment, was subsumed by an agenda based on comparing the effects of different types of ECT to one another. The part about comparing ECT patients to persons who haven't had ECT was dropped. Ten years on, although it still bore the same grant number, the project had little relation to the one originally proposed.

> There is a paucity of information on the effects of electrical dosage in patients who receive ECT. . . . This proposed study will use a random-assignment, double-blind, four-group design in 120 patients with major

depression to compare right unilateral ECT at three dosage levels: 50%, 150% and 450% above seizure threshold, with a bilateral group treated at 150% above seizure threshold serving as a standard. . . . The study will provide information as to which of these unilateral ECT conditions may be preferred in clinical practice. . . . This research is designed to address the questions of where in the dosing range unilateral ECT is optimized and, when optimized, how does this treatment compare to bilateral ECT.[17]

This type of narrow technical research, while it has had little to no benefit for patients, is of great interest to the companies that need new bells and whistles to add to their machines every couple of years in order to raise prices and best the competition. In essence, a device researcher like Sackeim can get paid twice; he is paid by the government to carry out research and then paid again when he sells his technical expertise to the device manufacturers.

In 2000, after nearly twenty years of public funding for this grant, Sackeim wrote an editorial touching upon the current status of research on ECT's permanent adverse effects. Writing as if at a distance, as if it had nothing to do with him, he mused: "Prospective patients, family members, and the public often want to know the frequency with which patients report substantial memory impairment following ECT . . . there is little objective evidence. . . . Indeed, our estimates of the probability of death with ECT are based on a more secure empirical foundation."[18]

To which, after about $8 million of taxpayer money had been paid for an investigation of the cognitive effects of ECT, there is only one response: Who is responsible for that?

There is one other NIMH grant that was intended to investigate the long-term effects of ECT: "Long-term Effects of Electroconvulsive Therapy," NIMH Grant No. 30723. Unfortunately, it is also in the hands of a strong ECT proponent with a long history of financial and career conflict: Richard Weiner of Duke University.

When he was first awarded the grant in 1978, Weiner promised the government (and the taxpayers) to investigate the long-term effects of ECT in a double-blind study. He said he would use controls and evaluate subjects after six months.

By 1978, as we have seen, Weiner was in charge of the APA's decades-long campaign to prevent a brain scan investigation by the FDA. It would have been impossible for him to maintain his political position that a safety investigation of ECT was unnecessary had he himself been engaged in such research.

So he rewrote his grant abstract. By 1984, although the original research questions posed had never been answered, the protocol for this grant had changed: it had become a comparative study of the effects of different types of ECT, with no controls. However, this time Weiner promised the government to use the money to assess the adverse effects of ECT at one year post-treatment.

But the question of what those effects were was never answered. There is no evidence that a one-year follow-up study was ever done. If it was, it has never been published.

By 1988, there were no more promises to do long-term assessments of adverse effects, but funding for the "Long-Term Effects of Electroconvulsive Therapy" grant kept flowing without interruption. And in fact, in the 1990s Weiner simultaneously received grant funding from the National Center on Research Resources (the arm of NIH that focuses on biomedical technology and instrumentation) "to determine the long-term effects of electroconvulsive therapy upon memory function, the EEG, and brain structure (as measured by MRI)."[19] That grant was never used for that purpose.

Rather than answering the questions he originally posed, Weiner's NIMH research has been all about endlessly comparing different ECT techniques. The abstract for Grant No. 30723 was revised to read, "There continues to be uncertainty regarding the optimal manner in which ECT should be delivered. . . . The proposed study will involve two components. The first, and most major, will be prospective comparison of two stimulus intensity dosing strategies. . . . A second smaller component of this protocol will investigate stimulus intensity effects on an intraindividual basis."[20]

As a lawyer might say, the very first sentence assumes facts not in evidence; that is, it assumes no uncertainty as to *whether* ECT should be delivered. It steamrolls over the question of what ECT does, right on to how to do it.

There's not necessarily anything shady about comparing different types of ECT to one another, if that's what you got a grant to do and you acknowledge that's all you're doing. However, the limitations of such a study are obvious. As Dr. Chris Frith, an ECT user from England, points out, this research design is "very likely to underestimate the deficit in relation to an untreated group."[21]

The problem is that such an approach necessarily presumes that ECT has been proven safe. They presume it to such an extent that many studies are done with custom-modified shock machines that put out twice as much more electricity as can be legally used in any other context besides research.[22] The theory seems to be since no amount of electricity can harm the brain, why not turn it up? But what if it isn't harmless? And since research dollars are limited, if the millions of taxpayer money earmarked for ECT gets spent on comparison studies, that means that basic research on the effects of ECT won't be done.

In fact, the three dozen published journal articles funded by Weiner's NIMH grant over the years aren't even limited to comparisons of ECT techniques, but go very far afield. They include a historical overview of ECT as it "celebrated" (his word) fifty years of continuous use; an investigation of how to make seizures longer by the use of intravenous caffeine; and a study of the effects of unilateral ECT on the heart.[23]

The studies by Sackeim and Weiner that focus on arcane technical details have shown no real benefit to patients. These grants have been renewed every time they asked for more money, and there is no reason to think the funding will not last as long as they want it. Currently, NIMH spending on Grant No. 35636 alone—which has been funded since 1981—is about $500,000 per year, the majority of which goes to salaries.

Tool of Bias #2: Compromise Financially in Every Way Possible

Back in the 1970s—"before there was a Mecta"—Weiner, who is an electrical engineer as well as a psychologist and psychiatrist, began his shock machine company involvement.[24] He's consulted for what became Mecta Corporation ever since, designing their machines, writing the instruction manuals, and making a promotional video for them. He also worked for Somatics Inc. (now Somatics LLC). This wasn't exactly a secret (Weiner's technical consultation is acknowledged in the Mecta and Somatics manuals), but it wasn't publicly disclosed, either.[25] In fact, in a 1996 television appearance Weiner flatly denied he was a paid consultant to the shock industry.[26]

His two-decade financial conflict finally became public later that same year, when the *Washington Post* did an exposé on shock and, in particular, "Experts' Ties to Industry."[27] But the *Post* had missed something: Weiner's patents on ECT techniques.

In 1980, the Bayh-Dole Law had made it possible for university recipients of federal grants to secure patents for their discoveries and to market them. This has been described as "farming out research to corporations" because of the influx of corporate money into university research.[28] As the chairman of the APA's ECT Task Force for over a decade—quite literally, the author of the book telling everyone else how to do ECT—Weiner was in a unique position to profit from the opportunity to develop patents.

In 1995, he filed a patent for an "electroconvulsive therapy method using ictal EEG data as an indicator of ECT seizure adequacy."[29] The ECT Task Force Report was revised between 1990 and 2001 to include a new section on "EEG seizure adequacy measures." The new section begins, "Recently, some ECT devices have included measures that convey information about EEG changes during and after the seizure." While stopping short of recommending such machines be employed exclusively, the section suggests that they may provide useful information. Certainly, those shopping for new shock machines would be encouraged to purchase those featuring Weiner's method.

The holder of this patent could license the method to any or all of the shock machine companies, of which there were four at the time. Because the patent had been developed with NIMH grant money, which is paid to an institution rather than an individual, Weiner could not legally hold the patent in his own name. It was licensed to Duke University.

In the 2001 APA ECT Task Force Report, Weiner belatedly disclosed this patent as well as his work for Somatics (which were not disclosed in the 1996 *Washington Post* article), but said he did not receive "royalties or personal payments," making it appear as if he had made a selfless choice not to hold the patent in his name.[30] In fact, he did not have that choice.

Now Duke makes money every time one of the new machines is sold. At the same time, Weiner's grant is paid directly to the university, as is all federal grant money. Should a university that profits from the sale of the machines simultaneously accept public money to do ECT research?

Holding the Line on Basic Research

Over the past two decades Sackeim has maintained, in several contexts, that research on whether ECT causes brain damage is scientifically uninteresting and unlikely to be funded.[31] He endorses the study done by Edward Coffey, Richard Weiner, and colleagues in 1988 as definitive on this issue. For him, it seems, there is no need to conduct further brain imaging studies.

Coffey et al. is in fact an MRI study, and has the distinction of being the first such study designed to examine brains before and after ECT.[32] It was funded by Richard Weiner's NIMH grant #30723 on "Longterm Effects of Electroconvulsive Therapy," meaning Weiner was the principal investigator. Coffey is an ECT advocate trained by Weiner.

Did Weiner's long-standing financial conflict of interest affect the results of this study? I had the opportunity to ask this question of Coffey personally at an APA meeting. To his credit, he did not try to deny the conflict. He said that it did not affect the results, because those on the research team who did the actual measuring, computing, counting, and other data crunching were not financially conflicted. But by definition there is no bias in counting and computing. The bias comes in the design of the study. If the flaws are built in—bias by design—the accuracy of the calculations doesn't matter. This is what happened in the Coffey study.

First of all, there were only nine patients in the study, which makes it statistically underpowered to tell us anything. There were no control subjects—without which it is scientifically impossible to draw any conclusions about causation. Of the nine patients, six had mildly to severely abnormal brain scans *before* ECT. Why, in such a tiny study, choose these over patients without signs of preexisting brain damage? After treatment, the patients were said to have a little more brain atrophy, or shrinkage—but they were studied only two to three days afterwards, which even the authors acknowledge was not enough time for possible ECT-related damage to show up. Despite these acknowledged and inherent limitations, Coffey et al. conclude (inconclusively) that "these initial observations need to be confirmed in a larger number of subjects."

Sackeim and others used the results of the Coffey study to redefine the question away from scientific investigation of ECT's effects. Their argument went like this: based on nine people, almost everyone prescribed ECT is coming in with serious brain abnormalities, but even if they had ECT previously, they can't be due to ECT since ECT doesn't cause them. Therefore their psychiatric conditions must be causing them. Thus, any changes post-ECT must be due to the natural progression of their mental illness.

Despite the issue of brain damage being settled for Sackeim in 1988, three years later Weiner and Coffey did a follow-up MRI study. This time they included thirty-five patients, still a small number for a scientific study. Fifteen of the patients had had ECT before their participation in the current research. Fourteen had cortical atrophy—brain shrinkage—on their pre-ECT scans. The researchers did not ask or reveal whether these were the same patients. In other words, they built into their research the assumption that ECT does not cause brain damage.

Several patients' brains showed increased abnormality post-ECT, but the authors attributed this to "cerebrovascular disease," not to ECT. They had to admit, though, that because of the absence of control subjects, this was no more than speculation.[33]

Tool of Bias #3: The Selective Review as an Alternative to Controlled Studies

If the question of whether ECT causes brain damage was too uninteresting to bother investigating scientifically with brain scans, that didn't stop Sackeim and Weiner from elaborating on it anyway—using their grant money to pay themselves to write selective review articles on the topic.

There are two types of review articles. In a selective review (such as that conducted by the FDA to support its position on ECT), the author picks and chooses from the literature, and may select only those articles that support his or her argument while omitting and not acknowledging the existence of those that refute it. In a systematic review, the author is constrained to consider and evaluate all the evidence on the subject. If an author chooses to write a review article, the systematic review is the scientific way to do it. But neither is a substitute for scientific research.

Richard Weiner chose to conduct a selective review rather than a brain scan study in 1984, when he published a lengthy article entitled "Does Electroconvulsive Therapy Cause Brain Damage?"[34] It consists of twenty-two pages of mostly omission, equivocation, and outright misrepresentation. A footnote explains why: it tells us the article is "an expanded version of material included in a device reclassification petition submitted to the U.S. Food and Drug Administration." NIMH money allotted for the scientific study of ECT's effects on the brain (Grant No. 30723) was being spent to augment and publicly disseminate a document produced for the political purpose of lobbying the FDA *against* a scientific investigation of ECT's effects on the brain.

Here is a typical example of how Weiner did this. Unable to debunk the findings of the Janis prospective study documenting permanent extensive amnesia, he simply dismisses the article, without explanation or footnote, saying "all forms of cognitive testing in such a patient population are now considered of questionable value." Even so, in the end, Weiner's conclusion is loaded with escape clauses: "For the *typical* individual receiving ECT, no *detectable* correlates of *irreversible* brain damage *appear* to occur" (emphasis added).

Ten years later, Sackeim did the same thing with his NIMH grant money: paid himself and his colleagues to write a review titled "Does ECT Alter Brain Structure?"[35] The authors specify no method for their review, leaving them free to editorialize, misrepresent, and omit. For instance, they leave out the results and conclusions ("a serious warning against the use of electroconvulsive therapy") of Colon's 1975 animal autopsy study, and then tell readers, without basis, that it is "statistically flawed." They then praise Coffey's work as "the most methodologically sophisticated." And again, note the legalistic language of their conclusion: "There is no credible evidence that ECT causes structural brain damage." And that is true, as long as you define all evidence that ECT causes brain damage as incredible.

In a survey of the most frequently cited articles on ECT from 1985 to 2001, Sackeim's review ranks in the top ten.[36] Since Weiner's was published in 1984, it wasn't included in that survey, but it has also been very widely cited. It is likely that few of those who cite to these articles are aware that they are only reviews, not scientific studies.

Selective reviews, easy to write and easy to manipulate, pay big dividends. For instance, Sackeim's review has been cited to reassure the general public of ECT's safety in everything from a high school psychology textbook to the Surgeon General's Report (see Chapter Fifteen).[37]

Tool of Bias #4: Make Yourself an "Expert"

Physicians are no less influenced by the lure of "fame and name" than are the rest of us. It's not a question of fraudulent reporting of results— although that has occurred—but rather that the very desire for success can distort the results, subtly and persuasively, often without one's being aware of it. In the great majority of cases—where results are presented prematurely, where success is overestimated and dangers underestimated, where there are biases in the selection of patients, and where failures are explained away as exceptions—the physicians responsible have been genuinely convinced of the validity of their conclusions. Self-deception is by its very nature difficult to guard against—almost impossible when fueled by unbridled ambition.

—Elliot Valenstein, M.D.

Funded research has many goals beyond advancing science and helping patients, and one of them is career building. How else but through research could Harold Sackeim, a man who is not allowed to treat patients, become unanimously hailed as the "world expert" on shock?

The first step: publish . . . and publish . . . and publish. Consider that at the time of the first APA Task Force, the ink was barely dry on Sackeim's diploma. By 1984, he'd shown himself useful enough to the industry to be hired as a consultant to the device companies. By 1989, his curriculum vitae listed 120 publications, most of them produced with taxpayer money, most of them on ECT. The more he wrote, the more he was considered an expert. In the late 1980s, the psychologist authored half of the 1990 APA Task Force Report on ECT, including the sections on adverse consequences and cognitive effects, and singlehandedly wrote its informed consent statement, which has been adopted for use for virtually every patient in the U.S.[38] The report also cites twenty-two of his articles.

He proved himself an "expert" by generating the maximum number of articles from each group of patients. Although only thirty to forty patients a year participate in the ECT research program at his institution, he's been able to produce twenty-five to thirty-five journal articles each year.[39] Such an extraordinary rate of production, even if it helps patients or science to some extent, benefits careers exponentially more. When the 2001 Task Force Report was published, Sackeim was able to cite himself more than sixty times.

By 1996, Sackeim had been appointed associate editor, or to the editorial boards, of influential medical journals like *Neuropsychiatry*. He was now himself a reviewer (that is, one of those who make the decisions as to who and what is allowed to be published) of about fifty medical journals, including most journals known to publish on ECT. Sackeim has served on the committee that was responsible for evaluating all the research applications that were sent in to NIMH on the subject of mental illness, and in particular, all the applications that had to do with ECT. If he didn't want a question asked or a project funded, he was in a position to kill it. He was also appointed the head of a "blue ribbon" NIMH panel whose purpose was to review and reevaluate the agency's overall mission, deciding if the work being done was in the important areas, and if not, what those areas were.[40]

The men who, like Sackeim, are able to successfully create and market themselves as ECT experts are in great demand as speakers, as highly paid expert witnesses for the defense in malpractice cases, and in the media. But the continued survival of the industry depends as well on their ability to influence the next generation.

Tool of Bias #5: Build a Dynasty

The shock promoters who are financially compromised are all involved in teaching and training future shock doctors—who then go on to teach others and become compromised themselves. This isn't unique to the shock industry, of course. Barbara Seaman has written about how doctors trained by surgeons who pushed radical mastectomies on women with breast cancer would have seen supporting less invasive treatments as "patricide."[41] But the ECT industry is so small and so tightly controlled that it is nearly impossible to gain entrance unless one is vetted by those who already belong.

There are two ways the industry transmits its values and ensures its survival. The first is from a well-known shock enthusiast to lesser-known contemporaries who already work in the same institution or, sometimes, different ones. The offer is tendered: if you want to advance yourself through ECT, I can help you. The second way is the more traditional teacher/student transmission of values from a shock doctor to a usually much younger student.

The American taxpayer pays for the old shock doctors to train the new. NIMH has special competitive grants (designated by the letter K affixed to the grant number) that have no benefit to patients or society, but simply pay for training to advance an individual's career. These are called Academic Investigator Awards or, in the case of younger doctors, First Awards or Scientist Development Awards.

The shock brigade has taken full advantage of this funding. For instance, W. Vaughn McCall at Wake Forest University in North Carolina, not far from Duke, received this grant to follow in Weiner's footsteps:

> This academic investigator award will provide the educational experience and mentorship necessary for the principal investigator to develop as a contributing clinical scientist in the areas of electroconvulsive therapy and depression in the elderly. . . . The primary side effect of ECT in the elderly is reversible cognitive impairment. The cognitive side effects can be reduced by using brief pulse. . . . The academic portion of this proposal will provide for class work in statistics and epidemiology. Further, this proposal will allow active study with . . . Drs. Harold Sackeim, Richard Weiner . . . who are experts in the areas of dementia, depression, ECT, and biostatistics cognitive testing.[42]

It's not just statistics McCall was learning, but a way of thinking about ECT according to the dogma of industry PR—cognitive impairment is a side and not a primary effect, impairment is reversible, brief pulse is the solution. He learned it well. After his training, he went on to hold a key position of power in the industry: editor of the *Journal of ECT*.

Other ECT doctors who were trained in the most advanced brain imaging techniques such as quantitative EEG, positron emission tomography

(PET), magnetic resonance imaging (MRI), single proton emission computerized tomography (SPECT), and brain energy activity mapping (BEAM)
include Mitchell Nobler at Sackeim's institution, Andrew Krystal at Duke,
and Charles Kellner at the Medical University of South Carolina. Kellner's
grant provided for "consultation with national experts" with the specific aim
of making Kellner himself an expert who would then train others throughout the Southeast.[43]

Kellner's $88,000-a-year training paid off handsomely. He, too, went on
to edit the industry journal. He became principal investigator on his own
research grants from NIMH (comparison studies of three different types of
ECT with no controls) while accepting funding from Mecta and Somatics.[44]
He is now the chief of psychiatry at a university medical center in the
Northeast, training still more shock doctors, and has become a prominent
media spokesman for ECT. On a television talk show, this expert in brain
imaging technology refused to answer when asked about his financial ties to
the device manufacturers, then told the audience, "There are now important
carefully controlled studies with MRI brain scans before and after ECT
showing conclusively that there is absolutely no structural brain damage."[45]
Despite all the grant money that has been paid by the government to train
Kellner and others in MRI, there is not one such study. None of these
researchers has ever used their taxpayer-funded expertise to answer the question of whether ECT causes brain damage.

The other ways a handful of self-appointed experts wield inordinate
influence over what other doctors believe to be true about ECT are through
teaching positions at prestigious universities and teaching hospitals and
through the continuing medical education (CME) courses where practicing
physicians earn credits they must have to maintain their licenses. In the informal, collegial setting of the latter—perhaps at a luxury hotel, with plenty of
coffee breaks—where most of the participants already work in the shock
industry, schmoozing is definitely on the agenda. As they hear about the latest trend in electrode placements, participants are being indoctrinated in the
ECT industry's culture of denial. The big-name speakers talk frankly about
such topics as how to use public relations strategies to promote the use of
shock and defuse criticism and how to defend against ECT lawsuits.

One such CME seminar took place shortly after I was contacted by telephone by the sister of a man who was scheduled to get ECT as one of Harold Sackeim's research subjects. He had signed up in order to get care for free (as all research subjects participating in clinical trials do), because he had no money, but he had misgivings about the treatment. One of the things I told her was that her brother had the right to speak to a patients' rights advocate from the federally funded Protection and Advocacy (P&A) program.

At that time a friend of mine, Laura Ziegler, worked for P&A. Anticipating a call from this patient, I discussed some details of his situation with Ziegler, without mentioning the man's name (which I didn't know). But no one from P&A could do anything unless the man requested their services, which he never did. That was the end of the story—in real life.

A few weeks later, at a CME seminar co-chaired by Harold Sackeim and Max Fink, a panel on "Drugs and ECT" devolved into anecdote, and Sackeim started talking about this patient—let's call him John—myself, and Ziegler, identifying us in such detail that he could not possibly have been referring to anyone else. In this story, after I spoke with his sister, John was approached by an "antipsychiatry organization" called "Committee Against the Psychiatric Abuse of the Mentally Ill." (There never was any such organization.) Ziegler—described as an "antipsychiatry representative" rather than a professional advocate—was said to have come to the hospital demanding to see him, forcing "very senior people at the institute" into tense discussions about whether to allow her access. In the end, a lawyer was said to have come to see John. The punch line of the story? When this lawyer saw how depressed he was, she changed her tune and talked him into shock, not out of it!

The students responded with appreciative laughter. They were totally duped by the story to the extent that it was followed by an earnest discussion about what they would have done at their hospital in such a situation.[46]

Ziegler and I were stunned that a professional in a classroom situation would fabricate a story based on real people, seemingly just for fun. Because this wasn't a college course, our only recourse was to refute Sackeim's account and express our disgust in a formal complaint to the American Psychological Association's Ethics Committee. Sackeim's made-up story, she wrote, was "practically encouraging his audience to see ECT candidates' attorneys—and their rights to due process—as cause for merriment rather than respect or concern."[47]

Tool of Bias #6: Own the Company

Richard Abrams literally wrote the book on shock. He is a student and protégé of Max Fink, and the author of the textbook *Electroconvulsive Therapy*, first published by Oxford University Press in 1988 and now in its fourth printing. It is the only textbook on ECT on the market, so when medical students learn about ECT, for the most part they learn from Abrams.

Abrams's ownership of Somatics, the company that makes half of the shock machines sold in America, was always public record. But no one thought to look. It took a shock survivor from Abrams's home state of Illinois, acting on a hunch, to expose him. Because she lived near Abrams, she was aware of how close his office was to Somatics's headquarters—"you could ride it on a bike"—and thought that couldn't be a coincidence. It wasn't.

Somatics sells the machines at around $15,000 each. It also sells various single-use ECT accessories such as mouth guards, conductive jelly, and disposable electrodes, for which Abrams holds the patents.[48] In an ad in the *Journal of ECT* in 2002, the company brags of having sold over a million of them. At the price listed, that is more than $2.8 million in sales just from the electrodes.

Abrams was the most-cited author in the 1990 Task Force Report, with sixty references to his articles. Yet he never disclosed his ownership of a shock machine company to the readers of the report or his textbook. In his books and articles, Abrams is in a dream position: he can recommend the use of machines and accessories that only he sells.

For many years, shock survivors including myself told reporters about Abrams's ownership of Somatics, but no one was interested. It wasn't until 1995 that reporter Dennis Cauchon broke the story for *USA Today*, citing a court deposition in which Abrams admitted that Somatics provided half of his income.

Somatics's co-owner, Conrad Swartz, is also a well-known and much published ECT doctor, with more than a page of references in Abrams's book. He told *USA Today* that his profits from Somatics were equivalent to an additional psychiatry practice (valued at $132,000 at the time) and that his financial conflict was a "nonissue." He then commented, "Psychiatrists don't make much money and by practicing ECT they can bring their income almost up to the level of the family practitioner or internist."[49]

Records show that Swartz does not disclose his ownership of Somatics when presenting workshops and CME seminars to other shock doctors. (Organizations that sponsor such workshops, including the APA, require disclosure of financial interests.)[50]

Abrams claimed that his publisher, Oxford University Press, knew he owned the company—a statement that surprised the publisher. "Wow," executive editor Joan Bossert told *USA Today*. "I did not know that. I really wish he'd told us."

It was "ridiculous," Abrams said, to think his ownership of the company created a conflict of interest.

Abrams left his job at the Chicago Medical School shortly after the *USA Today* article came out. He was fifty-eight. Was it retirement? If so, why does the 2002 edition of his book, published many years later, claim he still works there?

Tool of Bias #7: If You Don't Like Your Results, Throw Them Out

You might think that since the public pays for nearly all shock research, we ought to be able to scrutinize that research. Not so. It is true that anyone can submit a Freedom of Information request to NIMH. If they deem your request reasonable and if you pay all costs, you can get some general information pertaining to the project, such as how much money the researchers got. What you can't find out, what is made to disappear, is the raw data, especially those results the researchers do not choose to publish or disclose.

Not only can researchers choose to hide data from the public, but they can withhold it from their own subjects. Selma Lanes of New York City (a former distinguished author and editor of children's books as well as the definitive biography *The Art of Maurice Sendak*) was one of about 150 subjects in a 1992 research project to compare four different types of ECT. She didn't know she had been in an experiment, let alone what it was about, until I told her. Then she wanted to know what type of shock she had, and what type of testing Sackeim had done on her, and what the results were. She asked for her records and Sackeim refused, saying that because they were research records and not medical records, they belonged to him.

Lanes's cohort probably provided Sackeim with six or eight, or even more, published articles. Lanes's request to Sackeim for the journal articles for which she was a subject went unanswered. But nowhere in any of them can she recognize herself. Nowhere is there any mention that any subject ever suffered a permanent twenty-year amnesia, which is what happened to Lanes. Nor is there any mention in any Sackeim article ever published that he follows up patients one year after ECT, yet this was specified in the research protocol Lanes signed up for. Whatever deficits Sackeim found in his subjects a year after shock, he has chosen not to disclose them.

Similarly, Jonathan Cott—also, pre-ECT, an accomplished author, with fifteen books to his credit—was a research subject of Sackeim's in 1999. After ECT, he wrote a whole book about memory, describing how fifteen years of his life had been erased and his intellect permanently diminished.[51] Like Lanes, he didn't remember that he had been a research subject. To this day, Sackeim has never revealed that such extensive permanent amnesia and disability occurred in any of his subjects, ever.

Should he, or any other researcher, have the choice to simply "disappear" subjects like Lanes and Cott (and who knows how many others) in order to polish the image of ECT? Who's to stop him?

The Rise of the Special Interest Group

In his book about the psychopharmaceutical industry, *Let Them Eat Prozac*, psychiatrist David Healy writes, "One of the chilling things about this story is how a very few people in key positions can determine the course of events and all but shape the consciousness of a generation."[52] The drug industry is much larger than the shock industry, with a lot more money at stake. If a handful of people can shape policy and opinion in the drug world, it is all the more true in the ECT industry. This is true not only for one generation—but across generations.

The term "special interest group," long used in politics, is now an apt description for a group of scientists who share common financial interests and "are taking over control of science, acting to protect corporate interests in science by virtue of their medical positions."[53] What we are allowed to know and believe and do about shock is determined by these "self-selecting academic oligarchies," as they have been described so accurately.[54]

It is a great mistake, but one that many people make, to think that either academics or government employees are free of financial conflict simply because they aren't currently or directly employed by corporations. Today the university research center is no ivory tower, but one of the key players in the special interest group. In this vast and lucrative enterprise, the patients whose brains and bodies are on the line are forgotten. One patient advocate writes:

> Research stakeholders represent an interlocking directorate of self-interest: the biotech/pharmaceutical industry, university and free-standing research centers, bioethicists, government oversight agencies, and medical journal publishers. This confluence of self-interest groups tightly controls the conduct of research and the oversight process as individuals within the enterprise move freely from one to another position of authority. All of these players are financially and professionally interlocked. Independent public advocates are excluded from the process, thereby denying human subjects representation at any juncture.[55]

The oligarchs monopolize the federal grant money. They publish the articles that become scientific evidence. They decide who else is allowed to get grant money. They oversee grants. They act as editors and reviewers at the journals. They write the textbooks. They appear in the media and as expert witnesses in courtrooms. They testify to legislatures. They consult to government agencies. All of these activities enrich them directly or indirectly, and contribute to their ability to earn money as consultants to industry and/or owners or shareholders of companies.

The more they do these things, the more they are considered experts and the more they are allowed to do them. And as we enter the second generation of the PR era, they are training the younger ones to think and act as they do. There is no greater triumph for a PR campaign than for the workings of its machinery to become all but invisible, and for its pronouncements to be accepted as reality at the highest levels of society. The PR campaign to sell ECT has reached this goal.

13   *The Lie That Won't Die*

They [the practitioners of shock treatment] are on a crusade to convince other psychiatrists and the public that mental illness is a biochemical disorder best treated with electroshock. . . . The only real check on this campaign to bring electroshock back is the media, because those who consider themselves victims of electroshock tend to either go into hiding, or if they do speak out, they often lack credibility due to their illness. . . . The controversy illustrates the important role of the media in exposing potentially harmful activities and forcing politicians to find solutions.

—Vince Bielski of the *San Francisco Bay Guardian*, 1990

For the most part, the general public doesn't have the time or expertise to pore through original scientific research, or to investigate whether it has been biased by financial conflicts of interest. How, then, are we to tell good science from bad science, good advice on health matters from bad or biased advice? Whether we are deciding if we ought to avoid all fats in our diet, or if hormone replacement therapy is worth the risks, we make decisions based on what we see and hear in the media. But neither do the media look critically at what scientific research does and does not tell us. Instead, journalists rely on the pronouncements of those who hold themselves out as experts.

It's no accident that the men who get the most grant money are also the media spokesmen. Sometimes the media exposure comes first (it doesn't matter whether the spokesperson knows anything since there's a script), sometimes the grant money comes first. It's often a chicken-and-egg question. But with the rise of ECT research entrepreneurship and its lucrative offshoots since the 1980s, getting one's name and face in the media is like money in the bank. The institutions where ECT is a mainstay (or which would like to get into the business of ECT entrepreneurship) gain in prestige and funding as well from all the free PR.

The rise of the media psychiatrist, that hybrid of PR man and scientist, was news in the 1970s, as we have seen. But today it is a mundane fact of journalistic life that, as one commentator put it, "Public relations, whose birth early in the twentieth century rattled the world of objective journalism, has matured into a spin monster so ubiquitous that nearly every word a reporter hears from an official source has been shaped and polished to proper effect."[1]

By limiting reporters' access to a handful of carefully groomed, media-savvy shock doctors, the ECT industry makes sure that media coverage is favorable. It also shapes reporters' perceptions in not-so-subtle ways even before they are referred to the "experts." One reporter says that when Greg Phillips of the APA's media relations department took his phone call inquiring about ECT, Phillips immediately responded, "Is this about Scientology?"[2]

The veneer of science on ECT encourages reporters to believe that it is too technical for them to understand, and to rely on doctors to explain it, using the same script year after year. But once reporters extend trust to doctors in technical matters, they end up granting them carte blanche on the simple facts that would otherwise be the job of journalists to verify, such as the numbers of persons who receive ECT each year. This is why ECT's fake "comeback" continues to be, as it has been for three decades, a mandatory element of any story on shock.

In the PR era, reporters simply let the media psychiatrists point to their self-promotional efforts as evidence: "There are no nationwide figures of shock treatment cases over the past several years, but several factors indicate a resurgency, said C. Edward Coffey, a psychiatrist at Duke University. . . . Psychiatrists are publishing more articles about its benefits, colleges are offering more shock treatment courses for practicing psychiatrists and medical students, and medical supply companies are producing more shock treatment equipment."[3]

In 1995, the founder of the group Fairness and Accuracy in Reporting (FAIR), which challenges media bias and censorship, wrote a story exposing bias in ECT reporting, linking the fictional comeback to media hype and concluding that "rather than raising tough questions, news media have tended to cheerlead the resurgent shock technique."[4]

In fact, there has been no further attempt to determine how many people actually receive ECT since the small sampling studies of the 1970s. Each time a bill to collect that data on a state level has been introduced, the APA has lobbied against it, with the result that only three more states have successfully passed reporting bills: Texas, Illinois, and Vermont. Rather than looking for evidence, reporters just endlessly repeat the baseless 100,000 people per year figure that was used in 1985 to herald a comeback.

In the '90s and the '00s, with very few exceptions, media coverage of ECT whether print, broadcast, or online, retained its pro-shock bias and cookie-cutter homogeneity. Some papers, like the *Baltimore Sun* and the *Los Angeles Times*, have done more than one comeback story. The *New York Times* holds the record for the most; four so far, in 1987, 1990, 1993, and 2006, including one FAIR called a "pro-shock ad."

My own collection includes, as of 2006, around fifty near-identical comeback articles with titles like "A New Image for Shock Therapy," "Taking the Shock out of Electroshock," and "Shock Therapy Loses Some of Its Shock Value."[5] In a world in which media coverage feeds off itself, it now seems unthinkable that there could be any other way of covering shock in the mainstream media. Can it be that bias toward the ECT industry is built into the practice of journalism today, despite journalism's professed values of objectivity, balance, and fairness? Perhaps they aren't what they seem to be, especially when applied to science writing in general and to ECT writing in particular.

Objectivity?

> We all learned about objectivity in school or at our first job. Along with its twin sentries "fairness" and "balance," it defined journalistic standards. Or did it?
>
> —Brent Cunningham, *Columbia Journalism Review*

The notion of journalistic objectivity dates back only to the 1830s and has its roots in economics, not ethics. It was born of the need to sell the same story to ideologically diverse papers when the Associated Press was formed. At the same time, science was gaining currency as a basis for public policy and discourse, since it was thought to be value-neutral and uninfluenced by politics. The press aimed to emulate the scientific ideal, and to do so with the tools of objectivity, balance, and fairness. This must have seemed an achievable goal in an era before public relations was invented.

The irony of this attempt, as historian of science journalism Dorothy Nelkin points out, is that "this notion of objectivity is meaningless in the scientific community, where the values of 'fairness,' 'balance,' or 'equal time' are not relevant to the understanding of nature. On the contrary, scientific standards of objectivity require not balance but *empirical verification of opposing hypotheses.* Simply to balance sides gives readers little guidance about the scientific significance of different views."[6]

The physical concept of balance involves two forces counteracting each other, like scales balancing. But when truth is a power struggle between constituencies with unequal power and status, the scales aren't ever going to balance. They will always tilt in favor of the status quo. Furthermore, when two claims or opinions aren't equally valid, to balance them is to distort them to the unfair advantage of the claim that isn't supported by evidence, science, or logic.

If all objectivity requires is that one get both sides of a story, then the quickest, easiest way to do this is to rely on official sources—the "experts." Objectivity doesn't require that the sources, or the journalist, give *accurate* information.

The myth is that the journalist himself is free from bias: objective by virtue of his outsider status and his journalism degree. In reality, this is impossible, for all kinds of reasons. But even if it were true that someone writing for hire could be free of bias, no one who drops in on an issue briefly and then drops out to work on the next one can ever be wise enough to approximate real objectivity. A journalist can never know half as much as someone who has studied the issue for many years or who has made a lifetime commitment to it. This is especially true for a topic as complex as shock.

In the strange world of journalism, knowledge itself, especially personal experience, is suspect as bias. It's like jury selection, where those informed enough to have an opinion on the matter at hand are booted off because they can't be impartial. But there is a difference between knowledge and bias, between informed opinion and prejudice or hype, and between public relations spokespeople and real experts. In refusing to acknowledge this, and in not learning how to tell the difference, journalists often confuse ignorance with objectivity. Then, ironically, they ignore the biases anyone else can sniff out, such as the financial ties of the self-proclaimed ECT experts to the device companies.

The Tools of Bias

The tools of bias are as predictable and quantifiable in journalism as they are in medical research.

The journalistic concept of balance, unlike the commonsense version, doesn't require *equal* time or space. As one reporter put it, "As long as you don't fall into the trap of presenting just one side, you're playing ball."[7] Timing is also important, on screen and on paper. Who speaks first? Who speaks last? Whose words are left unrebutted? One of the first things they teach in journalism school is to put the least important part of your article at the end; if the article is too long, that is the part that will be cut. Similarly, what people read or hear first sets the tone for the whole article. So ECT survivors are often quoted at the end of an article or show that begins, "The new ECT is a safe and effective treatment."

The views of the less powerful would better be characterized as *ballast*. Their purpose is to weigh down the article or show so it doesn't sail off in one direction like a helium balloon; but there is never any question as to which way it wants to go.

Another less obvious tactic is what I have come to call "issue preclusion." Journalists get to decide not only who's allowed to speak, but who is allowed to speak on which issue. Why aren't the well-known shock doctors confronted with their fake statistics and misinterpretations of research? Because no one else is presumed able to speak on "the literature." Psychiatric survivors told many reporters, over a period of many years, that the one in two hundred figure the APA used as an estimate of how many persons suffer permanent amnesia was made up. That would have made a good story, if anyone believed it. But we weren't taken seriously. "Tell me why you got

ECT," the reporters would say. "Are you still depressed?" Trying to get the interview back on scientific matters is exhausting and usually unavailing. They want you for your personal experience, not your wealth of knowledge. If they want science, they'll go to a doctor.

But even when opposing doctors are featured, it is often a comparison of apples to oranges. If they are not addressing the same point, both seem to be right, and the audience must rely on subtle or not so subtle cues from the reporter as to their credibility. For instance, the words of the "anti" ECT doctor may be followed by the narrator's "But . . ." or a similar discreditor. It's not the subjects' fault that they're at cross purposes, nor can they do anything about it, because neither one is allowed to know what the other one said, or sometimes even who the other person was.

Another tool of bias that is largely undetectable to the uninformed eye is the flexible use of attribution. One perceived way to avoid responsibility for a controverted statement such as "there is no credible evidence of structural damage to the brain" is to place it in the mouth of a source with an M.D. I'd still hold any journalist responsible for knowing two simple things: that absent compelling evidence to the contrary, most people believe what doctors say, and that most people will assume the journalist printed the statement for the truth of it rather than the fact that it was said.

When the journalist puts the unverified words of an ECT proponent in her own mouth, stating as fact without quotation marks that "memory loss is temporary" or "the machines use much less electricity," the reader assumes and is meant to assume that she has done the necessary verification of that statement. When that is not the case—when she has simply taken the word of a perceived expert—the journalist has abused the trust placed in her.

In ECT journalism, the words of doctors are true and can be printed without attribution as facts, if they serve the writer's purpose, even if they mislead readers. But the words of former patients, if they see print at all, do so in quotation marks, as unsubstantiated opinions. This is standard practice in what are considered the highest echelons of journalism, though it would be unacceptable in a high school newspaper.

To give you just one example: Jennifer Hughes, a reporter for the Bergen (New Jersey) *Record*, wrote in a 2005 article that the 800 milliamps of electricity used in ECT is "about one-fifth the power you would feel if you were shocked through your wall socket."[8] Yes, the machines can put out 800 milliamps at each shock to the brain, as Hughes wrote in her article. But the claim that this amount of current is less than the brief zap you would feel through an electric socket in your house is quite misleading. It's an amount certified electricians would consider a highly dangerous—even lethal—exposure.[9] It is equal to the power you would feel if you stuck your finger in a wall socket for five seconds.

On the power of 800 milliamps of electricity, Hughes took the word of Charles Kellner, an ECT proponent who has disclosed financial ties to the device manufacturers. She also claimed to me that six other doctors from the ECT industry made the same statement about the amount of electricity used by the devices, and that she printed the statement (without comment or context) based on their word alone.

She didn't believe me when I told her the statement was false, that the shock doctors had understated the amount of electrical current used in their treatment. She wouldn't change it unless I sent her something "objective" in writing as proof. She hadn't asked Kellner, or any of the others, for any proof.

It would be absurd to say that the sameness and shoddiness of ECT reporting has to do with a sort of conspiracy or mass incompetence on journalists' part, or that all journalists are bad people. Most don't start out with the intention to lie, cause real harm, or write a bad article. Most think they are doing a good job. So what is going on?

The Middle Class Makes History

The press has the power to shape how people think about what's important, in effect to shape reality. But whose reality is being depicted?

—Brent Cunningham, *Columbia Journalism Review*

Journalists and psychiatrists share a class loyalty. They're all part of what used to be called the middle class but has been more accurately dubbed the professional-managerial class. This is because their class status depends not only on how much money they make, but on what they do and how much control and influence they have over their work and over others. Journalists and mental health professionals share the same culture and worldview, including the bedrock faith in professionalism itself by which the professional-managerial class defines and differentiates itself from the rest of the middle class.

These are the people who make the decisions and write the histories of and for the less privileged. But in speaking for others whose lives you don't understand and whose values you may not share there is the danger of error, bias, or outright deception. In the case of disenfranchised subjects like psychiatrically labeled people, journalists cannot help but be aware, as one writer put it, that "you're dealing with a population that has extremely limited resources for self-representation. They have no mechanism for holding folks accountable."[10]

With ECT, there is both opportunity and motive for purposefully distorting the truth because the interests of the speaking and the spoken-for conflict. When this happens, not only the truth of what we say, but plain facts (which would not seem to be in dispute) can be distorted.

For example, one of those standard comeback articles, published in a newspaper that is an icon of American journalism, contained the statement that of hundreds of ECT studies, none showed brain damage. Even one study showing brain damage would make her statement false. Unattributed, this statement carried all the weight of the newspaper's presumed credibility. I was, naively, flabbergasted to learn that such a respected newspaper hadn't checked basic facts. I called the reporter and asked her what had happened.

She became very upset. I'll never forget her words, which were more revealing than she probably intended. "Linda," she said, raising her voice, "do you expect me to believe that *doctors lie?*" Then she hung up.

Journalism in the Twenty-First Century

There are practical as well as philosophical constraints on the work of journalists today, none of which bode well for accurate reporting on ECT.

In March 2003, I got a call from a journalist from National Geographic television who was looking into doing a documentary on ECT. We had an initial conversation of about an hour, in which she told me something that no other journalist ever had. She told me that their rule was that before a statement could be aired—even if it were placed in the mouth of a subject and attributed to them—it had to be verified with three different sources. I had never heard of or seen journalism practiced this way in eighteen years of giving interviews.

A friend who went to journalism school in the '80s said yes, they used to teach students the three-source rule. "What killed it was CNN," she told me. When news networks went 24/7, they were desperate for stories and had to scoop everyone else, so fact-checking went by the wayside. Once this becomes standard practice, even journalists who have months to work on a piece don't feel any need to check facts.

With the explosion of news outlets, including the Internet, comes a relaxed notion of what constitutes a story. Today, the mere fact that a competitor has done a story on ECT *is* the story. Meanwhile, on the Internet, press releases of uncertain origin masquerading as news items (known as "e-spin") bombard the journalist on deadline looking for something to fill time or space. Some press releases come out looking like news on the websites of drug companies, hospitals, and universities, or accompany the publication of medical journal articles, spinning their findings; but they are no less public relations blurbs for all that. Fewer and fewer journalists see any reason not to run these items wholesale as news. They may state, "This story was adapted from a press release." They may not.

Censorship or Accountability?

At the same time that traditional ethical standards of journalism, like the practice of fact checking, are losing currency, there are fewer checks than ever on irresponsible journalism. There is no longer any official outlet for citizen complaints, no more National News Council or Fairness Doctrine. The News Council, opposed by journalism heavyweights like the *New York Times* and Walter Cronkite, ended in 1983 after only ten years. The Fairness Doctrine was eliminated during the Reagan years, in 1987, as a result of sentiment against government intervention. Discussions about whether press councils or the Fairness Doctrine should be revived invariably dead-end with the claim that any oversight body or mechanism spells the demise of "free speech." Journalists shriek that checks on their freedom to say whatever they want are just a form of censorship. Organizations of professionals spring up to fight against the threat of regulations or standards; some of these organizations offer free help to journalists threatened with libel suits.

Libel suits, they say, have a chilling effect on free speech.

This freedom of speech isn't what the framers of the Constitution had in mind.

Freedom of speech now has a new meaning, not the one it's had historically and not the one schoolchildren used to be taught in civics class. What it means now is freedom from responsibility, freedom from accountability. Freedom of the press has become immunity of the press.

To be invested with public trust and power without being held responsible: what is wrong with this picture?

Crony Journalism

This said, there is one check on the media today, and that is in the context of what I think of as relationship or crony journalism. That's when people who deal with the media regularly deliberately cultivate an ongoing, personal relationship with individual journalists in order to make sure their issues get covered the way they like.

People think news stories just happen. In reality, a lot of what's printed or seen is the end result of a two-way relationship with a journalist. This type of journalism (which I have never experienced) only happens when each needs something the other has. The reporter needs to fill his quota of marketable stories; the subject needs favorable publicity.

The seeds of these stories are planted long before they appear, with phone calls, lunches, and editorial meetings at which those who have insinuated themselves with individual journalists pitch ideas to the decision makers. The crony is never surprised by a businesslike phone call from an unknown, perhaps hostile, entity who's committed to doing a story on her topic with or without her. The crony already knows how the story is going to go, because she had a role in shaping it.

A crony relationship is unlikely to work out unless the journalist and source share a class identity and worldview. But when it does, it's more honest than other forms of journalism. There's no hidden agenda, no deception or false expectations. The relationship is not all give on the part of the subject and all take on the part of the journalist. Both parties benefit. Only the readers are duped, not realizing that the story didn't get into the paper on its merits.

Lobbyists for biological psychiatry and forced treatment (like lobbyists in other areas) are experts at crony journalism, with staff paid to cultivate the media. The media depend on them as sources on an ongoing basis, and any journalist who crossed them would risk losing access. That is the only leverage anyone has over the media these days: the knowledge that they still need you as a source and will call you again when they do.

Hit-and-Run Journalism

The type of journalism I have experienced routinely for more than two decades is far less pleasant. I call it hit-and-run journalism.

The relationship between the source and this journalist is, beneath the fake friendliness, adversarial. Journalistic ethics has nothing to say, as far as I have been able to figure out, about courtesy or responsibility to one's subjects. There is no ethical requirement that journalists be honest. They need not disclose information about their own biases that, if revealed, would negatively affect their subjects' willingness to be interviewed. For example, the reporter who became so upset at the idea of doctors lying was smart enough to realize that I had misgivings about the ability of her newspaper to cover the shock issue, given its abysmal track record. She told me, in more or less these words, "Hey, don't worry, I am no fan of doctors." She went on about a doctor who had treated her for a minor physical problem. She was not satisfied with the care he provided.

But there is a big difference between believing that a few bad apples make mistakes or provide poor care, and being willing to accept that doctors are capable of routine and deliberate lying. By any ethics deserving of the name, she had a responsibility to be as honest with me before writing the article as she was afterwards. But had she done so, she would not have gotten an interview with me.

Consider how odd it is that a total stranger asks you the most personal questions about yourself, requires you to answer every question he poses fully and truthfully (otherwise you will be suspected of hiding something), expects you to trust implicitly that he will not make any errors of fact or context when he publishes your name for thousands of people to see, and usually does not allow you to make any corrections of errors or misrepresentations either before or after publication. At the same time he will not tell you anything about his background, his motives, his opinions, whom else he has interviewed, or how he's decided to frame the story. Nor will he be responsible or accountable if his shoddy work slanders or libels you, maligns your work, or harms innocent people who make decisions on the basis of what they see and hear in the media.

This type of journalist makes himself inaccessible once the story is finished. He's driven off and takes no responsibility for the damage he's done to individuals or to the general level of public understanding of an issue. Why would he? He never intends to speak to the subject again. There's no one to hold him accountable for his actions.

Meanwhile, those who live with the issue every day, year after year, are left standing at the scene of the accident in disbelief, telling each other lamely, "If we hadn't talked with them, it would have been even worse," knowing that's not true, knowing that even if we did make their work slightly less awful, the harm that's been done to us outweighs that tiny gain.

A print article might be read by half a million people, a television broadcast seen by many millions. We know we'll be living with the fallout for a long, long time. Years of patient and unpaid work can be effectively undone by a journalist who didn't check her facts, intoned by a big name in network news.

Phil Donahue

"Hit and run" is how I'd describe what happened on the immensely popular Phil Donahue talk show in the spring of 1996. Or maybe "set up," one we couldn't have seen coming. Among the guests were an eighty-four-year-old woman who'd just had shock and her daughter. The daughter did all the talking, all about how wonderful shock was. The tiny, white-haired mother was led onto the set, sat with a frozen smile on her face and a lovely gold chain around her neck, and never said a word. Gradually the audience got suspicious.

"Let the mother talk," someone said. Applause! "No, I don't think so," said Donahue. The mother didn't even have a mike on.

"Can't she talk?" someone shouted again.

"Of course she can talk," said the daughter. "Mom, stand up." The old woman didn't appear to understand, didn't respond when her daughter tugged her arm.

"Look at that smile!" said Donahue. "Do you know we're talking about you?"

"Let's leave my mother alone. She's eighty-four years old."

Later on the same show, shock survivor Diann'a Loper appeared for "the other side." Loper lost many years of her life and her memories of her child's life due to ECT. The ECT also caused her to suffer spontaneous epileptic seizures at least once a day, which can be only poorly controlled with anti-epilepsy drugs. She's suffered permanent brain damage, and, understandably, she feels shock should be banned. She made her case to Donahue with passion and grace.

Richard Weiner added some showmanship to the standard APA PR line, telling viewers, "The type of electricity that's now used with ECT is modeled on the type of energy that is used within the brain itself . . . it's a more natural type of electricity that is now used," then answered "no" when asked if he was a consultant to the shock machine companies.

This farce was unmasked only after the lights had gone down and the audience had left. Backstage, the mother was no longer smiling and looked confused and anxious. Now, she seemed to be saying something I couldn't hear. But I heard her daughter repeating patiently, over and over, as if to a small child: "We're in New York, Mom. We just did the Phil Donahue show. We're going home now. We're in New York."

Meanwhile, Loper was in the next room rolling on the floor, quietly having a seizure.

20/20 Redux

In February 2001, I got a call from a man named Joel Bernstein, who introduced himself as a producer for CBS News's *60 Minutes II*. Would I be interested in talking to him? They were doing a show on ECT.

For my own safety, I tried to feel him out, but he would reveal nothing. How did he get interested in this topic? He was, he said, just intellectually curious about it. I could not get him to reveal anything about himself.

I didn't want to be on *60 Minutes II*, but I was morbidly curious to see if there was anything I might do this time to prevent the show from being a total train wreck. As a condition of meeting and talking with Bernstein, I got him to agree that if I were on the show, I would be asked the same questions as the pro-ECT spokesman, who predictably was Harold Sackeim. I would appear as an expert on ECT, not a mental patient.

We met at a place of his choosing, a downscale pub, where he bought me lunch and told me he wanted to do a program on the comeback of ECT. Patiently, I explained to him that this show had been done dozens of times, and that there was no comeback in actual fact. I tried to interest him in other angles, like the FDA classification issue, but I could see he had no interest. He wanted to do comeback. I said, "How can something be making a comeback for fifteen years?" and he did get the point, but it didn't seem to matter.

My impression of him was that he wasn't receptive to what I had to say. He had agreed to interview me on my terms, and we even made a date for the interview, but then he told me "other people" wouldn't allow it.

He was also speaking to a colleague of mine named Juli Lawrence, an ECT researcher, survivor, and proprietress of the popular Web site www.ect.org. We both sent him, and he accepted, a list of questions for Sackeim. They were the type of tough questions any investigative journalist ought to love.

Joel Bernstein was not that person. He didn't use any of the questions. The show followed the APA's PR script to the letter. The hook was, "The procedure that was considered barbaric has made a significant comeback and is now given to more than 100,000 Americans a year." Deadline pressure can't explain why Bernstein didn't check this claim with three sources, or even one source; he had months to put the show together.

The segment included clips from *Cuckoo's Nest* (twice). It featured one of Sackeim's patients, and Sackeim himself on camera for much of the show. Peter Breggin spoke, sandwiched between Sackeim clips, for a total of fifty seconds. In a thirteen-minute segment, this was ballast, not balance.

It was *20/20*, that nightmare from 1985, all over again, with the same players. Breggin was allowed to say only that he believed shock should be banned (followed by a disclaimer that "most psychiatrists" find him "old-fashioned"), while Sackeim was allowed to address the questions of memory loss and brain damage with sweeping denials that sounded scientific but weren't based on science. "Most patients" believe the memory loss is a small price to pay, he claimed, and those who experienced devastating memory loss are "extremely rare." These lines are straight out of the APA Task Force Report, where they aren't footnoted to any studies or evidence, because there isn't any.

Four people who had had ECT were interviewed. Those who had positive things to say about it got three and a half minutes of air time. Diann'a Loper played the role I'd played in 1985, the token "unhappy" patient, with ninety seconds to tell of her brain damage and amnesia. Her words were followed by the mandatory "but" and a rebuttal by Sackeim.

The only difference between the 2001 debacle and the 1985 show was that I'd now had sixteen years of direct personal experience working to educate the public about the nature and risks of ECT. I knew how many others had worked even longer and harder than I had. But all our efforts had failed, if you judge by what the public is still being told about shock.

Like the overwhelming majority of journalists I have known, Joel Bernstein took on a completely different personality after his piece was done. The facade of professionalism was gone, replaced by hostility and contempt. In a tone of voice I had never heard before, he said he didn't want to talk to me. I was, he said, paranoid and irrational. I had wasted his time. When I asked him why he hadn't told his viewers of Sackeim's financial conflicts, he replied that he didn't think it was important, that it didn't belong in his piece, and that he didn't have enough time to include it.

Only then did Bernstein admit he had withheld information from me about his own standpoint. He had done the show on the suggestion of a personal friend of his, a psychiatrist. By definition, he'd be seeing this friend again; it was important that the show meet with the friend's approval, as I'm sure it did. Who was I? Someone whose opinion didn't matter, someone he never expected to hear from again; just someone who lived this issue every day, every year.

CBS set up an Internet forum where people could discuss the show. When someone posted that Sackeim worked for the shock machine companies and that CBS knew this and did not disclose it, there was general disbelief. *60 Minutes II* enjoyed such a reputation for quality journalism that people felt betrayed by its failure to tell the whole story. Clearly, viewers did not share Bernstein's stated opinion that Sackeim's finances were not important.

The Atlantic Monthly

The single worst piece of journalism I have ever read or had the bad fortune to be associated with appeared in February 2001, in one of the universally revered icons of the American media, the *Atlantic Monthly*. As with the *New York Times*, the more public trust a media outlet enjoys, the more a reporter is free to abuse that trust with complete immunity.

A young reporter named Daniel Smith, writing his first feature for the magazine, took full advantage of that immunity. I agreed to an interview with him on one condition: that Smith himself agree to be interviewed by me, after publication, about the process of writing the article. I hoped in this way to gain some insight into why ECT articles end up the way they do, and thus to keep our interaction from being a total loss should the article turn out badly.

Even the way Smith dressed for our interview was designed to reveal nothing about himself: I recall him wearing the plainest of button-down shirts and pants. He didn't answer any of my questions as to who he was or why he wanted to write this article. We spoke for three hours, and he taped the interview.

More than a year later, I got a call from the magazine's fact checker. His questions, and the proposed wording of the statements he read off, truly alarmed me and were my first hint that something was seriously wrong. First of all, though I'd discussed this at length with Smith and given it to him in writing as well, he had gotten the mission statement of the Committee for Truth in Psychiatry wrong. Our mission is not hard to understand. We do one thing and one thing only: advocate for truthfully informed consent to ECT. The fact checker clearly wanted to print that CTIP wants to ban ECT. "No," I said, "you can't say that because it's not true."

There were other factual matters that Smith had gotten wrong, and I corrected each of them with the fact checker. Smith had written that I told him I was committed to a mental hospital several times. Although I was coerced and held against my will, I have never been committed. Smith also wrote that I showed Harold Sackeim my medical records. That was not true. Then there was the matter of my participation in what he termed psychiatric conferences, which I took to mean conferences of psychiatrists, like the American Psychiatric Association's annual meeting. Was it correct to write that I was "hardly ever afforded time to speak?" That wording struck me as very strange and confusing, since it implied that I should have been "afforded time to speak," which is not the case for anyone who attends these events. I couldn't shake his determination to keep that exact wording. He got me to admit that, while misleading, it was not technically false. I couldn't understand why this small point was so important to him.

My last words to the fact checker on the phone were: "It's very important you get this right."

It was gut wrenching to get the phone call from a friend that morning in January 2001. She was the first to see the article and wanted to warn me it was as bad as it gets.

The most salient fact about the Committee for Truth in Psychiatry, that all members had experienced permanent memory loss without having been informed that this was possible, was left out of the article, so that the reader was led to believe that the organization was a bunch of "fanatics" (the *Atlantic*'s word) who just wanted to ban ECT out of hatred for psychiatry.

But it was worse than that.

Smith had carefully concealed from me that one-third of the article was to be about Scientology. Had he asked me, I would have told him that CTIP has nothing to do with Scientology. It's true that Scientology is opposed to psychiatry on principle, including ECT. What is not accurate, what is deliberately and calculatedly false, is lumping CTIP together with Scientology and Peter Breggin as "an unlikely trio of activist groups" who are trying "to ban the procedure outright": "These groups have agitated for the complete elimination of ECT. They have pushed legislative attempts to limit or ban ECT. They have initiated and supported lawsuits against psychiatrists, hospitals, and ECT device manufacturers. They claim that ECT is authoritarian, violent, and representative of everything that is wrong with the profession of psychiatry."[11]

While this is true of Scientology, it is not true of CTIP, and Smith knew this. Later, in the letters column, Smith would claim: "Nothing in the section of my article concerning CTIP states that CTIP's mission is to abolish electroconvulsive therapy or that the organization files lawsuits. . . . Andre may have taken this to mean that every group is engaged in all the activities."[12] But only two groups were mentioned in the article, CTIP and Scientology, so any reader would have necessarily taken "groups" to mean both of us.

All of the other facts the magazine had been informed were false were printed. The context in which the fake facts appeared made it sickeningly clear why Smith wanted to print them. They were necessary to the central thesis of the article. Boiled down from eight thousand words, the theme is this: shock is safe. Therefore, all opposition to it is irrational. Critics can be lumped together and dismissed as beyond the fringe in one way or another.

Thus, the false claims that I had been committed and "re-committed" served to depict me as dangerously crazy. The false claim that I showed Sackeim my medical records lent credibility to Sackeim's conjecture that a "psychotic break," not ECT, caused my amnesia and loss of IQ. That strangely worded sentence about not being "afforded time to speak" was followed by, "More often, she simply rises from the crowd," which made me look disruptive as well as dangerous. (I had told the fact checker that I rose from the crowd only in the sense of getting up and walking to the microphone during the official question-and-answer period following a lecture.)

Missing from Smith's article, which opined that "there is no way to know for sure whether ECT was the culprit in Andre's loss of IQ and memory," was the fact that he knew that there was such a way—neuropsychological testing—and that the doctors who evaluated me attributed my brain damage to ECT. But facts and science could only trip up Smith's argument, which, insofar as it focused exclusively on ascribing motives to its characters (independent of the characters' own stated motives), was not and didn't even pretend to be a scientific argument, but a moral one.

Because there had been a tape, because there had been fact-checking calls, at first I thought I might have some recourse. As my phone calls and a long letter to the magazine's editor-in-chief Michael Kelly went unanswered, I began to understand: it was precisely because of, not despite, the power of the *Atlantic* that Smith could get away with such blatant misconduct, and that the editor could back him up. When I tried to reach Kelly by phone, his secretary hung up on me. That wouldn't have happened if they hadn't been sure no one would believe me.

The magazine's statements about CTIP and me, in particular the part about being committed several times, seemed to me to be textbook examples of libel. I went looking for legal advice, and discovered that while it is easy to find lawyers and even organizations to represent defendants (the media) in libel actions, lawyers who will represent plaintiffs keep a lower profile than those who defend drunk drivers and murderers. There seems to be a great stigma attached to even legitimate libel lawsuits because the media have been successful in depicting them as, by definition, attacks on the First Amendment. Because of the power and wealth of the media, it is almost impossible to win such a lawsuit, and nobody will take one on contingency. The lawyers I consulted believed I had a case and agreed to represent me— for a $20,000 retainer. Then it would cost tens or even hundreds of thousands before it was over.

Nothing before or since has so vividly or painfully brought home to me that "free speech" in America means simply that those with money and power get to say what they want to, while those without are silenced.

So there was no lawsuit against the *Atlantic*, and there were no retractions, and no consequences for Smith or the magazine. Readers shocked and outraged at Smith's tactics posted more than eighty responses on the magazine's Web site. Only a few comments were in his favor.

After stringing me along for months, Smith reneged on his promise to let me interview him.

14   *Erasing History*

Besides the media, the public generally gets its opinions about shock and other treatments for mental illness from official sources, trusted authorities like the federal Center for Mental Health Services, the National Institute of Mental Health, the Surgeon General, and state departments of mental health. All of these have taken positions on ECT during the PR era. If you've heard or read anything of what these authorities say about ECT, it's likely to have been dumbed down to the size of a sound bite reassuring you that shock is safe. Virtually no one reads the original reports, but even if you had, you would be getting less than half of the story.

You just have no idea what could have been, or almost was. And the reasons for "almost" are as stereotypical as a tabloid's headline about a psycho killer. They have nothing to do with facts or science and everything to do with who has the power to enforce a particular version of the truth. Make no mistake, whenever a government entity takes on ECT (or any other topic, such as the effects of psychiatric drugs on suicides), these are hotly contested *political* statements, and the process by which they are developed is a political power struggle. Different constituencies fight for input, and the playing field is not level.

In order to show how this plays out in real life, I have chosen three recent stories from the front lines. In each case I was directly involved in the years-long process of trying to shape the final documents: the "Background Paper on Electroconvulsive Therapy" put out by the federal Center for Mental Health Services, an agency of the Department of Health and Human Services, in 1998; the U.S. Surgeon General's Report on Mental Health released in 1999; and the state of Vermont's official informed consent form adopted in 2000.

In the beginning of this book I talked about the ways in which mental patients are seen as less than human and deprived of fundamental rights in daily life. That type of attitude does not disappear when we show up at the courthouse, the statehouse, or at a place like the Carter Center, which hosted a meeting to promote the Surgeon General's Report on mental health in 1999.

I vividly remember a lunchtime conversation with a bureaucrat from the Center for Mental Health Services (CMHS), where she was working on the center's position paper on ECT. I tried to explain to her that shock can permanently impair a person's ability to work. I thought she might care about the economic consequences of shock, even if she didn't care about mental patients.

Her response: "But *those* people would never be able to work anyway."

These types of stereotyped *attitudes* of exclusion are played out in stereotyped *mechanisms* of exclusion. These are not specific to psychiatric survivors but are used successfully with other disenfranchised or dissident groups. First, the group or person is structurally excluded from participation by formal or informal rules. For example, a person can be excluded because "only" doctors, certified experts, or state residents are allowed to participate. These rules may or may not actually exist, but as long as someone with authority says they do, the person is usually dissuaded from challenging them.

Second, the group or person may be procedurally excluded. Information or access is withheld in an informal manner that seems careless or accidental, and thus difficult to challenge, but usually is not. For example, letters and phone calls from the excluded persons are simply ignored (for years on end if necessary), and no details are revealed about the process that could allow them to figure out how to get involved. Procedural exclusion can also mean giving the appearance of meaningful involvement to some groups—allowing them to speak at meetings—but disregarding their input. It also encompasses tokenism, when an organization or government agency selects one person who is nominally a member of the excluded group but who is or can be convinced that it is in his or her own best personal interest to go along with what the government wants to do rather than what the group wants.

It is important to note that it is not really necessary to *do anything* for structural and procedural exclusion of a powerless group like ECT survivors to occur, nor does it necessarily involve malice or bad faith on the part of any of the actors involved. The most powerful mechanism of exclusion is simple: the status quo. Survivors have always been excluded from a voice in research or policy, while industry spokesmen have always (at least for the thirty years I am calling the PR era) made research and policy.

What I am really talking about in this chapter is how social change occurs. Much of what I will describe is applicable to all struggles for social change; some is specific to the shock issue. ECT is unique in that it is hard to think of another public debate where the money, power, and influence of one group so exceeds that of the other. No two groups seem more unequal than psychiatrists and former ECT patients.

But change is not impossible. Sometimes, stronger friends and allies help out; sometimes, just plain luck or quirk of individual personality makes all the difference.

The Center for Mental Health Services' Report on ECT

In March 1998, the federal Center for Mental Health Services published what it called a "Background Paper on Electroconvulsive Therapy." It had been commissioned because of the media uproar over the threatened forced shock of eighty-year-old Lucille Austwick in 1993. Austwick, a resident of a Chicago nursing home who suffered from dementia and was labeled depressed, had adamantly refused her doctors' recommendation for ECT. So had her state-appointed guardian, yet her doctors sought a court order to force it on her. After national news outlets reported on the case, the doctors backed down, claiming Austwick no longer needed shock. An Illinois appellate court went on to decide the case anyway, given its importance, and ruled against the psychiatrists. Patients' rights advocates demanded a response from the federal government: What was its position on involuntary ECT? After all, Medicare and Medicaid pay for it.

For four years the Committee for Truth in Psychiatry had tried to convince the Center to allow us to have input into the paper, which was to include interviews with "organizations with particular interest in ECT." They refused. (Marilyn Rice had passed away in 1992, so I was now the informal director of the group, and coordinated the campaign for inclusion in the CMHS report.) After three years of not returning our calls or answering our letters, director Bernie Arons finally allowed me to be interviewed. But in the end the entire interview was censored, and CTIP wasn't included as an interested organization. The material the government had decided was too hot to publish went into our newsletter, *Shockwaves*.

The newsletter prompted an editorial response from a Mental Health Association advocate: "What is it about our system which cannot seem to tolerate dissent?"[1] What indeed, when CMHS's official position is that decisions about mental health policies and services should be made with input from those of us with psychiatric labels? Arons never gave us a straight answer as to why he censored the input of shock survivors, but he said that it was done at the insistence of NIMH, which has the ultimate say over federal mental health policy.

As Arons and his staff reminded me in heavy-handed kiss-off letters at the end of our four-year battle, federal agencies are accountable only to their parent agencies, and ultimately only to Congress: "Individual citizens and private organizations do not formulate Federal Government policy. Federal policies are based upon Federal laws and court interpretations of Federal laws. However, Federal agencies are ultimately accountable to the public for implementation decisions, policies, and practices. Individuals can lobby the Congress to change laws and policies and disseminate critical assessments of both, but the Federal Government speaks for the overall will of the people, and does not allow private interests to speak in its name."[2]

But the distinction between public and private interests is not as clearcut as Arons would have us believe. Government officials, politically appointed, move fluidly from the private sector to the public sector or between related public posts; this is the interlocking directorate described in Chapter Thirteen. Often those serving as regulators of an industry just came from, or are about to go back to, a highly paid position in the same industry. Sometimes they leave a government post and are hired back as a consultant. Or they might hop from a position at a nonprofit to a government gig.[3]

People don't change their views and values as they switch jobs. This is why people who move between the public and private sectors—for example, an FDA drug evaluator who leaves the agency for a position at a pharmaceutical company—are best described as "gatekeepers of corporate interest within public institutions."[4]

Marilyn Rice would have had the most succinct answer to the question about why the mental health system can't tolerate dissent. She always used to say, "No one's bread is buttered on the side of exposing the truth about ECT."

In the end, without acknowledging the existence or input of a national organization of former patients who'd experienced permanent amnesia, the CMHS report could only say, "The issues regarding brain damage and memory loss have not yet been fully explored or understood."

The Surgeon General's New Clothes

On December 13, 1999, the U.S. Department of Health and Human Services released "Mental Health: A Report of the Surgeon General."

Five years later, an Internet search for that title returned about 18,400 hits. You've never heard of it? Then the plan failed. Surgeon General David Satcher and his team had aspired to nothing less than to reach every home in the U.S. with its chosen message: *Seek help if you have a mental health problem.* The help they wanted to sell you included ECT.

The PR person behind this ambitious late-century attempt to sell mental health treatment was Celinda Lake, who was simultaneously orchestrating the Gore 2000 campaign. She extensively test-marketed the predetermined messages of the report, like "Mental illnesses are a set of diseases like physical illnesses" and "Half of the people in any given room are affected by mental illness." Polls showed that most people already believed most of the messages. They were, however, ambivalent about the message that "effective treatments exist for most mental illnesses," so that became the theme the report really hammered home. The weapon of choice was "science": not actual science, but the repeated use of the word.

> Q: How can we make sure the Report is not *perceived as* a Gore 2000 election tool but is, in fact, *received as* a science-based, evidence-based look at mental illness and mental health? [Emphasis added]
> A: From our research, I do not think that will be a significant problem. No one we surveyed or talked to in focus groups, for example, doubted that one in five people were affected by mental illnesses, or that 50 percent of the people or their families could have an

experience with mental illness, or that mental illness was a major problem in our country.

—Question by Bill Emmet of NAMI to Celinda Lake[5]

Science, then, wasn't necessary to sell the public on the illness metaphor for troubled and troubling behavior; the challenge was to sell the perceived solutions—drugs, shock, and therapy—as science based. And the biggest challenge would be selling shock, where there was no science supporting the industry's claims.

Networking over the Internet, mental patients and survivors of psychiatry first became widely aware that the Surgeon General's Report was in the works in 1997. Shock survivors knew it would have to include a section on ECT. The report was being developed by CMHS (along with NIMH, though we didn't know that until later). We began contacting them, asking to be involved. But just as with the Background Paper on ECT, emails, letters, and phone calls were simply ignored. We wrote to our congresspeople and to the report's managing editor and senior scientific editor. To the extent that we got any response, it was this: "If we included ECT survivors in the report, we'd have to include *everyone* . . . we'd have to include *Holocaust survivors* too!"

Eight or ten mental patients had been carefully chosen by CMHS to work on a selected part of the Surgeon General's Report—the part about the consumer movement—but this was not inclusion; it was tokenism. CMHS seemed confident that those few people could be trusted to keep their mouths shut and do as they were told, and not to let the rest of us in on what was going on.

They miscalculated by one.

Joseph Rogers was the original conservative mental patient, or consumer. His organization, the National Mental Health Consumers' Self-Help Clearinghouse in Philadelphia (originally the National Mental Health Consumers' Association), was the first mental patient group to take money from the government and has been continuously funded since 1986. Rogers was slated to be one of the senior reviewers of the report, and so was able to see a draft of the ECT section. Outraged, he leaked the four paragraphs to the public. Thanks to the advocacy community and to Rogers's ability to generate media coverage, a firestorm broke out.

"Federal report praising electroshock stirs uproar," wrote the *New York Times*. The story was also picked up by Reuters, *The British Medical Journal*, and other general and mental health media.[6]

The draft called ECT "safe and effective" twice. In a report that repeatedly claimed to be based on cutting-edge neuroscience, not a single scientific research study was cited in support of that or any other claim. For instance, the assertion that research showed that ECT does not cause brain damage was backed up by a survey of the use of shock in the elderly. Mostly, the report referenced Weiner's review article and a textbook chapter written by Sackeim and psychiatrist Matthew Rudorfer. Rudorfer is a key member of the ECT fraternity, administering and overseeing grant money at NIMH. He is the "scientific officer" assigned by NIMH to address scientific concerns about Sackeim's long-standing research grant. We knew him for his authorship of several pro-shock puff pieces.[7] Not surprisingly, we soon found out that the section of the report in which ECT was discussed, the chapter on "Adults and Mental Health," had been edited by Rudorfer.

Basically, it followed the standard PR line: "Decades ago, patients underwent ECT without anesthesia ... those now antiquated procedures contributed to the negative portrayal of ECT in the popular media. . . . Its use declined until the 1980s, when use began to increase amid growing awareness of its benefits. . . . Adverse cognitive effects of ECT have been reduced by modern advances in treatment technique, including oxygenation, reduction in the electrical dose by the use of brief pulse stimulation, and unilateral electrode placement." This was followed by the standard denials of brain damage, permanent memory loss, and cognitive deficits.

Rogers put this all in context, publicly saying that Richard Nakamura, the NIMH deputy director in charge of the ECT section, was "very pro-electroconvulsive therapy, and I think he is looking for the Surgeon General's Report to give better legitimacy to electroconvulsive therapy and a clearer and more definitive statement on electroconvulsive therapy."[8] He likened the response of the Surgeon General's spokesman to the media exposure to "what it's like when you turn on the light in a room full of cockroaches and they scurry for cover."[9]

As a result of the overwhelmingly negative publicity, as well as all the creative ways people across the country had expressed their displeasure with the Surgeon General (such as sending him the snipped-off plug ends of electrical cords with the message "Pull the Plug on ECT!"), Joseph Rogers was able to put pressure on NIMH. Nakamura and Rudorfer agreed to meet with Joseph's co-worker Susan Rogers, myself, and a representative of the National Mental Health Association (NMHA). Since Ms. Rogers and I were both conversant with the scientific literature on ECT, we bombarded Nakamura with references that had been left out of the report. We challenged them to provide one single scientific study to support their claim that ECT is "safe." They could not, yet at the same time told us that the wording of the report was "non-negotiable."

I left the meeting knowing I'd impressed Nakamura, yet sure that it wouldn't make any difference. Meanwhile, I continued my phone calls to the psychiatrist who was the report's senior scientific editor. I'd been calling for several months, but he never answered the phone or returned my calls. Having an assistant or an answering machine is the simplest yet most effective method of exclusion ever devised. In his case it was the latter, and it let me speak at length.

There came a day, though, when he accidentally answered his phone. The call was brief. As soon as he heard who was calling, he started talking over me loudly: "Your organization does not have credibility as scientists!" I would have liked to continue the conversation, but he hung up.

What he didn't understand was that we weren't the only ones outraged by the government-approved exclusion of survivors and critics of ECT. The industry PR line that all criticism of ECT comes from Scientologists and antipsychiatrists was about to be resoundingly debunked, as the mainstream rallied against the report.

Surgeon General David Satcher wrote on his Web site at the time: "I would most like to be remembered as the Surgeon General who listened to the American people and responded to what they said. I encourage all of you to write to me."[10] And we did. Even the tokens—those conservative former patients appointed by the Surgeon General, most of whom held respected positions in nonprofit or government agencies—wrote to him expressing a unified position on ECT: "We believe the Report should include all the research on this controversial issue including that which indicates serious side effects."[11]

At Alternatives '99, an annual conference for current and ex-patients and advocates funded by CMHS, over 300 people signed a petition calling on the Surgeon General to work with the Committee for Truth in Psychiatry to develop a statement accurately reflecting the risks of ECT.

Thanks to the efforts of Joseph and Susan Rogers, four major national organizations of impeccable credibility (National Association of Protection and Advocacy Systems, National Mental Health Association, International Association of Psychosocial Rehabilitation Services, and the Clearinghouse) joined forces to express "serious concerns" about ECT in a two-page letter to the Surgeon General. The letter cited research studies documenting the risks of death and memory loss, and asked that the report be revised to include more research than a few references to Richard Weiner.

There was never any response.

Though we were told, indirectly, that the ECT section had been revised, we were not allowed to see it and we feared the worst. There was one last opportunity to make our voices heard in a very public way.

The "Rollout" Circus

A two-day "Rollout Meeting" for the Surgeon General's Report was scheduled at the Carter Center in Atlanta on November 17 and 18. Former first lady Rosalynn Carter would host and call it her annual Symposium on Mental Health Policy. Susan Rogers had been invited and somehow wangled an invitation for me. We both wrote letters to Carter explaining the ECT situation, and Rogers asked to be given time on the formal program to present to the audience. She planned to hand the Surgeon General the three hundred-signature petition asking him to work with CTIP. And we would try to make sure every participant got a copy of the Clearinghouse's letter asking for their help in assuring that the report "is accurate and meets recognized standards of scientific objectivity."

On the first day of the meeting, we set up the copies on a table, and also began handing them out to participants as they walked in. It wasn't long before Lei Ellingson, assistant director at the Carter Center, told us, "You can't hand those out here." Rogers stood her ground. Ellingson said that if we continued to distribute our material on private property we would be removed. We were free to hand out anything we wanted out on the highway—a long distance away. The message was clear: no criticism of shock treatment was allowed at the Carter Center.

To this meeting were invited all manner of mental health workers from psychiatrists to psychosocial rehabilitation practitioners; benefits managers; hospital administrators; epidemiologists; alcoholism and drug abuse counselors; policy fellows; lawyers; chaplains; sociologists; mental health commissioners; industry bureaucrats and lobbyists . . . in short, everyone who makes money off mental patients, but very few of us.

For that reason, I suppose, everyone but us was willing to sign up to promote the Surgeon General's Report without having read it. We were put in small groups to brainstorm promotional strategies. It was like an organizing meeting for a political election campaign; do volunteers sit around arguing over whether they agree with everything their candidate says, or do they concentrate on getting her elected? The actual report wouldn't be released for another month. All we were getting were campaign slogans, repeated over and over: Mental illnesses are real. Treatment works. More people needed to be treated. And the most jarring slogan of all, from the keynote speech by Deputy Surgeon General Kenneth Moritsugu: "Science is truth!"

But real science doesn't need a rollout meeting.

Her request for time on the program denied, Rogers stood up during the public comment period and read the letter the Carter Center had tried to censor. And then she added: "When Dr. Moritsugu referenced 'the best science, the best available science, and solid science,' he could not have been including ECT for it constitutes bad science. It is not 'safe and effective,' as the report has said. . . . Part of our problem with the report was process. If people with psychiatric disabilities had been involved from the beginning in a representative and adequate way, I do not think we would be seeing the problem with the section on ECT."[12]

But we were overruled by psychiatrist Leon Eisenberg of the Carter Center, although his words unwittingly reinforced our key point: "We must not get stuck arguing over the details, rather than recognizing the opportunity to have a national policy enunciated on behalf of a group that has been left out and is still being left out."[13]

On the shuttle bus to our catered dinner, I found myself quite accidentally sitting next to Dr. Nakamura. He was cordial enough, making small talk about his family while I listened politely. But he was still worrying at what I'd said at our meeting. "You said you had memory loss?" he began.

"Yes, about five years. . . ."

"Now, think back to that time. What happened to you? Did you fall off a ladder? Are you sure you didn't trip and bang your head? Maybe you had a boyfriend who hit you . . . try to remember."[14]

I felt a slow burn of horror. Just as he would never have expected me to say, "Are you sure you have two children? Maybe it was only one," I would never have expected another human being—much less a scientist—to question my authority over my own life. *You are lying*, yes, I might have expected that. *You are crazy*, shorthand for the same thing, sure. But *You do not know what happened in your own life?* And to try to tell me, based on nothing but his own beliefs about ECT, some story about what must have really happened?

Instead of trying to understand and learn from what happened to me, putting it together with information from other sources to see if he could draw some conclusions, Nakamura was attempting, like a defense lawyer in a malpractice case, to punch holes in it. That, he obviously thought, was what science was about. It was nothing but the old (and very male) doubting game. Nakamura was looking for a reason, any reason, to support what he already believed: that ECT can't cause permanent amnesia. It was my job to prove to his satisfaction that nothing else in the world could have damaged my brain, not his job to investigate whether ECT had done it.

Had this definition of science been applied to other areas of medicine, we'd never even have gotten to the point where one previous Surgeon General had been able to prove that smoking causes lung cancer. This future director of NIMH—and everyone behind the report—seemed to me to have his own definition of science: What we who call ourselves scientists want it to be.

"The Best Available Science"

We got the news on the morning of December 13. I cried, remembering how hard Marilyn Rice had worked to inform people about the risks of shock, thinking I'd somehow let her down. I wondered what it was that we could have done that we hadn't, while Susan Rogers tried to convince me it was really OK, because the report no longer used the specific phrase "safe and effective."

But the safety claim had snuck back in: "ECT may be the safest treatment option for severe depression." (The reference for this was the textbook chapter by Sackeim and Rudorfer.) The new version had been expanded from four paragraphs to ten, with seventeen sources instead of five, but the reliance on biased and financially conflicted industry sources hadn't changed. There was now only one cite to Richard Weiner, but there were *fourteen* references to Harold Sackeim. Rudorfer cited himself twelve times, and they were all to the same two sources: the textbook chapter he wrote with Sackeim, and the editorial praising shock he wrote to accompany Sackeim's article. Here it was: the "best available science" the Surgeon General of the United States could come up with.

The section telling people ECT can't cause brain damage had been expanded with more references. But they weren't to "decades of methodologically sound studies," as the reader was led to believe; they were to Sackeim's and Weiner's reviews, to the NIMH Consensus Conference, and even to the CMHS report from which survivor input had been censored. The report now endorsed "maintenance" shock (that is, giving persons shock once a week to once a month on an ongoing basis).

The section on cognitive deficits had been made worse with the unsupported claim that "most patients return to full functioning." Previously, there had only been the claim that adverse effects had been reduced compared to the old shock. And readers were also assured that severe memory loss was "clearly the exception," though no one tried to back this up with even a fraudulent reference.

The claim that ECT now uses "one-third the electricity" hadn't been corrected, though Nakamura had been given the references to do so. The neuropsychological test results, the amnesia studies of Squire and Janis, all the other studies—it was as if they hadn't existed.

The day the report came out, Joseph Rogers issued a press release, titled "Surgeon General's Relative Caution on Shock Treatment a Victory for Advocacy Movement." I thought I understood. There was no longer any chance of a good outcome, so he might as well make the best of a bad one. To criticize the report further would be futile in the light of the onrushing tidal wave of preplanned positive PR.

In the end, all our efforts vanished. We worked ourselves silly, while the status quo simply stood pat. Denied, ignored, delayed, excluded. Today the Surgeon General's Report is just another footnote (along with the NIMH Consensus Conference Report and the CMHS report) appended to the statement that "ECT is a safe treatment."

A Trip to Vermont by Way of Texas

Vermont has a long and proud tradition of mental patient activism. Bills to ban shock have been introduced with regularity, as recently as 1985 and 1990. In the mid-1990s Vermont Protection and Advocacy (P&A) seriously looked into the feasibility of banning shock. Proposed legislation would have given patients deemed competent the absolute right to refuse shock, and prohibited it entirely for incompetent patients unless they had previously signed a power of attorney giving consent. At the least, some Vermont advocates wanted a ban for children under sixteen, a step already taken by several other states.

By the 1999–2000 legislative season, it was looking good for some kind of shock legislation; the only question was, what kind.

Advocates were encouraged and inspired by what had happened in Texas in the 1990s; the shock industry must have dreaded a replay. There, legislation to ban shock completely had not only been introduced but had come close to passing. In the end, the state not only passed a law requiring that statistics be kept, but banned shock for minors and beefed up the statewide consent forms to warn patients of "the possibility of permanent irrevocable memory loss." And five years after the original reporting law was passed, the state looked at the statistics on death rates, which were about one in two hundred for elderly people, and amended the consent form to remove the word "remote" before "possibility of death" in the consent form.

A major force behind this move was two shock survivors, Doug Cameron and Diann'a Loper. Cameron, as we saw in Chapter Six, was able to debunk the industry's claims of "less electricity" using mathematical formulas.

Even after ECT caused her to suffer daily epileptic seizures, Loper was a successful and highly paid lobbyist, and she put her skills and contacts to impressive use to ban shock. A shock survivor of great credibility and eloquence had direct and frequent access to legislators and was able to convince many of them to do what she wanted.[15]

That scenario had been a nightmare for the industry, and it was about to happen for the second time in five years with Anne Donahue.

Donahue comes from a wealthy and established family in Vermont, and prior to her shock treatment, had practiced law. In 1995 and 1996, when she was around forty years old, she received two courses of ECT, thirty-three sessions in all, for severe, recurrent depression. Though the shocks relieved her symptoms temporarily, she was left with devastating memory losses going back nine years. "While the more distant incidents may be random events, they are hardly insignificant ones: hosting and driving Mother Theresa for a full day visit to Los Angeles in 1989; the dinner reception for my National Jefferson Award in Washington, DC, in 1990, where I met and sat beside my co-honoree, General Colin Powell; my brother's wedding in 1991—the list goes on, and keeps growing as people bring up references to the past in casual conversations."[16]

She had extensive neuropsychological testing done, just as I had, with the same results: permanent and significant cognitive deficits and a thirty-three point reduction in IQ. The industry might have created another Marilyn Rice, I thought, another highly educated, well-spoken, dedicated crusader against fraud and deceit, someone who could talk back to it in its own language.

I was particularly impressed with the draft of an article she had written and sent to me around 1997. It described the nature and extent of ECT amnesia and its effects on her life in great clarity and detail, making points I'd never seen in print before—like how we tend to underestimate the extent of our amnesia because you can't know something is missing from your memory until someone else tells you about it or you accidentally discover it. And a lot of other good points like that, plain as salt to me but eye-opening to people who haven't been shocked.

And heresy to shock doctors. I said to her at that time: "If this article ever gets published, I will eat it." I meant it.

Donahue described her article as "the beginning of my battle to push for informed consent protections," and she was serious about publishing it. She sent a copy to Harold Sackeim and he took notice. He even invited her to meet with him and, I imagine, sized her up the way he had me in 1990— damage control, a routine part of his job. I'd come up short, a flea to be brushed away, but Donahue did not. She was not only a lawyer, but a player in mental patient politics; she edited a statewide newspaper for mental patients and was the board president of Vermont P&A. Anyone meeting her would be struck by what some would call confidence and others, arrogance. It seemed likely she'd get her paper published somewhere with or without Sackeim. In short, Donahue was a force Sackeim couldn't dismiss.

He promised her he'd publish her article, as long as she made some revisions that would make it more suitable for the *Journal of ECT*. He kept her on this hook from 1997 until June 2000, when the article was published. (It arrived in my mailbox accompanied by a knife and fork and some salt, which made it quite tasty going down.)

Even edited, it still packed a punch. "My long-term memory deficits far exceed anything my doctors anticipated, I was advised about, or that are validated by research. To the contrary, either I am one in a thousand, a complete anomaly, to be able to document memory loss still remaining after 3 years and extending as far back as incidences eight to nine years ago, or the profession in general, after all these years of ECT, has still failed to identify and come to grips with the true potential risks."[17]

Donahue wrote an article in her newspaper, *Counterpoint*, praising Sackeim as a reformer who was working to fix the problems with ECT just as fast as he could. He'd only "just been awarded a $5 million grant for a comprehensive study of the long term effects of ECT," she gushed. "Finally— after 60 years—it is going to happen."[18] She was apparently unaware that this was a renewal of a grant he'd had for nineteen years without ever doing such a study.

Like the APA, she didn't think that shock should ever be banned for anyone, even children or persons deemed incompetent. So she drafted her own shock bill and took it to her local legislator, who introduced it as H.12. From behind the scenes Sackeim kept in touch with developments through Donahue, telling her, "I admire your efforts to stay true to convictions, and negotiate between the medical establishment, extreme ideological positions, etc."[19]

The bill as introduced had some protections for patients. It specifically required that any consent form adopted by the state had to inform patients that "there exists a division of opinion as to the efficacy of the proposed treatment, why and how it works and its commonly known risks and extent of side effects," a protection also contained in Texas law. Patients also had to be told about "the degree and duration of risks of memory loss, including its potential irreversibility," that "research is incomplete regarding cognitive side effects," and that "there exists minimal research on the effect of ECT on a developing brain." However, the bill explicitly permitted the use of shock on children under fourteen.

When hearings on the bill began, it attracted national attention as shock bills always do, but despite being in constant contact with advocates on the ground in Vermont, I had difficulty even finding out when the hearings were going to be. I asked to testify for the Committee for Truth in Psychiatry, but was told that no one from out of state would be allowed to speak.

That turned out to be a lie. Sackeim, who'd been heavily promoted as an expert to the legislature by Donahue, was flown from New York to Vermont, and Donahue personally escorted him to a hearing in front of the combined House and Senate Health and Welfare Committees. He testified for an hour and a half, telling legislators the proposed informed consent requirements were "misinforming" and "simply wrong," that he opposed legislation, and that the state should use the APA guidelines. Though hearings went on for days, the legislature heard mostly from ECT practitioners; less than a handful of speakers were psychiatric or shock survivors.

I wrote up twenty-three pages of testimony and sent it to that black hole where papers go that no one ever reads.

In her testimony, two weeks after she'd submitted her article to the *Journal of ECT*, Donahue said she now felt that that shock practitioners should be given a chance to regulate themselves. She no longer thought her bill was necessary.

The Department of Developmental and Mental Health Services (now renamed the Department of Mental Health) announced that it would convene an ECT study committee made up of representatives from the local hospitals that did shock, representatives of the department, and Anne Donahue. This worked to appease the legislators, at least temporarily. In March 1999, they agreed to table the bill while the committee worked to develop a uniform informed consent document for the state.

Meanwhile, despite having told the legislature, "I don't have any interest in money," Donahue proceeded to sue the hospital where she was shocked for half a million dollars.[20] Although she didn't have a lawyer, she described her hopes for a settlement as "skyrocketing" because Harold Sackeim had signed on as her expert witness.[21]

Under Vermont law, she couldn't sue for being misinformed about shock unless the correct information would have changed her decision, and she steadfastly maintained that she would have chosen shock even knowing what it would do to her memory and IQ. But by now she espoused a major plank in the PR platform: that permanent massive losses are due to poorly performed (old or outdated) ECT, not any inherent risk in the treatment itself. Her treatments had been performed only four years earlier, and at an internationally renowned hospital associated with Dartmouth College. But because she now complained they'd been done wrong, she could still bring a lawsuit. In her complaint, Donahue claimed that her doctors committed medical malpractice because they didn't follow the APA guidelines.

As the appointed committee met to draft informed consent materials, Donahue (now on a first name basis with Sackeim) would forward the drafts to him, and he'd respond in the form of friendly emails ("I hope your summer has been good. Harold").[22]

While all of this was going on, we advocates did all we could to avoid being shut out of the process, asking for minutes of the meetings, asking that they be taped since they were supposed to be open to the public, even those who couldn't be present. There was no response.

Sackeim suggested about fifteen changes to the proposed consent document, and all but one were dutifully made by the committee. In particular, they took out the warning that "different kinds of memory problems are one of the side effects and that these can range from minor to very severe . . . some amount of memory loss could be permanent." Most of the changes made to the model form they'd started out with, itself a derivative of the APA form, were minor and meaningless. The more substantial changes were to the detriment of truthful information. The original form had mentioned brain damage as a possible consequence of treatment; that warning was deleted.

One of the most bizarre chapters in the history of ECT had been written: a survivor who'd been plucky enough to get her own permanent cognitive deficits confirmed by neuropsychological testing had endorsed a consent form which tells future patients "testing shows that many parts of thinking are improved by ECT."

Vermont psychiatric survivor Cindy Haggett put it this way: "I have tried to understand what her motive may be and the only one I can think of may be her need to justify that her choice of ECT for herself was the right one. She lost a great deal, it is clear, and so if she can prove that was the only way for her to regain her emotional health, then perhaps she can accept the cost. Unfortunately she will never know, as she did not choose any other way."[23]

Because the committee formed to develop the proposed statewide informed consent materials had so blatantly excluded everyone except ECT proponents, advocates of the original H.12 bill were able to go back to the legislature and convince them that more input was needed.

Donahue could hardly advocate for her bill now; to do so would be to acknowledge that the consent form she had spearheaded wasn't enough to protect patients. And it would have alienated her from the doctors, who were so outraged that the bill had come back that one of them was threatening to boycott the consent form. In last-minute discussions before the House Health and Welfare Committee, Donahue now argued that to mandate state oversight of ECT would undermine "the whole intention of the bill" and "turns it into a political issue where it doesn't belong."[24]

As passed on May 2, 2000, the bill provided that Vermont's commissioner of mental health could oversee ECT, but left wide latitude as to how to do that. The state had to develop a uniform consent form and materials, but there was no longer any direction about what must be included. A second ECT study committee was to be convened to make recommendations and to issue a report on the consent materials developed by Donahue and the others on the first committee, but it had no teeth; there was no requirement that the state incorporate those recommendations. The bill specified that twelve organizations were to be represented on this committee, but only three included psychiatric survivors, and Anne Donahue was on the boards of two of them.

In an email to the chair of the newly formed committee, who was also the chief counsel for the Department of Developmental and Mental Health Services, Donahue was blunt: "It is only input which can be disregarded."[25]

Survivors and concerned citizens from outside the ECT industry were now in a (depressingly familiar) high stakes battle against the structural exclusion of our input. Laura Ziegler and I lobbied our hearts out, she on the ground in Vermont, me by phone and mail. Ziegler had found two medical experts, a neurologist and a neuroanatomist from outside the industry, who were ready and willing to testify. But the legislature had refused to hear them. Donahue told Assistant Attorney General Jennifer Myka, "In terms of a medical or research expert knowledgeable about ECT to present the 'other side,' none exist."[26]

No one had more access to the members of the committee or sent them more written material than Donahue. Not only did she besiege them with her own material, most often her summaries of ECT research by Sackeim, but she tried to tell them what to think about what they read or saw by putting her own spin on it.[27] In mid-2000 she responded to feedback and criticisms by others, including the Committee for Truth in Psychiatry, in a dense thirteen-page paper. She didn't allow that any of the criticisms were valid. In her paper she cited Sackeim twenty-three times, the Surgeon General's Report thirteen times, and the APA Task Force Report twenty-three times.[28] I could see through this, but I was sure most committee members would simply be dazzled or overwhelmed by it.

After months of lobbying the ECT study committee, they finally allowed me to speak for twenty minutes. Peter Breggin got thirty. By this time Harold Sackeim had already testified *three* times to the legislators (no time limits for him), had been specifically asked if he had financial ties to the shock machine companies, and—seeming to hesitate just a couple of seconds—told them he did not.

While some on the committee clearly had a vested interest in ECT, many others were new to the issue and put forth their best and most honest efforts to make sense of the sea of conflicting information—that is, the information that they were allowed to see and hear. In the face of deliberate obfuscation—Donahue's tireless promotion of Sackeim, Sackeim's denial of his industry ties, the director of ECT at a local hospital telling them that it would be "unethical" for the FDA to conduct safety studies—and with no history or context and very few opposing viewpoints to rely on, the majority of the committee members did what most people would do: trusted what they were told by those who had placed themselves in positions of public trust.

In the end, as Donahue had predicted, none of it mattered; the meetings, the comments, the testimony, the final report of the ECT study committee in January 2001. None of it changed the practice of ECT or the informed consent process in Vermont from protecting doctors to protecting patients. In November 2001 the state of Vermont made it official: "DDMHS has selected *The Practice of Electroconvulsive Therapy, Recommendations for Treatment, Training, and Privileging*, Second Edition, published by the American Psychiatric Association (APA) as the basis of the standards of practice."[29]

A few final changes were made by the department to the Vermont consent forms. The part telling people that ECT would improve their memory was rewritten according to Donahue's recommendations to make even less sense than it already did: "Some patients report their learning and memory is improved after ECT; testing shows that some people experience improvements to pre-illness levels."[30] If ECT did not have a *permanent* deleterious effect on learning and memory, then *all* patients would return to pre-"illness" levels once their "illness" was gone. "Testing shows" is a blatant lie, since there has never been a study in which ECT patients were tested pre-"illness" to establish their baseline status; patients are always tested in the hospital shortly before shock, when for understandable reasons they are not functioning well. In fact, this is how the industry got the idea in the first place to claim that "ECT improves memory"; the fine print on this, which is never included, is that their memory (function, not recall) "improves" (if it does, which is not always the case) only from the subpar performance that would be expected on any test of anything from someone miserable enough to be waiting their turn for ECT.

To confuse patients even more, later in the document they are told that some people "experience a return to improved thinking and memory." The phrase "return to" was added by Donahue because, she said, "misinterpretations would later result" if it wasn't; but how is it possible to experience a *return* to improvement?

Patients are then told some should expect "memory loss for which there is no known treatment"—a change in the direction of greater honesty—and that they will be getting a referral for follow-up of memory loss (a possibility that's not even hinted at in any other consent form.)

If former ECT patients were really referred to neuropsychologists outside the shock industry for help, the citizens of Vermont would indeed be ahead of the rest of the nation. But this doesn't happen, because no such referrals exist in the entire state. In at least one case when a badly damaged patient found out that he was entitled to a referral for assessment of memory loss, he was somehow put in touch with Anne Donahue, who told him to see—who else—Harold Sackeim.[31]

The Blood and Flesh of Christ

The industry had dodged a bullet, lost nothing, and gained a great deal. It had convinced a severely damaged survivor of what everyone would call "modern" ECT that the only problems with shock were "past abuses, different techniques from the past, or information not grounded in methodologically sound and up-to-date research."[32] The PR line had shown itself elastic enough to define the past as "anything that happened before we figured out the right way to give shock, which we are doing right now."

Sackeim, in an editorial accompanying and carefully defusing Donahue's published article, conceded no more and no less than he had to in order to maintain control of the situation, namely that it was possible for "exceptional" patients to experience permanent (he calls it "sustained") and substantial amnesia. However, he said, only certain patients could be believed when they claimed permanent amnesia: those, like Donahue, "who believe the treatment was valuable, even life saving." In other cases, it was still OK to attribute reports of amnesia to unresolved psychopathology or "natural progression of an underlying illness."[33]

Because Donahue kept mention of her IQ loss and other documented neuropsychological deficits out of her article, not only was no concession necessary on these points, but Vermont could keep on telling patients ECT might cause "improved thinking."

But even Sackeim's small and strategic concession was too much for others in the industry, who weren't used to conceding anything. In an editorial in the *Journal of ECT*, and then in the updated 2002 edition of his textbook *Electroconvulsive Therapy*, Somatics owner Richard Abrams viciously denounced Donahue:

> Ms. Donahue's personal belief is no more subject to scientific investigation than is the belief that the Eucharist is composed of the blood and flesh of Christ. No amount of scientific testing of wine and wafer can determine the composition of the blessed sacrament, because dogma specifies that in the miraculous transubstantiation all properties of flesh and blood are lost. Likewise, no amount of memory or cognitive testing, in association with even the most advanced imaging techniques, can ever prove or disprove Ms. Donahue's claims, because they partake exclusively of the essence of pure subjective experience, the validity of which is, by definition, inaccessible to the scientific method.[34]

He proceeded to attack Sackeim as well for his "personal conviction" that ECT could cause permanent memory loss. "This is puzzling, because the author . . . is not known for making unsupported, faith-based claims in his research articles." But he wasn't done yet; the shock machine company owner went on to claim that not only does ECT improve memory by 71 percent, but it grows new brain cells. His breathless conclusion was: "All claims that brief-pulse ECT can induce, or has induced, permanent memory loss must receive the Scotch verdict: *unproved.*"

Despite this extraordinary public rift between the Mecta and Somatics camps, things might have ended up a lot worse for the industry, at least in Vermont. Anne Donahue was elected to the Vermont House of Representatives and now serves as the Republican representative from Northfield.

15   *The Triumph of Public Relations over Science*

In its public relations campaign, the APA has successfully reshaped perception of the nature and risks of shock for a whole generation of doctors, patients, and the public. In doing so, it has subtly redefined the very meaning of words like "informed consent" and "competency" to its advantage. The result is that the ECT industry has found a foolproof way to get around the laws protecting patients' rights to full disclosure and to refuse treatment. As well, it has been able to insulate itself from potential liability for damages. Patients today often have, in reality, *fewer* rights and less recourse than they had before the PR campaign. How did this happen?

The PR Line for the Twenty-First Century

Beginning in the 1990s, the industry began to formulate a novel public relations solution to its enduring problem of shock patients who continue to allege brain damage. It now claims that mental illness causes brain damage. Since everyone who has had shock was labeled mentally ill at some point, this theory serves as a convenient smokescreen for reconceptualizing brain damage as the result of intrinsic disease rather than an outcome of treatment. (In one fell swoop, the estimated fourteen million Americans who are labeled depressed have been defined as brain damaged—a story no one in the media has picked up on yet.) By the rules of the doubting game, the onus is now placed on others to prove that depression does not cause brain damage, not on the industry to prove that it does. Meanwhile, a brand new answer to the embarrassing question of how ECT exerts its therapeutic effects is offered. According to Harold Sackeim and others, not only does shock not cause brain damage, it causes patients to grow new brain cells.

I first heard Sackeim talk about this at the beginning of the 1990s. This was in the context of an interview that was to have been a discussion of ECT research, but instead, he wanted to talk about his new explanation for why

ECT survivors report brain damage and memory loss. They were mistaking the effects of psychiatric conditions for the effects of ECT.

He tried to tell me that my massive loss of intelligence post-ECT was caused by psychosis. But I was never psychotic. He had nothing to hang this theory on. Nevertheless, he continued to elaborate on his theory that mental illnesses are literally toxic conditions that damage the brain. Depression, he said, is a progressive cerebrovascular disease, and any changes in the brain are due to this ongoing degenerative disease process, not ECT. That was why, according to Sackeim, there was no need for a brain scan study looking at people before and after shock. It was in the best interest of humanity, he concluded, that scientists were investigating this new theory of depression, rather than that tired and boring old question of whether ECT causes brain damage.

During a 2001 conversation, he repeated the claim he first made to me ten years earlier. I queried him on all angles, so that there was no chance of misunderstanding him. Depression itself, period, causes permanent brain damage, he said, even when it's successfully treated, even if the person recovers and never again has any symptoms. In my case, he said, a single episode of depression lasting a few months, sixteen years earlier, must have damaged my brain severely enough to cause permanent cognitive problems. This was true even though I hadn't had any of these cognitive problems while I was depressed, only after the ECT when I was not.

In support of his theory, Sackeim—who speaks in literature citations whenever possible—threw out some names, dates, and journal references. I read the articles, but they didn't say what he claimed they did. Intrigued, I got in touch with the scientists themselves. All do brain research. None of them do ECT. Some work only with animals, not humans. None were aware of Sackeim's attempts to hitch his theories to their research. All were willing to discuss their work with me in detail.

Scientists Respond to Sackeim

All of the researchers told me, in no uncertain terms, that Sackeim's "depression causes brain damage" theory was not supported by the science.

The scientist Sackeim mentioned most enthusiastically as supporting his theory was psychiatrist Yvette Sheline of Washington University in St. Louis,

Missouri. Sackeim even said he was Sheline's mentor, a claim she denies; they didn't meet until her career was well established.

Since about 1995, Sheline's work has involved brain imaging studies of persons with psychiatric histories, especially women with recurrent depression. In the work Sackeim cited most often, she measured the hippocampus of a small number of women who'd been depressed for many years. (The hippocampus is a tiny structure deep within the brain, associated with learning and memory, and long known to be sensitive to the effects of shock. It is the brain region most vulnerable to neuron loss from seizures.) She found that, on average, the depressed women had smaller hippocampi than controls.[1]

The jump from that finding to "depression causes brain damage" is one only a PR man, not a scientist, could make, as Sheline and her research team emphasized to me in personal communications. Sheline's colleague, a nurse, laughed out loud at that claim, then went on to explain several points. The differences between the brain scans of patients and controls are so minute they can't even be seen except with the most high-tech equipment. They do not come anywhere near the threshold of "brain damage," but might be within the limits of normal variation. And these brain differences do not cause any differences in function. No one with a slightly smaller hippocampus reported any cognitive deficits, memory disability, or sudden severe amnesia.

Most importantly, there is no way to know whether the brain differences are causing the depression, or the depression is causing the brain differences. As Sheline carefully summed it up to me, that there are differences between the brains of patients with a history of depression and those with no history of depression neither proves nor disproves that depression causes changes in the brain. She added that she had never seen in her depressed patients anything like the extent of memory loss shock survivors commonly experience, and that hippocampal volume loss definitely did not cause IQ loss.

No subsequent research has changed this conclusion; for instance, in a 2003 literature review Sheline wrote: "Depression per se may produce structural brain changes, but this is an unproven hypothesis."[2]

The work of other scientists who influenced Sheline, such as Bruce McEwen of Rockefeller University and his student Robert Sapolsky at

Stanford, suggests that depression, by itself, does not cause brain cells to die. But it may make the brain more vulnerable to loss of cells caused by neurological insults like seizures, even possibly lowering the threshold of what type of insult will cause neuron death. And like every doctor outside the shock industry, Sapolsky and McEwen are clear that seizures cause brain damage.[3]

What this suggests is not that ECT can't damage the brain; it suggests that the likelihood of brain damage from the dual insults of seizures and electricity is high, because the depressed person's brain is so fragile.

That is exactly what was found in the study Sapolsky co-authored on ECT. People who had the highest levels of stress hormones prior to ECT (and most research suggests that only about half of depressed people do have elevated levels of these hormones, called glucocorticoids) had the largest declines in cognitive and memory function post-ECT.[4]

McEwen summed it up like this: "There's certainly enough evidence in neurology about seizures causing brain damage. On the other hand I think the evidence is very up in the air that depression causes brain damage."[5]

Sapolsky was even blunter about what he thought of the claim that a single short episode of depression could cause permanent brain damage: there was "zero evidence" for such a claim, and the person making it "should be publicly flogged."[6]

What about the role of ECT in causing any atrophy seen on the brain scans of formerly severely depressed patients? Has anyone even thought to ask whether these people had had ECT, and whether that, rather than depression, might be responsible for hippocampal atrophy?

Yvette Sheline allowed her research subjects to have had as many as two courses of ECT previously on the assumption that since ECT has no permanent adverse effects, these women would not differ from depressed subjects who had never had ECT. She drew the line at three courses. But there is no basis for the arbitrary cut-off point and the assumption that it takes three courses of ECT for any permanent adverse effects to occur. In her published articles, Sheline doesn't always reveal how many of her subjects had ECT previously, or separate them from non-ECT patients when she gives us the results of their brain scans. That means she can't rule out the possibility that

ECT caused or contributed to their outcomes. However, when she reanalyzed her data leaving the former ECT patients out, she still saw slight but significant differences between the depressed subjects and the normal controls.[7]

Another study by P. J. Shah et al. in 2002 found that structural brain changes in the hippocampi of persons with chronic depression were correlated with the cumulative number of ECTs these people had received. The authors concluded: "It could be argued that the differences were the result of ECT . . . the possibility that the findings are ECT-related could not be discounted." Nevertheless, they tried to dismiss that possibility by citing Sackeim's 1994 selective literature review as evidence that ECT cannot cause brain damage. These authors also found that persons who had previously experienced depression, but no longer did, were not any different, brainwise, than controls who had never experienced depression—refuting Sackeim's claim that depression results in permanent brain damage in persons who are never again depressed.[8]

Additionally, there are studies similar to Sheline's in which researchers looked for relationships between depression and brain atrophy but found none.[9]

Brain Regeneration or Brain Damage?

The speculation about neurogenesis—the growth of new brain cells from neural stem cells—and the role of this process in brain function and in biopsychiatric treatments in humans is based on animal studies. These studies seem to show the proliferation of brain cells in some areas, in particular the dentate gyrus of the hippocampus, as a result of electroconvulsive or antidepressant treatment.[10] But most of these studies focus on trying to find a way to prevent or reduce this proliferation (for instance, investigating whether the anesthetic used for ECT could help prevent it).[11] Why? Because, for one thing, no one knows whether the new cells are a good or a bad sign. No one knows what they do, or if they will grow up to be neurons (the kind of cells lost in brain damage), and if so, how long they live or what their function might be.

The studies purporting to show brain cell proliferation from ECT may in fact be showing evidence of brain damage, neuroscientist Richard

Nowakowski of the Robert Wood Johnson School of Medicine told the *Los Angeles Times*. (He developed the cellular techniques used in those studies.) "It's not clear in these studies whether they're seeing proliferation or something else," he said. As far as what the changes actually mean, "Anyone who tells you they know doesn't."[12]

It has been shown in animals that ECT causes proliferative sprouting of mossy fibers—a type of neural connection. Mossy fiber sprouting is seen in epilepsy and brain damage. According to scientists who spoke with the *Times*, it's very unlikely that the type of neural connection that results in enhanced functioning would happen instantaneously, with an electric shock.

Talk of mossy fiber sprouting confused the rank and file at the 2004 APA conference, where Sackeim and his protégé Sarah Holly Lisanby presided over packed talks about "brain stimulation" and their newly invented "magnetic seizure therapy." Hardly a word was said about ECT that year in their enthusiasm to sell their new treatments; but in the process of promoting the latest "new and improved" versions of shock treatment, ECT came in for some indirect criticism.

Lisanby showed slides of mossy fiber sprouting in monkey brains, saying electroshock causes it but magnetic shock treatment doesn't. This sprouting and the associated new synaptic connections were related to ECT's cognitive effects, she said.

An audience member had a logical question: Why had she said ECT is not neuropathological when it causes mossy fiber sprouting? Sackeim took over on that one, dismissing mossy fiber sprouting in a generalized way, saying that everything causes changes in the brain and that change isn't damage.

No one would have dared to contradict him. After all, he'd just been hailed by the chair of the panel as "a giant in maintaining the science of ECT."[13]

No sooner had the industry begun marketing the "depression causes brain damage" line than the media began lapping it up. The narrator of the *60 Minutes II* shock segment told millions of viewers, "Depression itself kills brain cells and lowers IQ." Joel Bernstein said he got that from Bruce McEwen, though he never talked with McEwen, only Sackeim. McEwen was unaware of the media's distortion of his work and could only account for it in public relations, not scientific, terms: "When an idea gets into the popular mind, like we're losing brain cells, it's very hard to get it out. Somehow people want to believe it."[14]

The New Meaning of Competence

The new PR claims—like the old ones—are being used to persuade the public and decision makers that shock is harmless. In the face of all the evidence of brain damage and memory loss, the industry is covering its bases in a new way—saying that there is no such damage, but even if there is, it's not from shock. It's setting up this theory the same way it has approached the question of brain damage throughout the PR era: not by scientific controlled studies, but by assertions from perceived authorities and selective reviews. Meanwhile, as we have seen, the existing science is distorted or ignored.

One of the results of the new campaign, as far as we are able to determine from the limited data available, is that it has become easier for doctors to convince judges to order involuntary ECT.

It's always been true that shock can be done forcibly by court order, except perhaps for the brief period in the 1970s in which the first *Wyatt* decision required explicit consent without exception. (And even then, as we've seen, psychiatrists paid the decision no mind.) That is, shock can be done by court order as long as a patient has been deemed incompetent to consent for herself.

Technically, an incompetent (sometimes called incapable) patient is one unable to make *any* decision for herself. In the case of someone who is unconscious or in a coma, or someone labeled catatonic who is unable or unwilling to communicate, the need for substitute decision making, if a decision must be made, is clear. The justification for state intervention is that she cannot get treatment without it. Theoretically, having a decision made for her by a court or representative is not overruling her wishes, but trying to approximate what they would be if she could express them. Medical advance directives or living wills can provide guidance in these cases, although they are not always followed.

Parents make medical decisions for their minor children all the time, of course, as do some parents of adult children—for instance, the parents of a severely retarded thirty-year-old who is unable to understand why she must undergo a complicated or painful medical procedure. But helping the helpless to get treatment they would want, or do not object to, is quite different from forcing people into treatment they strenuously object to.

What's changed in the case of forced ECT is the type of patient being shocked against her will. The perceived lower risk of the procedure is redefining the meaning of competence, with the result that judges are deciding that people are incompetent largely on the basis of their objection to treatment. In fact, the new "incompetent" mental patient is not one who cannot make a decision, but one who makes a decision her doctor disagrees with.

Let Them Go Shock Themselves!

Lucille Austwick. Kathleen Garrett. Adam Syszko. Michael Matthews. Dina Hernandez. Joan T. Paul Henri Thomas. They are ordinary people whose names made headlines for the same reason: they said "NO!" to shock loudly and clearly, and then their doctors took them to court to shock them against their will.

Two of these people—Austwick, who had dementia, and Hernandez, who was mentally retarded—would likely have been classified as incompetent by pre-PR-era standards. But each woman was able to say no, and in each woman's case her relative or guardian said no as well, and then the doctors went to court to shock them anyway.

For every case that makes headlines, every bit of evidence we have suggests that there are thousands that don't. For instance, in the state of New York, court-ordered electroshock increased 73 percent from 1999 to 2000.[15] An investigation by that state's mental disability watchdog agency found that 40 percent of the shock that took place in state-run hospitals in 2001 was involuntary.[16] The vast majority of these patients, convinced they couldn't win against the state, didn't even try to fight the orders.

The above-named persons were spared forced shock only because of the publicity surrounding their cases. But if the state really had a compelling interest in forcibly electroshocking these people for their own good, a few newspaper articles wouldn't have changed that.

The case of Paul Henri Thomas, which received the most media attention, illustrates that what's really fueling the push for forced shock is the best interests of an industry that believes, as ever, that customers won't buy its product of their own free will.

Competent If Yes, Incompetent If No

If a patient were really incompetent in the old sense of the word, she'd be unable to consent to treatment, as well as to refuse it. Courts might be asked to overrule an incompetent patient's decision to undergo shock. But that's never happened, because doctors who order shock never question the mental competence of a patient who does what they want. It is, quite simply, a logical and statistical impossibility that every person who says yes to ECT is competent, while every person who says no is incompetent.

Paul Henri Thomas, an inmate at one of New York State's public psychiatric facilities, Pilgrim Psychiatric Center, originally consented to shock in 1999. His competence was not questioned. After three shocks he decided he didn't want any more. The hospital took him to court and shocked him by force, approximately sixty times. But they never stopped trying to get him to consent, using pressure and threats, long after he had been declared incompetent. As his supervising psychiatrist later testified, "The staff would ask him, are you going to consent or are we going to have to go back to court?"[17] Had he ever succumbed to the pressure to "consent," he would immediately have become, in their eyes, legally competent, without any change in his alleged mental condition.

In court in 2001, Thomas's lawyer asked his treating psychiatrist, Andre Azemar: "If Paul had said yes, would you have tested his competency?" Azemar looked baffled and didn't answer the question. "If they say no, we have to do it," was his response.

The day before his doctor signed a petition for forced shock, Thomas was considered by his psychiatrist to be legally competent. He even signed a legal document, an advance directive, with his psychiatrist as witness. The doctor testified that Thomas became incompetent the day of the forced shock petition.

Dr. Azemar was asked: What constitutes capacity? And he replied, "Understanding what the treatment is about; he understands the consequences of the treatment, and has the ability to assess benefits and risks."

Both Azemar and supervising psychiatrist Robert Kalani said that Thomas was incompetent because he "is unable to assess the risks and benefits of ECT."

Thomas had already had dozens of treatments. By what standard did he not understand its benefits and risks? Questioning from Thomas's lawyer clarified the situation. He asked the doctor, "Did he understand what *you* thought were the benefits and risks?" Yes, the doctors said. Thomas was perfectly capable of hearing and understanding what his doctors were telling him. He just didn't agree with them.

Ironically, Thomas's doctors themselves did poorly on the witness stand on "understanding what the treatment is about." Kalani testified that the FDA had "approved" the machines used to give shock. As we've seen, the devices never had to go through the approval process, because they were on the market prior to 1976. He also testified that the FDA had conducted animal trials of shock and that there have been "lots of" before-and-after MRI studies proving that ECT doesn't cause brain damage. Wrong again.

Patients and doctors have always disagreed about the nature, risks, and benefits of electroshock. They always will. But only the doctors get to define the "right" answers. Controlling *perception* of the nature, risks, and benefits of ECT is the key to shocking patients without informed consent, or without any consent at all. Because the industry has been so successful at shaping these perceptions, the informed consent and right to refuse laws against which it protested so loudly beginning in the 1970s have never had the predicted effect of eliminating or even decreasing the use of shock.

Today lawyers, judges, and rank-and-file public hospital psychiatrists like Kalani will spout some version of the current industry line without the least idea, or concern, about where it came from or whether it's accurate. The more they perceive shock as harmless, the less compelling the state's interest need be in forcing it on citizens, and the easier it is to shock us. As the judge in *Price v. Sheppard* said at the dawn of the PR era, "As the impact increases, so must the importance of the state's interest."[18]

The Success of the PR Campaign

One way we can measure public perception of electroshock, and thus gauge the success of the PR campaign, is by comparing the pronouncements of judges in the pre-PR era with those of today. It is clear that in the 1970s, judges could imagine rational refusal. As we have seen in Chapter Five, their rulings were peppered with strong warnings about the known or suspected serious adverse effects of shock.

Compare that with the decision summarily ordering forced electroshock of Kathleen Garrett of Missouri twenty-five years later. Using the same language preprinted on the form the state uses to petition for court-ordered shock, the decision says: "There is a strong likelihood that electroconvulsive treatment will significantly improve/cure the aforenamed patient's mental disorder for a substantial period of time without causing her any serious functional harm."[19] The judge reached that decision after hearing testimony from both Mrs. Garrett and her son that the shock she had previously received had caused permanent memory loss. Her psychiatrist convinced the judge that he could minimize memory effects by using the unilateral technique. He testified that he had never seen any medical literature critical of ECT.

Dr. Laura Fochtmann, Max Fink's protégé, contributed to an amicus brief submitted on behalf of the New York State Psychiatric Association.[20] She painted a picture of a treatment with virtually no risk using selective citation. In a paper with fifty references, she managed to cite to Sackeim, Weiner, and the APA thirty-seven times. The statement that "the majority of patients state that the benefits of ECT outweigh the problems with memory" had not even a fraudulent footnote to support it, but simply saying it under the Psychiatric Association imprimatur was sure to be enough to convince the judge. Any lingering memory or cognitive problems, Fochtmann assured him, were due to drugs or mental illness, and therefore couldn't be due to shock. She cited Sapolsky's work in support of her claim that ECT is harmless. When he learned about this, he called it "bizarre and unsupportable logic."[21]

Fochtmann didn't have a single study to rebut the evidence that convinced judges in the 1970s that ECT could cause brain damage. But she cited one of Sackeim's selective and misleading review articles and called shock safe. Not only are there no permanent adverse effects of shock, the brief said, but "if anything, ECT induces growth of new nerve cells."

In the end Judge W. Bromley Hall ruled against Paul Henri Thomas, denying the risks of brain damage and memory loss: "The risks of the treatment are from the anesthesia and increased blood pressure during the seizure. . . . Although it is accepted without dispute that the procedure is unpleasant, every safety measure is taken to minimize risks."[22]

Laurie Gatto, attorney for the State of New York, was blasé about winning the Thomas case; for her it was just business as usual. "The intensity of the objection by Mental Hygiene Legal Service [which represented Thomas] is the only thing that was surprising," she told a reporter.[23]

But the state did not win, in the end. The order for forced shock was stayed. The doctors who had sworn that there was no alternative but shock for Thomas, no drug or therapy that could help him, were proven wrong. While his appeal went forward, the hospital decided that—without any shock at all—Thomas was well enough, after two years of being held against his will, to be released. Like Kathleen Garrett, Lucille Austwick, and so many courageous patients, he made not only a competent decision, but the correct decision.

"Come in for Evaluation"

In 2001, the publicity generated by the Paul Henri Thomas case led to public hearings on shock in the New York State assembly. The legislators had proposed four new ECT bills, including one that would have required the state to keep statistics on shock use and another designed to ensure informed consent. All of the bills were ultimately defeated. Sackeim testified in opposition to any regulation of ECT, as he has in so many other forums. This time, he may have gotten a little carried away. Whether he intended to or not, he made the following statement to the assembly: "I've never seen a case where there has been a permanent effect of ECT on anterograde amnesia, and I invite anyone in the country who believes ECT has had a deleterious effect on their cognition to come in for evaluation."[24] (Anterograde amnesia, in this context, means permanent loss of one's pre-shock facility for learning, retaining, and remembering information, not the wiping out of one's past that is known as retrograde amnesia.)

People took him seriously, writing and emailing him, relieved that a professional was listening, hopeful that he might offer help. At least 175 people wrote to him.[25] I was one of them. Since I helped coordinate efforts to make people aware of Sackeim's offer, I was often cc-ed on their emails. I also know that most of these people never got any response at all.

No one, not one person, was invited to "come in for evaluation." The responses, in the few cases where Sackeim responded at all, consisted of emails or phone conversations in which Sackeim tried to elicit information he could use to blame something, anything but ECT, for the person's problems. One person who had had insulin shock was told that the insulin shock, not the electric shock, must have damaged his brain. Another who was on psychiatric drugs was told the drugs, not shock, caused her cognitive problems, as well as the onset of epileptic seizures after ECT.

In my case, Sackeim had a tougher time, because I have not taken any psychiatric drugs since shock, nor have I had any mental illness. Sackeim's so-called evaluation of my anterograde amnesia consisted of nothing more than almost an hour of him arguing that depression causes brain damage, that this was a better explanation for my memory and cognitive deficits—including loss of intelligence—than ECT, and that he didn't need to test me to know this.

I said I would like to come in for an evaluation. He replied that he saw no point in that. Although he had specifically invited ECT survivors to "come in" for evaluation, now he claimed that he hadn't said he would see people in his office or do any formal testing. And he summarily dismissed the idea of brain scans, saying he wouldn't pay for them.

Nevertheless, survivors of ECT, taking Sackeim at his word, continue to this day to write to him, asking for the promised evaluation. Under oath, Sackeim was asked what he did with all the communications from these people.[26] He said he threw all of them away, along with all the hundreds of other communications he'd received in other contexts over the past twenty years from persons who reported long-term adverse consequences of ECT. The obvious question was asked: Why? Sackeim answered, "I average maybe 400 e-mails a day so I don't necessarily want to keep a lot of that stuff."

The other reason he threw them away, he said, was to avoid "somebody wanting in this context to talk about it"—that is, I inferred, so he wouldn't have to disclose the contents of the communications when he was hired to defend doctors against claims of memory disability and brain damage.

In his role as a government-funded researcher who had accepted millions of dollars to study the adverse cognitive effects of shock, Sackeim should have welcomed this wealth of evidence on his topic, evidence he himself had asked for. But in the PR era, protecting the industry takes precedence over protecting patients, and certainly over advancing science. As we have seen, it is only by carefully defining and limiting what is "known" about ECT that the industry can continue to survive and grow. It will do this by any means necessary, hijacking real science to its cause while refusing to conduct any scientific investigation of its own. In the end, any assessment of ECT— what it is, what it does—breaks down over the lack of real science behind it, forcing us to ultimately evaluate it in entirely different terms.

16   *Should ECT Be Banned?*

THE MORAL CONTEXT

Morality is the silence in which one can hear the unheard voices.

—Simone Weil

It is impossible for anyone—doctors, patients, the public, the media—to discuss shock without speaking about it in moral terms. Questions such as, how much risk is justified for how much benefit? what should patients be told or not told? and whether forced shock can ever be justified—these are by their very nature moral questions, to be decided based on values and principles. At the same time they cannot be answered without the valid scientific evidence to answer other questions: Does ECT cause brain damage? How much permanent amnesia, how much permanent cognitive disability does it cause? For how many people?

If shock has no permanent adverse effects, then some may say it's permissible to force it on unwilling patients; if it causes permanent brain damage, then many may agree it's not acceptable to use it, ever. What you think should be done about shock will depend on what you believe to be true about it.

The problem is that what passes for evidence has already been skewed by the moral choices made by the industry, choices not questioned because we are not even aware they have been made. These choices make it difficult for the rest of us to think clearly about traditional moral issues like help and harm, and for us as a society to decide what to do about ECT.

Dishonesty, self-dealing, and deception—and the means and motive to tightly control information—pervade the practice of ECT and contaminate the moral discourse. Therefore, it is necessary to step back, before we can even try to reason morally on this issue, and ask how the myriad choices made by industry stakeholders every day over the years affect what it is possible for us to "know" about shock.

- A researcher with a sincere interest in ECT but who is not known to the industry and has not been trained by anyone in the industry finds that a federal grant review panel turns down his request to do a before-and-after CAT scan study.[1]
- In a questionnaire designed to measure anesthesiologists' "knowledge" of ECT, their answers are scored as correct if they are deemed "pro-ECT." If they express the view that ECT causes permanent memory damage, they are said to be "lacking knowledge."[2]
- During a lecture on ECT at a professional meeting, a financially compromised proponent of ECT, recognizing a former ECT patient in the audience, refuses to acknowledge her or allow her to speak—though she patiently raises her hand in the air for thirty minutes when the floor is opened for questions.[3]
- A shock proponent simultaneously provides consultation to a shock machine company and to his state's Office of Mental Health to develop an "informed choice" packet for patients on the risks and benefits of shock.[4]
- A member of the APA's Task Force on ECT lobbies against and defeats a bill that would have required her state to collect and disclose information on memory loss and death due to ECT. She receives an award from her state Psychiatric Association for her efforts.[5]
- A research team studying the cognitive consequences of ECT routinely administers a test of cognitive function to patients who received ECT but never publishes the results of the testing or even discloses in any of their published articles that the test was given.[6]
- Value judgments about the veracity of former ECT patients are subtly but unmistakably conveyed in the industry literature. Reports of devastating memory and cognitive deficits are dismissed as "complaints" (as if they were speaking of a bad haircut), and their amnesia is described as "subjective."
- A shock machine company is sued seven times by patients who suffered permanent adverse effects, but its owners never report the injuries caused by its products to the FDA as required by law.[7]

Each of the above decisions reduces the amount of information available to the rest of us, the duped, without our ever knowing it. Every day the industry makes many more choices that are designed to, and do, alter the climate in which we aspire to make our own (free, voluntary?) moral choices. And whether you are a doctor with no financial investment in ECT trying your best to do the right thing for a patient, a depressed person desperate for relief of emotional pain, or a judge who must decide whether to order shock against a person's will, they do not alter it in the direction most of us would choose.

And yet the industry is quick to attempt to justify what it does in moral terms.

The Moral Argument for ECT

Shortly after the *New Yorker* published Berton Roueché's account of Marilyn Rice's ECT experience, "As Empty as Eve," he received a letter from Rice's referring psychiatrist.[8] Ironically, there is no indication that the writer, Dr. Peter Mendelis, recognized that the "very ill woman" in the article was his own patient. He refers to her as Mrs. Parker, not Marilyn Rice. But he was the psychiatrist who talked her into ECT; and in fact no one was more aware of the full extent of her memory loss, since she continued to see him for months after ECT.[9]

This letter is significant not just because it comes from the psychiatrist without whom there would have been no Committee for Truth in Psychiatry, but because it highlights the key moral arguments the industry uses to justify its practices and existence. Mendelis, like every other pro-ECT psychiatrist, defends shock by claiming that people will kill themselves if they don't get the treatment. Since nothing else can be done for these people, they must be kept in the dark about ECT's harmful effects—for their own good, since otherwise they might not have ECT.

Just as important is what the industry's moral argument doesn't allow to be said. Although Mendelis says that the article is well written, nowhere does he respond to what it says; nowhere does he acknowledge the irreparable damage that was done to his patient. Instead, the *actual* and profound harm that was done to her, and that is done systemically to others, is ignored and disregarded because of some *theoretical* help that shock might bring (but might not) others like her. He takes Roueché to task for scaring people away from ECT and thus pushing them over the line into suicide (he has no evidence for this claim.) The writer, he says, is encouraging death, and should feel guilty for what he's done.

Here, it's quite clear that this tactic allows Mendelis to escape his personal responsibility. The doctor feels he's done nothing wrong. Nothing's on *his* conscience. The harm's been caused by a man who never pushed a button on a shock machine, only a typewriter keyboard.

But the argument serves the industry as a whole as well as the individual doctor. By saying that ECT saves lives (of which there is no evidence) and ignoring the ways in which it has destroyed lives (for which there are decades of evidence) it says, in essence: we won't take any responsibility for the bad outcomes because they couldn't have been caused by ECT, but we will claim credit for the good ones because they were caused by ECT.

That's not just faulty moral reasoning; it's faulty reasoning, period.

Ends and Means: Assessing Benefit and Harm

> Moral mandates appear to lead to the legitimization of any procedure so long as the mandated end is achieved.
>
> —Linda J. Skitka and Elizabeth Mullen,
> "The Dark Side of Moral Conviction"

The bogus argument that ECT saves lives relies on the traditional moral principle that it is permissible to inflict a certain amount of harm if that harm is necessary to achieve a greater good; in other words, the ends justify the means. For instance, cancer patients suffer the pain and nausea of chemotherapy in order to achieve remission of their disease. But cancer patients know what they are getting into.

If honest, rigorous, financially disinterested studies and publication based on scientific merit were the rule, and if we had the statistics and the reporting laws the industry so opposes, we could do a kind of moral calculus. We could quantify the percentage of patients who experience permanent harm and the degree of harm, as well as the costs to patients' families and to society. Then we could weigh these factors against the percentage of patients helped and the extent of the help they received.

One of the reasons this hasn't happened is that another kind of calculus is tacitly going on all the time. In this one, the value of mental patients' lives (worth very little, as we have seen, financially and otherwise) is weighed against the perceived hopelessness and burden to society of mental illnesses, and then multiplied by the perceived lack of any solution besides biological psychiatry. By this calculus, there is no reason not to use shock, even if it's harmful. And there's no other choice anyway except to do nothing. Our society prefers even wrong action to inaction in the face of a perceived social problem. Historically, the unspoken imperative justifying even admittedly brain-damaging treatments such as lobotomies has been that it is always better to do something than to do nothing for psychiatry's lost souls.

But even if we reject these false but widely held premises, we still cannot do a genuine moral calculus. That is because the information we need to make our decisions not only as individuals but as a society is withheld. The benefit to be expected from ECT is vastly exaggerated, while its risks are denied. The "lifesaving" claim, a moral argument based on a lie and masquerading as a scientific argument, continues to be made despite all evidence to the contrary, because it has nothing to do with evidence. The industry promulgates made-up figures on the death rate from ECT (1 in 10,000), using its political clout to make sure actual data are never collected.[10] Meanwhile, the few statistics we do have consistently tell us it is far, far greater; one in two hundred for the majority of patients who are elderly, a rate that hasn't changed since the 1950s.[11]

What we know for certain is that ECT has one potential benefit, relief from distressing feelings and thoughts while the brain recovers from acute organic brain syndrome, and that this is very short lived. The 1985 NIMH Consensus Conference finding that ECT's benefit lasts no more than four weeks stands uncontroverted.

But even this benefit may be overstated. In February 2004, Sackeim et al. published their second NIMH-funded, multicenter study of ECT's effectiveness.[12] This time, they looked at patients who had been shocked in community hospitals with the devices in standard commercial use. They found ECT to be even less effective than in their previous study (where patients were shocked by customized research devices putting out twice as much electricity).

Sixty to 70 percent of patients got no benefit from ECT at all. And even among the small number who did respond, 64 percent relapsed within six months. Those who did not respond to ECT initially did only slightly worse in the long run; about 75 percent of them were symptomatic six months later.

This raises the question of whether ECT may be, for the majority of patients, a treatment with only potential harm and no benefit at all even in the short term—a situation that profoundly affects our moral calculus. In fact, if it is more likely than not that there is no benefit to a procedure, then there is no need for calculus at all.

Besides misleading patients about the good to be expected from ECT, the industry continues to ignore, distort, or conceal the evidence for permanent harm, refusing to investigate the question (or to publish what it knows) and controlling the resources to do so.

After Weiner's 1986 finding of significant permanent amnesia, there was an eerie silence in the research literature that lasted more than two decades. The study begged for replication. But it seemed that now no one was interested in doing long-term follow-up studies. Meanwhile, the industry continued to reassure a generation of patients that ECT had no long-term adverse effects. There can be no scientific justification for this collective choice. It was a moral decision. In fact, we now know that it wasn't a decision not to conduct research; it was a decision not to make the results public.

Sometime in his first decade of research funding, Harold Sackeim conducted studies following up his ECT patients at one year, three years, and five years.[13] Yet in twenty-five years of federal funding to investigate the cognitive consequences of ECT, he never published any data following up patients longer than two months after shock. (Those studies consistently showed that patients were amnesic.)[14] It's an easy out on the question of permanent amnesia; if you've never published your results, it's as if you've never seen it. It's much the same as his throwing out all evidence of permanent anterograde amnesia (memory dysfunction) and then swearing he's "never seen a case" of it.

We are justified in presuming that Sackeim's long-term studies of the 1980s and 1990s showed permanent memory and cognitive deficits. This would be consistent with what's now known about selective publication of research on antidepressant drugs, in which studies showing negative or questionable results of drug treatment are either not published or published in such a way as to falsely convey a positive outcome.[15] It would also be consistent with his own long-delayed published admission of permanent harm.

In January 2007, the Sackeim team finally published what they called "the first large scale, prospective long-term study of cognitive outcomes following ECT."[16] As ECT studies go, it was one of the largest ever, including about 250 patients from seven hospitals in the New York metropolitan area. In one of their only studies to use normal controls, they found "substantial" memory deficits in shocked patients at six months even with Sackeim's self-designed (and inadequate) memory questionnaire (the AMI) and the grossly inappropriate measures used to assess cognition (for instance, the Mini-Mental State Exam, which was designed for use in dementia patients). However, data on how the controls compared with ECT patients on tests of cognitive function was withheld.

The researchers also allowed their subjects to have experienced ECT previously, thus building in to this six-month follow-up study the assumption that ECT's adverse effects resolve within two months; about half of the subjects assessed "before ECT" had actually already had shock. Despite all this, the authors were forced to conclude that "the adverse effects can persist for an extended period, and characterize routine treatment with ECT in community settings."

Sackeim then backhandedly criticized all his prior work, saying, "Empirical information about ECT's long-term effects derives mainly from small sample studies conducted in research settings, with follow-up intervals frequently limited to two months or less . . . these studies could not adequately assess the severity and persistence of long-term deficits." It was effectively an admission from the industry's top researcher that its reassurances to patients and the public over the past generation about the harmlessness of ECT had been based on absolutely nothing but hubris.

Fifty million people worldwide, according to Sackeim's own estimate, have received ECT over the generation it took him to officially admit that shock routinely causes permanent amnesia, without being warned of this possibility.

Moral questions look different when all the evidence, not just industry spin, is considered. How much harm is justified for how much benefit? How many years of memory should a reasonable person be prepared to sacrifice for the chance of one month's respite from depression? How can a patient even make this determination when there is no way to predict the extent of permanent amnesia in any particular individual? What about the patients who experience no benefit at all? Is it acceptable to wipe out their past? What about patients who depend on intellect and memory for their livelihood—is it moral to try ECT, knowing they may lose their ability to earn a living? What if there is no one to support them should their mental abilities never return? What of the responsibility of the doctor who subjects his patient to such risks to provide those most damaged with evaluation, rehabilitation, and compensation? How many patients constitute "acceptable losses" for the industry? Should the amount of money made by the industry factor into this calculation? What about the amount of income lost over the lifetimes of persons disabled by ECT?

We as a society don't have a formula for this, even if we had good data.

British researcher Lucy Johnstone has suggested cautiously: "If up to a third of people will suffer a serious adverse psychological reaction to ECT, and if there is no way of identifying those individuals in advance, the ratio of costs to benefits may begin to seem unacceptably high."[17] Just a few years later, a scrupulous systematic review of the literature on permanent memory loss found that *at least* one-third of ECT survivors experience this loss, and that "many" rather than "rare" individuals claimed by the industry had years of life (even decades) wiped out. This extraordinary development in the history of ECT will be discussed in detail in the next chapter.

Are All Bets Off If It Is Brain Damage?

"Does ECT cause brain damage?" is a question that can only be answered by unbiased scientific research. But as we've seen, there is little of this available, thanks to industry control of the research agenda and dollars.

In a 1982 review of the existing evidence on brain damage, neuropsychologists Donald Templer and David Veleber noted: "A wide array of research and clinical based facts that provide suggestive to impressive evidence in isolation provide compelling evidence when viewed in composite fashion . . . the fact that many patients and subjects suffer no demonstrable permanent effects has provided rationale for some authorities to commit the non-sequitur that ECT causes no permanent harm." They concluded: "ECT has caused and can cause permanent pathology."[18] A decade later, updating the review for a book called *Preventable Brain Damage*, Templer had no reason to revise this conclusion.[19]

Psychologist Andrew Reisner, struggling with the limited and biased data available in 2003, wrote in his review article: "In this writer's professional experience with patients who have undergone an informed consent procedure for ECT . . . not a single patient has reported that he or she was told of the controversy concerning ECT and brain damage. . . . Given the enduring uncertainties and disagreements regarding this issue, this author would suggest that part of the informed consent process should include at least a discussion of the brain damage controversy."[20] However, as he notes, the American Psychiatric Association specifically recommends that mention of brain damage be excluded from the informed consent process.

"What should be done about ECT if it is brain damage?" is a moral question. The industry has lobbied against brain scan studies as if its very life depends on it, but that's not necessarily the case. We as a society could—as one psychiatrist put it back in 1944—make a moral decision that "a socially adaptable individual with a little brain pathology is preferable to a psychotic patient with no demonstrable brain changes," and decide to continue to allow brain damage for mental patients.[21] As neurologist John Friedberg wrote at the beginning of the PR era, "Assuming free and fully informed consent, it is well to affirm the individual's right to pursue happiness through brain damage if he or she chooses." But, he pointed out, this raises another moral question: "Whether we, as doctors sworn to the Hippocratic oath, should be offering it."[22]

An open acknowledgment like this, while good for patients and society, would be very bad for electroshock's image. In the PR era, according to the industry's moral calculus, its image takes priority over patients' rights to determine what happens to their brains.

Can Lying to Patients Be Justified?

There is nothing in the Hippocratic oath, or in other codes of medical ethics, about lying to patients. Paternalistic lies like those told by doctors to patients even outside the shock industry are often held to be harmless, even morally justifiable. After all, the doctors are acting only out of altruism, and they are lying for the good of the patient. Isn't this what happens when patients are told shock is harmless?

This type of lie assumes that patients can't be trusted to make their own decisions because they would not make the decision the doctor wants, and that the doctor knows best. In the case of shock, the lying is to all patients, not just those who are thought to be too mentally incapacitated to make their own decisions. It is never moral to deceive an entire group of people simply because they belong to a group and are assumed to share certain characteristics.

The motivation for paternalistic lies seems to be altruism, but to assume this ignores the complicated motives of the liar and the benefits that accrue to the individual and the system from the lie. Individuals maintain the power and sense of inviolability that comes from duping others and getting away with it; by simply maintaining the lie in the face of all evidence to the contrary, they escape personal and legal responsibility for their actions. The industry never needs to worry about profits declining because potential patients know about the risks of shock. Even if patients didn't reject shock en masse, it would be the worst sort of public relations disaster for the industry as a whole to be found to have concealed the risks for decades. The damage would accrue not just to the individual doctor and the shock industry, but to the general fabric of public trust in the medical profession.

The picture changes when the lies are seen from the perspective of the duped patients. There is real harm to the lied-to. The patient is never aware of the deception (until it is too late) and is denied the opportunity to evaluate risks and benefits for herself and the chance to make a different choice than what his doctor wants. She may be left with brain damage and disability she never would have risked if she had known they were possible. She and those around her suffer harm that was entirely preventable. And should she seek redress, the entire profession shields itself with the paternalistic lie she was told at the outset.

"Retroactive Consent" and the Needs of Psychiatrists

Given that lying is generally held to be immoral, those who tell paternalistic lies feel the need to seek justification for their actions. They sometimes claim to find it in the gratitude of former patients. Gratitude is interpreted by the professional as retroactive consent, justifying not only deception but coercion and even force: See, it's OK; she liked it; she would have had it anyway.[23]

Rarely do individual patients who have experienced severe adverse effects have the courage to confront their shock doctors. But demonstrations against shock by organized ex-patients, such as those that occur at psychiatry conferences, are common and very public displays of ingratitude. Upon being handed a frying pan filled with brains on a bed of dollar bills at a shock doctors' seminar in 1991, "a rather embarrassing experience for somebody like myself," Max Fink was momentarily flustered. "You sort of feel, Well, what have I done wrong? Do I deserve this? Maybe I do."[24] (The brains—of a cow—were from the local butcher shop.)

The industry's need for grateful shock patients and the ways it uses them to justify its practices can be seen in the way it courts those few patients who say, after the fact, that they are glad they had shock. While hundreds of patients who speak publicly about permanent amnesia and disability are ignored, silenced, or told they are lying, those few patients who speak out about similar disabling effects *and* say they would have chosen shock anyway are rewarded with speaking engagements, awards from the APA, publication, and citation. They are even allowed to comment on, and acknowledged in, the APA ECT Task Force Report. For instance, in 1995 Martha Manning, a psychologist who experienced memory loss as well as temporary relief from depression with ECT, wrote a memoir about depression in which ECT played a small part. In her book, she stated flatly, "I will never be the ECT poster-girl."[25] But once it was published, she didn't say no to all the media interviews, speaking engagements, and awards that came her way (as long as she praised ECT). Manning became the darling of the industry.

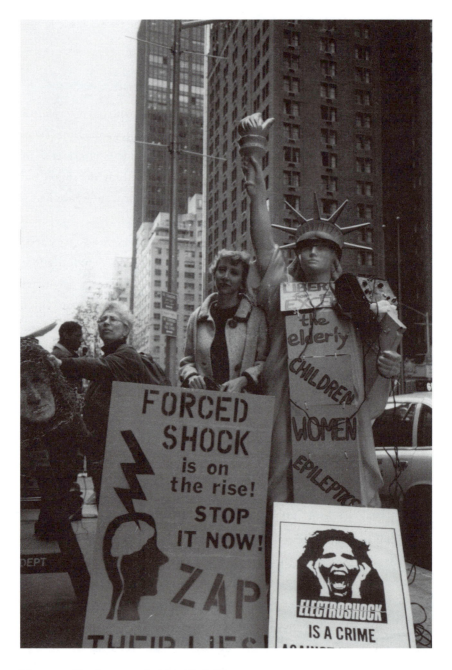

Figure 6. Shock protest in New York City, 1991.
(Reproduced courtesy of Michael Susko.)

However, after the reporters and photographers had left, her depression returned again, and again. She has quietly had at least two more courses of shock, leaving her with memory function so poor she's grateful to be able to read a newspaper.[26]

Anne Donahue's eloquent descriptions of amnesia were just like mine, just like Marilyn Rice's and so many others', but were acceptable to the industry because of this disclaimer: "I remain unflagging in my belief that the electroconvulsive therapy I received in the fall of 1995 and then the spring of 1996 . . . may have saved not just my mental health, but my life. If I had the decision to make again, I would choose ECT over a life condemned to psychic agony, and possible suicide."[27]

But in fact ECT didn't save her from psychic agony; like Manning's, her depression returned after ECT.[28]

It is important to note that expressions of gratitude do more than prop up shock doctors' self-esteem; they may ward off costly legal challenges to the practice of uninformed consent. In Donahue's state of Vermont, if a patient states after the fact that she would have consented even had she been given truthful information, she may not sue for lack of informed consent. However, in most states, retroactive consent is not legal.

For some patients with catastrophic losses, saying they would have chosen the losses may be an attempt to salvage the autonomy and dignity denied to them in the consent process, and to reassert control over their lives. (And to the degree that they are rewarded professionally and/or financially for their statement, it may actually result in greater control.)

However, none of these patients (and none of the hundreds I have met or read about) has ever expressed gratitude for being lied to. Not one has ever said, even in retrospect, that she or he preferred being deceived to being truthfully informed.

Far from justifying paternalistic lies, grateful patients who say they would have chosen shock's adverse effects of their own free will show the lies, in their cases, to have been unnecessary. The lies aren't for them; they are for the vast majority who the industry fears would say no if told the truth. The lies are for the good of the industry, not the patient. They fail every test for justifiable paternalistic lies.

Patient gratitude serves many of the needs of psychiatrists: to feel useful and needed; to have their competence affirmed; to relate to their patients in other than a mechanical way as objects; to resolve any lingering reservations about deception or coercion. This is why "grateful" ECT patients are practically canonized. But as ECT survivor Dr. Sylvia Caras reminds us in a treatise on the complex meanings of gratitude in psychiatric patients: "We should not determine the needs of others by our own needs."[29]

First, Listen

The guiding principle of medicine has long been held to be "First, do no harm." On the front cover of Max Fink's book on the ethics of ECT is a quote Fink attributes to Hippocrates: "I will use treatment to help the sick according to my ability and judgment, but I will never use it to injure or wrong them."[30]

But how is a doctor to determine whether he is harming, or has harmed his patients? Is there any other way than by listening to them? Isn't refusing to listen, and dismissing what one hears despite one's unwillingness to listen, itself a profoundly moral choice? It has harmful consequences for individuals, society, and science.

Fink starts his moral discussion from the presumption that ECT has no permanent adverse effects and only trifling, rare, temporary ones. He then proceeds as if the only moral issue is that ECT is not used enough or sooner or more; also that the stigma against it is unfair. He praises the use of coerced and involuntary ECT, saying that it is often unethical *not* to use shock against a person's will.

But you can't base a valid argument about ethics and morals on false premises. Fink's presumption is false, a lie maintained over the years as all lies are: by moral choices. All evidence that is contrary to what he has long ago decided to believe (and has taught to countless others) is ignored or dismissed. The experiences of Marilyn Rice and Anne Donahue are mentioned in Fink's book, but he gets the basic facts about their lives wrong and then dismisses them in two paragraphs.

What of the physician's duty—his or her moral responsibility—to attend to, to listen to, patients, especially when the patient says something other than "Thank you, doctor?" There is a moral perspective that can recognize that a physician's responsibility to a patient involves more than treating the person as a diagnosis or an object, and that his or her responsibility doesn't end with the last shock. Like the different ways of knowing discussed in Chapter Eleven, there are different moral orientations associated with men and women, say feminist scholars.[31] Whether or not this is true in the world at large, I have seen ample evidence in the world of shock, where the female point of view is nearly nonexistent.

Fink's book is written entirely from the *justice* perspective. This is moral decision making based on abstract principles, rules, or laws. All people are to be treated the same, regardless of their circumstances; that's justice, by this reckoning. Someone who reasons from this perspective doesn't ask, Who is this person? What does she want? He asks, What rule or principle should apply to our decision about what should be done to her? What does the law allow? From this perspective, it's not only unnecessary to listen to the patient, it's not necessary to get her consent. The only duty is to abstract principles. This sensibility is said to be predominantly male.

In contrast, a morality of *care* owes a duty to the individual and places her at the center of determining right and wrong for her. This perspective, more likely to be associated with women, focuses on nurturing, caring, maintaining relationships, and avoiding harm—including the harm that is always done to the patient and to the doctor/patient relationship by coercion, deception, or force.

From a care perspective, examples of wrongs would be trust betrayed, relationships damaged, people not being listened to, or not attending to those who've been harmed. This moral outrage is vividly portrayed in the accounts of both Rice and Donahue.

From a justice perspective, wrongs are violations of laws, principles, or protocols. What's right is what the authorities say. Think of a shock doctor on the witness stand, for instance, invoking the APA Task Force Report; nothing was done wrong as long as those guidelines were followed. I can still hear the voice of my own shock doctor at her deposition. Asked to account for her decisions, which destroyed my life, she never used the word "I," but only repeated in a mechanical voice, "It was the usual custom and practice of New York Hospital at the time. . . ."[32]

Rather than ask whether anyone was hurt and whether it could have been prevented, a justice perspective asks only if the usual rules were followed.

The act of not listening—even to the point of silencing, defaming, and personally attacking those who attempt to speak—may not be recognized as a conscious moral act by those who hold, or would hide behind, a justice perspective. Dismissing persons who experience permanent adverse effects from ECT as unable to accurately perceive reality has become as standard a part of the industry tool kit as rewarding those ex-patients who say they were pleased with the outcome of their treatment. Today the dismissal may go far beyond denying that a disastrous outcome was caused by ECT, as Dr. Nakamura did to me; it is a denial that anything really happened to the person at all. In this scenario, there is merely the person's "belief" that something happened, a belief with no validity because the person has no validity. Anyone with an M.D. or Ph.D. may claim authority over the facts of her life. Fifteen years after her death, Max Fink published an article claiming that Marilyn Rice (and others like her) imagined her amnesia because she was mentally ill.[33] And a recent book promoting ECT by denying any permanent amnesia accounts for Leonard Frank and Rice by saying that Frank "believed" his education had been wiped out, while Rice only "believed" she had lost her memory.[34]

When a shock doctor says or implies in print that a person he has never met (or who is no longer alive to defend herself) made up a story about having amnesia because she was crazy, that isn't a medical judgment or a professional opinion. It's plain old hate speech.

On the face of it, even if Rice or Frank, or any of us, actually had a psychiatric condition, there is no logical or medical reason why we couldn't experience permanent, extensive amnesia from ECT as well. But of course what the shock proponents really mean when they call us mentally ill, and what is always understood, is that we are liars. In disparaging the sanity and veracity of its former customers, the ECT industry exploits prejudice against mental patients in the the service of its own agenda, just as eugenicists and Nazis did in the early part of the twentieth century.

ECT survivors are justifiably and endlessly outraged by being told that we don't know what we know. If we are not competent to know what happened in our own lives, or the contents of our own minds, then what can we know? Quite simply, this is a global invalidation of the person. If empathy is the foundation of morality, it is a grave moral violation to invalidate another person's experience by denying that it ever happened. It's not only that the shock doctors lack empathy, remaining totally unmoved by the human suffering their treatment causes. They feel the need to go far beyond lack of empathy for their former patients—routinely heaping calumny on any of us who (as they see it) threatens their economic interests.

But the act of not listening has far greater consequences than the considerable hurt it causes those individuals who are not heard, who are ignored, who are called liars or crazy just for saying what happened to them. To close one's ears and mind to those who have been seriously harmed; not to listen, not to empathize, not to acknowledge, not to allow, not to publish: this is the opposite of, and the undermining of, real science and genuine medicine.

Paternalism versus Autonomy

We like to think we know what's best for our patients.

—Max Fink

The history of ECT is notable for men who were attracted to shock treatment and used it to take authoritarianism, sexism, and paternalism to unethical and even illegal extremes. Male ECT practitioners continue to be admitted to the pantheon that includes H. C. Tien and Gary Aden. For instance, there's Dr. Christian Hageseth III, who sold promotional videos in the 1990s for his own bizarre brand of "compassionate ECT" (it involved infantilizing patients by dressing them in cartoon-character gowns and giving them teddy bears to hold), lost his license for having sex with a patient, and then was prosecuted when he prescribed drugs over the Internet that led to another patient's suicide.[35] Ewen Cameron's misdeeds occurred in the 1950s but were only brought to light recently. In work funded by the CIA, he gave his subjects so many consecutive shock treatments that they forgot their entire lives, even their names, and had to be completely "reprogrammed."[36]

And then there is Max Fink, who has done more for the PR image of shock over his long lifetime than anyone else. He is an unabashed proponent of what he calls good old-fashioned paternalism. Fink has spent some time wrestling with the industry's fundamental PR problem: if shock doesn't cause any permanent memory loss or brain damage, if it only restores the mind as he claims, why do so many people report that it is damaging? Why do some oppose it and keep trying to get it banned? Why, despite his lifetime of effort, does it still—yes—sometimes get bad press?

Fink blames it on Vietnam. "The war made it very difficult for all the people in our country. We began to challenge all authority, not just the authority of our President and the Congress that had forced the war on people, but we also challenged the authority of physicians and medicine."[37]

In this way he's able to trivialize the movement against electroshock as nothing more than a fad, like bellbottoms—while unwittingly getting to the very heart of the matter. Yes, it is about challenging those in authority who make choices for us without our consent and without telling all they know. No, it has nothing to do with Vietnam.

There really is no compromise possible between those who want to reserve for themselves the right to decide when and whether other people can make their own decisions about what happens to their brains and bodies, and those who believe there is no qualifying that right for some people without endangering the rights of all people.

We are back to the fundamental question with which we started this book; the fundamental *moral* controversy that launched the public relations era in the first place. Do mental patients have the same rights as other human beings, including the right to say no?

Should Shock Be Banned?

The argument that electroshock sometimes helps people is in our view a non-valid argument. We live in a civilized society in which not all the things that help people are allowed, because some of them violate the ethical values of our society. For instance: hitting people may be very effective in the short run but is nevertheless not allowed. Lying to people may be very helpful but here again it is not in accordance with the ethical values of a civilized society. Our opinion is that electroshock should be banned for the same reason.

—Ed van Hoom, letter to the FDA

Even in a free world it is appropriate to issue warnings commensurate with the evidence. Warnings are what guarantee relative freedom.

—David Healy

ECT is currently banned in Slovenia, in some cantons of Switzerland, and in part of Italy. It was banned in the city of Berkeley, California, for forty-one days in 1982. The Vermont, California, West Virginia, Utah, Texas, Florida, and New Hampshire legislatures considered full or partial bans. Several states ban the use of ECT on children.

Americans like to say proudly, "It's a free country." And yet we in the United States ban an ever-growing list of behaviors and procedures that cannot be made safe, like driving without a seat belt, or while talking on a hand-held cell phone, or after too many martinis. Why do smokers now stand huddled, shivering on street corners in the dead of winter when they'd much rather be inside with an ashtray on their table? Because freedom is not absolute. Because the price of their freedom to smoke (to *knowingly* choose to endanger their own health) is not to endanger the health of others.

In the case of ECT, a minority of the people who get it may be helped to feel better temporarily and an even fewer number of these may by virtue of their own personal circumstances or temperament not mind the degree of permanent memory loss or cognitive disability they experience—but only at the cost of serious permanent harm to a majority of patients who are either not helped at all or only so fleetingly that they may not even remember it. And as the FDA letters tell us, when people are disabled by ECT's effects the cost is always multiplied by more than one: teachers no longer teach, nurses no longer nurse, families become strangers and break up.

In short, those people desperate for temporary relief from depression cannot have a chance for a brief respite at the cost of permanent disability for others, even if they escape or don't mind such devastation themselves.

Anne Donahue believes ECT might have saved her life. What would have happened to her if she hadn't had shock but had other treatment or no treatment, no one can know. But what can be shown is that ECT has caused many people to die who would not otherwise have died, those who suffered heart attacks or strokes or brain hemorrhages from shock. It can also be shown that people kill themselves after ECT just as much as or more than people who haven't had it, and that some of those who did made it clear that ECT's effects or fear of further ECT was the reason they had chosen to end their lives. Ernest Hemingway, who could no longer write after ECT erased his memory, is only the most famous example.

Even knowing all this, some people would choose to have ECT, as some choose to smoke. But people aren't allowed to know. This is the strongest argument that ECT is immoral, and it makes a ban not only deeply consistent with the American values of freedom, choice, and autonomy, but the only way—at this point in history and given the choices the industry has made— to protect those values.

Truthful informed consent would be another way, if it were possible. It seemed, back in the 1980s, as if it were. Marilyn Rice used to say, "I'm not against shock." She'd pause a beat to let that sink in, in case her listener had read somewhere in the media that the Committee for Truth in Psychiatry was an "anti-ECT" organization. Then she'd say, "I'm against *lying* about shock."

Rice died in 1992 no closer to her goal of truthfully informed consent. In some ways the situation for patients has gotten worse as the industry PR complex has grown bigger, more powerful, and more brazen. The triumph of PR over science these last thirty years seems absolute and irreversible.

There is no way to make shock safe, there is no way to warn people that it isn't safe, and so it must be banned.

17   *Where Do We Go from Here?*

Despite the success of the public relations campaign, the battles over shock, primarily between doctors and patients, show no sign of subsiding. There are some subtle but hopeful signs that people who have experienced ECT and those who have the critical thinking skills to see through the industry propaganda may yet shift the balance in favor of truth and science.

The saga of the ECT device at the FDA is not over, and there continues to be a role for ex-patients and the public to play in determining what happens next. The APA's petition to reclassify the ECT device languished in limbo for thirteen years following the FDA's proposal to grant it. The FDA neither reclassified nor rescinded its proposal. On April 22, 2003, the FDA quietly withdrew the proposed rule, simply because so much time had passed since it was issued.[1]

But it's not correct to say that nothing happened over those years. It did, but through the intervention of Congress, not the APA. The FDA was still under pressure to comply with its own laws requiring that untested, pre-1976 Class III devices eventually undergo the same scrutiny—premarket approval—as new devices. That a backlog of 189 devices remained that had neither been tested nor reclassified was an embarrassment to the agency.

Shortly after the FDA published its proposed rule to reclassify the ECT device, Congress passed the Safe Medical Devices Act of 1990 (SMDA). Its purpose, among other things, was to ease the FDA's burden of investigating the backlog of pre-1976 Class III devices by making it easier to reclassify them. Frustrated by the inability of any manufacturer of a Class III device to come up with a "performance standard" as required for Class II status, the FDA had dropped that requirement in the new law. Now, all that was needed to reclassify to Class II were "special controls." Special controls could include a standard, but didn't have to. They were somewhat loosely defined and included labeling, guidelines, recommendations, and postmarket surveillance. The last aimed at shifting the responsibility of ensuring device safety from the FDA onto doctors and the public (in FDA-speak, from premarket to postmarket). The new law set up a registry, called MedWatch, through which doctors and patients could report, after the fact, serious adverse outcomes from medical devices. But neither doctors (who are legally required to report) nor the public are generally even aware the program exists, and only a small fraction of bad outcomes are reported. The database does contain reports about ECT devices.

The SMDA established deadlines for the FDA to meet in making final rulings on the remaining Class III devices. All of them had to be either reclassified to Class II or I, or, if they were to remain in Class III, the FDA was required to call for premarket approval applications (PMAs). The devices were divided up into groups according to how suitable the FDA thought they were for reclassification. The ECT device was placed in Group 2, those the FDA considered "strong candidates" for Class II.

Section 515(b) of the Food, Drug and Cosmetics Act already required the FDA to call for PMAs on all devices remaining in Class III, but a new section, 515(i), established an intermediate step before calling for PMAs. Class III device manufacturers would now have to provide the FDA with all safety and effectiveness information known or available to them, specifically including adverse safety and effectiveness information.[2] Based on this information, the FDA would decide whether to reclassify to Class II.

On August 14, 1995, a 515(i) was issued for the ECT device and published in the Federal Register.[3] The manufacturers had two years, until the deadline of August 14, 1997, to submit the required data.

Here was the opportunity for which the shock industry had been waiting for years: a chance to get around the PMA procedure. If the manufacturers had submitted anything at all, no matter how half-baked, the FDA would surely have turned a blind eye to its inadequacies and reclassified the device. All they had to do was slap a response together; a few citations to Sackeim and Weiner, and the whole FDA mess would be over.

The manufacturers submitted nothing. They ignored the FDA's call.[4]

It wasn't supposed to be optional. By law, according to FDA counsel, the device should have been taken off the market. If manufacturers don't respond to a 515(i) they are not allowed to market their device, because it's considered a misbranded device.[5]

Nothing happened. The manufacturers weren't prosecuted. The devices continued to be sold. The manufacturers continued to develop fancier, pricier models, filed 510(k)s claiming they were equivalent to the pre-1976 models, and sold those.

The FDA had missed every deadline set by Congress and every timetable it set up for itself for dealing with the ECT device. By its own law, it couldn't stall forever, yet it was stuck. It had no basis for reclassification, but leaving the device in Class III was simply not an option, because the manufacturers had demonstrated that they could not (and more than that, *would* not) respond to a call for PMAs. What was the FDA to do? How could it avoid taking the ECT device off the market? Because that was simply unthinkable. The APA would never allow it.

Nor could the APA write and submit the PMA itself, standing in for the absent manufacturers as it had in filing its petition. Any person or organization can petition the FDA; only the manufacturer of a medical device can file a PMA, because an approved PMA is literally a license to market the device.

After it became clear to the FDA that the manufacturers were not interested in participating in the regulatory process, and clear to the manufacturers that the FDA was not willing to use the law to enforce their participation, the agency began trying to find a way out of its sticky situation. Its solution was unheard of: the FDA would take on the manufacturers' task of convincing the agency that their product was safe. It would do this, not by conducting safety studies or independent scientific investigations, but by picking through the published articles on ECT in a selective literature review—the same tactic it had used to justify granting the APA's petition.

In the words of Steve Hinckley of the FDA's Office of Science and Technology in the summer of 2000: "We'll just do another literature review and reclassify." Toward that end, the agency convened an internal committee, as it had in 1988, to review the literature. But this was very different from the task of deciding a petition. This was a case of the agency (historically lacking in the initiative to do even the minimum that it is required to do by law) allocating its inadequate resources to do something it didn't have to do.

Does the FDA have the legal authority to reclassify a device on its own initiative, without a petition from the manufacturer or anyone else, without any submission of evidence from the manufacturer, on the sole basis of data it has sought out and selected for the purpose of supporting a reclassification? I asked this question of device evaluator Steve Hinckley and never received an answer.[6]

I then framed the question a little bit differently. Has the FDA ever before reclassified any medical device on the basis of nothing but its own selective literature review? This time, I got an answer: a clear no. A selective literature review does not meet the FDA standard for "valid scientific evidence," upon which reclassification must be based.

I asked another FDA official if the agency had ever reclassified any other medical device in the complete absence of any submission from its manufacturer. The man who answered me had been at the FDA for over twenty-five years. He thought for a while, and then said no, he'd never known of any such case.[7]

A Stone Wall, and a New Petition

Phone calls and letters to the FDA asking for information on the proposed reclassification went unanswered for nearly a year. Because organized ex-patients had no names of anyone directly involved, we had written to everyone in a position to know about medical devices, including the FDA director. We didn't get any acknowledgment, not even a brush-off letter, from anyone. This would be understandable, if deplorable, if we had written to a private corporation. But this was our government—unacceptable.

Meanwhile, I discovered that Max Fink's protégé Laura Fochtmann had been appointed an independent consultant to the FDA's Neurological Devices Advisory Panel. Any proposed reclassification of the shock machine would have to be reviewed by this panel, and the FDA generally does what the panel tells it to do. The ECT industry was anticipating such a proposal and was ready for it.

But Fochtmann should have been disqualified from serving on the panel once she revealed her career conflict of interest due to her position on the APA ECT Task Force, inherited from Fink, as well as any financial ties she may have had to the manufacturers. Clearly, a person in a key position of authority in a group with a twenty-year history of lobbying for reclassification should not serve on the panel that would decide on reclassification. By law, the FDA is supposed to screen panel members for potential ethical conflicts, and can disqualify those with such conflicts. This means that either Fochtmann failed to disclose her work for the APA, or the FDA allowed her to serve despite her conflict of interest.

On December 10, 2003, the Committee for Truth in Psychiatry filed a new citizen petition with the FDA. The petition, given the docket number 2003P-0555, asks the FDA to maintain the ECT device in Class III for all indications. In support are appended six hundred pages of evidence overlooked by the FDA in its previous selective literature review, as well as new evidence of the risks and lack of efficacy of the device. As with the APA's petition, this one serves as a vehicle for any interested person to comment on the safety and efficacy of ECT. All comments become a public record.

The FDA did not go so far as to grant the petition, but claimed in a letter of September 3, 2004, that "the agency has no plans to reclassify the electro-convulsive therapy device at this time."[8]

Yet the agency cannot leave it there. For two decades, the FDA has never wavered from its intent to declare the ECT device safe without a safety investigation. There is no reason to think it has changed its mind now. The law is still clear that the FDA has only two options: call for PMAs, or reclassify. To do the former will unleash the full fury of the ECT industry upon the beleaguered agency. To do the latter is to abdicate its responsibility to protect patients in favor of a powerful special interest. We have seen, historically, what happens when the interests of psychiatrists and mental patients collide.

The Good News

It is possible to end this complex, long, sad history on a note of hope for the future. That wouldn't happen if we ended the story in the United States, where the industry has an iron grip on research funding, the "scientific literature," the media, and the government.

In the United Kingdom there is no shortage of proponents of ECT, but they lack, at least as far as anyone can tell, the same crude financial ties that motivate the main players in the United States. The Royal College of

Psychiatrists is that country's equivalent of the APA. Like the APA, they issue guidelines on the use of ECT. Their 1995 "Fact Sheet on ECT" assured patients that ECT is safe, effective, and sometimes life-saving. It claimed that "people . . . report that it makes them feel 'like themselves again' or that 'life is worth living,' " and that "memory loss goes away within a few days or weeks although some patients continue to experience memory problems for several months. As far as we know, electroconvulsive therapy does not have any long term effects on your memory or intelligence."[9]

Their Institute of Psychiatry is roughly analogous to our NIMH, a prestigious research institute funded by the government. But it has a component NIMH lacks—the Service User Research Enterprise (SURE). (Service users is the British term for consumers, survivors, or plain old mental patients.) In 2001, as a part of a larger review of medical treatments by the British government, SURE was commissioned to review "consumers' perspectives" on ECT. The government specifically requested a systematic review. Two of the researchers who worked on the report had experienced ECT themselves. Others providing input or consultation were psychiatrists (including ECT enthusiast Chris Freeman), patient advocacy groups (of which there are many in the United Kingdom), and academics.

A systematic review of the literature on what patients say about ECT had never been done before. Unlike the selective reviews so beloved by ECT proponents, which choose between studies in order to support a predetermined viewpoint, this one had to include all existing studies. But because of the nature of their topic, they went way beyond that. They included in their review all the firsthand accounts of ECT they could find: on Internet sites, in public testimony, in print media, and on video.

Amazingly, in the U.K. three patient advocacy groups had conducted surveys on ECT that included large numbers of former patients.[10] While a clinical research study on ECT typically includes about a dozen people (it's unusual to find more than twenty-five), each of these surveys included two to four hundred people, providing a much broader picture than could possibly be found in even a busy research facility that might shock fifty people in a year.

And while SURE found only seven research studies that follow up ECT patients even as long as six months, probably because of the presumption that the adverse effects of ECT resolve quickly, many of the people in the British surveys were years postshock. Putting these surveys together with the data from the small group of clinical studies that passed methodological muster yielded a far different picture than that painted by the Royal College.

Although the review did not set out to study memory, memory loss quickly established itself as the main theme of all the literature: "In all types of information gathered for the Review it is evident that memory loss is a persistent side-effect for at least one third of recipients of ECT. For some, this memory loss profoundly affects their lives and sense of self."[11]

The one-third was not an average of all studies; in most of the evidence, the percentages were higher, far higher. The reviewers were being very cautious, instead taking the lowest number they could find in the professional literature as a floor or lowest estimate of permanent amnesia. By doing this, while adding "at least" to convey that more loss is possible, they made their conclusion unassailable.

The report makes clear that the amount of time permanently lost is not limited to the weeks or months immediately before ECT, as generations of patients have been told: "Many people describe how several years of their lives and occasionally as much as 15–20 years have been wiped from their memory, whether or not they feel helped by ECT."

SURE found no evidence of any long-lasting or permanent benefit from ECT in the studies or testimony by former patients.

Another major conclusion that emerged from the review was that voluntary and informed consent to ECT is an illusion. At least half of the former patients did not receive adequate information about ECT before having it, and they specifically related this to not being informed about permanent amnesia. One patient quoted described "being like a baby, waiting for the never to be realized promise that your memory will come back after a couple of months."

Involuntary ECT is a reality in England (where 20 percent of patients are shocked by force) as well as in the United States, but court orders are not the only effective way to force unwilling patients into "consenting" to shock. One-fifth to one-half of ECT patients, depending on which study results you look at, felt they had no choice but to sign for ECT because of coercion, threats, or an overwhelming sense of helplessness and powerlessness. MIND, England's largest mental health charity, whose survey of 418 former patients was included by SURE, put it this way: "It seems difficult to understand how, in such circumstances, people can be said to have 'consented' to treatment."

British Survivors Make History

These findings from the eighty-five-page report made their way into the mainstream scientific literature with the publication of two summary articles: in the *British Medical Journal* in June 2003, and the *British Journal of Psychiatry* in 2005.[12] And so the pooled knowledge of former patients, so long denied and dismissed as anecdotal, now counts as science.

In 2004 another historic study, co-authored by Diana Rose, was published in the *Journal of Mental Health*.[13] It was the first prospective study ever to utilize a questionnaire designed by persons who'd experienced ECT. In a prospective study, subjects are chosen before ECT and then followed up at some later time. Usually, the subjects are all the people who have ECT at a particular hospital during a chosen time frame. But by definition, survivors of ECT don't have access to hospitalized patients, which makes a prospective study impossible unless professionals and institutions agree to collaborate. This had never before happened.

This study was done by the "user" group Communicate at London's Maudsley Hospital. They designed a questionnaire to assess former patients' views on their satisfaction (or lack thereof) with ECT and the adverse effects experienced. This was the first published study where people were asked whether ECT had caused loss of intelligence, and 40 percent of them said yes. Forty-five percent reported permanent memory loss.

That the findings of this prospective study confirm the results of the retrospective studies suggests that the findings are robust and not the result of sampling bias. And the results of all the studies are consistent when former patients are asked about coercion as well. About a third of the people in the Communicate study said they felt forced to "consent" to ECT even though they were not legally compelled.

Having asked for information from ECT patients, the British government had to act on it. In April 2003, its National Institute for Clinical Excellence

(NICE), a part of the National Health Service that evaluates health-care technology, issued a report on ECT. Its conclusion was that, given its risks, the use of ECT should be limited. The report specifically notes:

> It was apparent that the nature of cognitive impairment experienced by users was variable and often long lasting to such a degree that it ⁻ outweighed any perception of benefit from ECT treatment. . . . It [the Committee which authored the report] was also concerned that the potential for cognitive impairment following ECT be highlighted during the consent process. These factors featured significantly in the Committee's deliberations, and specifically in its decision to restrict the use of ECT to situations where all other alternatives have been exhausted or where the nature of the mental illness was considered to be "life-threatening."[14]

However, the report leaves it up to the individual doctor to decide what patients should be told about cognitive impairment. In addition, NICE also noted that there is no evidence of the usefulness of ECT in schizophrenia, or as a maintenance treatment, and that its usefulness in depression is limited to the short term.

The industry was furious. In the United States, Richard Weiner's protégé W. Vaughn McCall, in specific protest against what he called NICE's "sharp restrictions," churned out a quick study (using NIMH money) designed to show that ECT improves "quality of life." But he had to set the bar so low to ensure the results he wanted—for instance, asking whether patients could go to the toilet by themselves as a measure of life quality—that the results were unintentionally comical and likely unavailing.[15] Royal College psychiatrist Chris Freeman led an appeal of the NICE decision, claiming it was "perverse." The report was upheld.

The Royal College, bound by the findings of an agency of the British government, decided to delay and rewrite its own forthcoming ECT guidelines. In Britain, the previously unthinkable had happened: hundreds of ECT survivors, speaking as one about severe and permanent shock damage, had forced the government and the industry to hear us.

However, it is premature to say the industry is listening. When the Royal College of Psychiatrists issued a revised edition of its ECT handbook for practitioners in 2005, its recommendations were contradictory and confusing.[16] The chapter on "Adverse Effects of ECT" assured readers (without any supporting evidence whatsoever) that "ability to learn new information and non-memory cognitive functions (intelligence, judgment, abstraction, etc.) are not affected." It also warranted that ECT amnesia is "reversible," though "a small proportion of people complain of persisting memory difficulty." The author of this chapter left out all the new British survivor research; of her sixteen citations, all but three were to financially conflicted American shock doctors.

Yet in other places the new ECT handbook advises psychiatrists "to be particularly careful to discuss the topic of retrograde amnesia" and strongly recommends that "the possibility of both short-term and long-term cognitive impairment" be discussed with the patient and family. And the suggested consent form—much less chatty than the APA's—tells patients that memory loss, "possibly permanent," is one of ECT's "serious/frequently occurring risks."

In the face of the new reports, when it issued an updated information leaflet for patients in 2007 the Royal College simply gave up on trying to sell ECT as a treatment based on science. Instead, it seemed to be saying, what's true about ECT depends on whom you choose to believe. Different "opinions" or "views" are presented in a way that seems, at least in spots, more honest about the adverse effects: "People against ECT say it 'works' by concussing and damaging the brain. . . . Those in favour of ECT say it is an effective treatment, especially for severe depression." But no evidence is given in support of these claims. Instead, ECT is presented as a topic on which people simply disagree strongly, and the prospective patient given no basis for deciding what to believe: "There are many areas of disagreement about ECT, including whether it should even be used at all. The main areas of disagreement are over whether it works, how it works and what the side effects are." The permanence of memory loss, the leaflet says, is one of many areas that are "not clear."

Beyond Denial

There are signs that it is becoming possible for professionals to move beyond denial of ECT's permanent adverse effects, toward not only acknowledgment of damage but help for ECT survivors. In 2006 and 2007, the British journal *Advances in Psychiatric Treatment* (put out by the Royal College of Psychiatrists) published two groundbreaking articles on ECT. The first, by Americans Harold Robertson and Robin Pryor, incorporates the voices of survivors (from the FDA files and the British studies) into a discussion of the different types of memory and cognitive disability caused by shock.[17] The authors further discuss how best to assess these deficits with the type of neuropsychological tests used on persons who have experienced other types of brain injury. They criticize the tests commonly used by ECT proponents as much too simple and not relevant to ECT. Finally, they propose a model of informed consent that describes rather than denies what we know.

> Patients can be told that permanent amnesia is one of the "common" (Sackeim, 2000) or "serious/frequently occurring" (Royal College of Psychiatrists, 2005) effects of ECT and that it affects at least one-third of patients (SURE, 2002; Rose *et al.*, 2003). Such amnesia may be presented as having multiple dimensions: the amount of life lost, the temporal gradient, the nature of what is lost, and the effect of memory erasure on the individual's life. The amount of life lost to amnesia cannot be predicted; patients should be warned that it has been known to extend to 10–20 years (Pedler, 2001; SURE, 2002). It should be made clear that amnesia is not limited to information about discrete events or to facts that are easily regained, such as dates and telephone numbers, but that it encompasses all thoughts, feelings, personal interactions and relationships, learning and skills associated with the erased time period, and thus there is no simple or easy way to recapture what is lost. Since the temporal gradient of ECT amnesia is the opposite of normal forgetting, patients should be warned that the most recent months or years will be most affected.

The authors say that true informed consent must include warnings about permanent cognitive disability as well. "Patients should be clearly told that ECT may have serious and permanent effects on both memory ability and non-memory cognition. These are best described in everyday terms: 'the ability to plan and organise and get things done' rather than 'executive function.' Intact memory and intelligence are highly prized in our culture. The more valuable a possession, the more important it is to know about even a small chance that it may be permanently lost."

The next year, Maeve Mangaoang and Jim Lucey (a psychologist and psychiatrist from Ireland) built on Robertson and Pryor's work in the first article ever published to address the issue of how best to help rehabilitate those who suffer memory and cognitive disability: "Cognitive rehabilitation techniques that are used with brain-injured patients should also be considered for use with patients experiencing memory and/or cognitive disability following ECT."[18] I've described in Chapter Eleven the efforts of myself and other survivors to access neuropsychological testing and the type of rehabilitation they describe. These authors propose that ECT providers should be the ones to initiate such referrals; Robertson and Pryor say this is unlikely to happen due to their fears of being held personally liable for damages. It is not clear that the very real unmet need of ECT survivors for assessment and treatment of brain injury will ever take precedence over these concerns. Mangaoang and Lucey's article seems destined for the oblivion that has befallen virtually every published article critical of ECT. Nevertheless, their conclusions deserve to be widely disseminated.

> What is striking from the literature in this area is the lack of routine, formal assessment of patients' neuropsychological performance following a course of ECT, despite the long-known risk to memory function. . . . All patients should undergo cognitive assessment before their first ECT session. . . . Reassessment should be scheduled after a sufficiently long interval (more than 6 months after treatment) so that persistent cognitive and memory deficits can be identified. . . . It should now be clear that documenting neuropsychological deficits is not enough; a specific programme of cognitive rehabilitation should be designed and made available to all patients following ECT, and details about this treatment should be included with the information that patients receive prior to treatment. . . . Cognitive rehabilitation following ECT offers a constructive way of treating and managing the most common side-effect, which is currently left untreated. Over time, this acknowledgment of the presence and impact of

cognitive disability in ECT-treated patients, together with the education of patients, families and mental health professionals about ways to deal with these difficulties, would lead to better overall adjustment by patients and the development of a new sense of self.

Denial of, and withholding help for, injuries caused by ECT is not only bad for patients, they argue, but ironically ends up subverting industry PR as well. "Failure to attempt to rehabilitate patients may reinforce the negative public image of ECT specifically and psychiatry in general."

The Search for the Holy Grail Continues

Although there is absolutely no suggestion from the SURE work or other reports that anyone's ECT was done improperly, or that any adverse effect corresponds in any way to how or when ECT was done, and although persons who had ECT with all types of techniques and in all eras report the same damages, the Royal College is grasping at the only straw left to it.

Rather than draw the obvious logical conclusion—permanent memory loss and cognitive disability happens when you put electricity through the brain and it cannot be prevented—they borrowed a page from the American PR book. The problem, they decided, must be that ECT just wasn't done right. The solution was to raise the standards, and teach everyone to do it correctly, and check up on them to see if they were doing so. It wasn't that ECT causes damage, only that poorly performed ECT might do so.

The counterargument is quite simple. It's this book; it's history. As we have seen, such a claim has been made over and over since the very early days of ECT. And each so-called refinement or modification of the shock box or the electrode placement or the accompanying drugs and anesthesia has failed to eradicate the serious, permanent adverse effects. The simple reality of biology and neuroanatomy won't be fooled.

What is the Royal College's solution? Unilateral ECT, invented back in the 1940s and abandoned: "The balance between immediate benefit and longer term risk of distressing retrograde amnesia can be moved in favor of benefit by the use of unilateral ECT." It noted that "many practitioners in the UK were sceptical about unilateral treatment because of earlier experiences of limited efficacy," but went on to suggest, citing Sackeim, that this only meant the electricity hadn't been turned up high enough before.[19]

It also set up a new program to audit and monitor ECT, called the ECT Accreditation Service (ECTAS), and invited hospitals to sign up (for a fee). ECTAS, a project of the Royal College's Research Unit, has its own ECT guidelines. Compliance is entirely voluntary, but the idea is that the guidelines are supposed to ensure good outcomes. A brochure for the service asserts, "If ECT is ever legislated against or falls into disuse it will not be because it is an ineffective or dangerous treatment, it will be because [of a failure] to supervise and monitor it correctly."[20] The guidelines provide no clues as to what patients are to be told about the nature and frequency of ECT's risks, other than that "consent is to be obtained by a psychiatrist with adequate knowledge of the nature and effects of ECT."

After generations of denial of these effects and their nature by organized psychiatry on both sides of the Atlantic, where would that psychiatrist be found?

The Inevitable Conclusion

Perhaps the most important lesson is that we do not have enough of the right kind of evidence to resolve the debate over the appropriate contemporary use of ECT. One desirable outcome would be the instigation of relevant collaborative research between patients and prescribers into the short-and medium-term benefits and risks of ECT in depressive illness. This would be in everyone's best interests, but only time will tell whether it happens.

—Dr. A.I.F. Scott[21]

This statement by the editor of the latest Royal College ECT Handbook, while admirable in its call for collaborative research, leaves the reader wondering: What is *enough* information? What is the *right kind*? Who is this *we* who gets to decide these things?

If history tells us anything, it is that answers to these questions cannot be left to those with a financial, professional, or career stake in the procedure. Those of us who had everything—our brains, memories, intellects, and lives—at stake, and lost, say that seventy years is enough and that the "right kind of evidence" is and always has been all around us.

If any other medical treatment had admittedly been done incorrectly for seventy years (while, at periodic junctures, the manufacturers and users of the equipment had proclaimed "Now we know how to do it!" and been proven wrong) . . .

If the manufacturers and users had admitted, after seven decades, that they still didn't know how to do it, and meanwhile seven decades of accumulated evidence showed that large numbers of patients had been harmed, permanently disabled, or killed . . .

What would we, as a society, do?

Would we say to the doctors, "OK, keep trying everything that hasn't worked in the past. We'll be your guinea pigs"?

Would we say nothing and look away, betting our lives that the treatment will never be used on us but only on people who don't matter quite so much?

Would we let it be used for another lifetime?

Epilogue

> The challenge [in writing history] is to get the reader beyond thinking
> that things had to be the way they turned out and to see the range of pos-
> sibilities of how it could have been otherwise.
>
> —David McCullough

Even in a book this long, so much has had to be left out. For this I apologize
to those whose stories got told only in passing or not at all. I had difficult
choices to make. Two of the most important stories left out were those of
the citywide ban on shock in Berkeley, California, in 1982, and the period
from 1991 to 1993 when shock was nearly banned in Texas. I chose to focus on
Vermont instead of Texas because I had more primary source material available to me, and had been more directly involved in the legislative process in
Vermont. My choice throughout the book was to focus on one typical
example in great depth (such as the Thomas case) as a way of better understanding a great big important issue (forced shock).

One might reasonably conclude from this book that there is little hope of
protecting persons who end up one way or another at the wrong end of a shock
machine from the tragedy of permanent brain damage and disability. After all,
a theme in the history of electroshock is that it repeats itself over and over. The
same lines, the same actors, the same plot; shock is "new" in 1945 and in 1985 and
in 2005; the New York legislature becomes Texas becomes Vermont.

And yet, another theme is the central and unpredictable role played by
individual personalities, personalities drawn into the shock issue either by
personal proclivity or horribly bad luck. Anne Donahue couldn't have been
made up or foreseen. And as the industry czars age and pass on—in the trans-
fer of power from Fink to Fochtmann, Sackeim to Lisanby—the ground will
shift slightly, or not so slightly.

The ground trembled in 2007, with the publication of Sackeim's article
finally admitting that ECT routinely causes substantial permanent memory

deficits. Meanwhile, the "comeback of ECT" campaign has entered its thirtieth year. The first comeback article of 2008 contained one sentence obliquely referring to the article: "Cognitive problems from ECT may be more problematic than was recognized even 10 years ago."[1] But nothing else in the PR script has changed. Sackeim's admission may be too little, too late to make a difference for patients.

The prestigious journal that published his article, *Neuropsychopharmacology*, did not reveal that Sackeim had been paid by Mecta while conducting this research. That wouldn't be surprising, except that the editor of the journal had just been forced to resign after a firestorm of publicity over his and other authors' undisclosed financial conflicts.[2] That firestorm had been building for years.

Since about 2001, I and so many others have watched in amazement as a few dedicated individuals took the psychiatric drug industry, and much of medicine as we know it, to task. Slowly but steadily, they've exposed the fraud and deception that looks so much like that of the shock industry: the financial dirty dealings of those pretending to be objective researchers, including those we trust with our taxpayer dollars at NIMH; scientists skewing their research any way they like through fraudulent design and withholding data without, until now, anyone ever knowing about it; respected medical journals publishing articles without revealing that authors had financial interests in the companies whose products they researched; peer review that was supposed to ensure the scientific integrity of published research but in reality was often little more than an old boys' network. The Food and Drug Administration, supposedly the watchdog of public health, was revealed to be as corrupt and pro-industry as all the other stakeholders in the enterprise. In short, none of the safeguards we assumed were protecting the public from shoddy science and deadly products were working, and people were being needlessly hurt and killed as a result.

At first there were just a few voices, most notably those of Vera Sharav and David Healy, then others joined until there was such a groundswell that the media got hold of it and didn't let go. There was so much dirty laundry; it made a great big juicy story because the pharmaceutical industry is so big and so powerful, and almost everybody knows someone on psychiatric drugs.

I would never have believed this could happen, but in the U.K., their equivalent of the FDA banned most psychiatric drugs for children, citing the lack of evidence that the drugs work, combined with research—previously suppressed by the drug makers—showing they increase the risk of suicide and violent behavior. And in the United States on October 15, 2004, the FDA ruled that antidepressant drugs must be labeled with a "black box" warning that they have been shown to increase the risk of suicide in children and adolescents. (Three years later, after examining more data, it extended that warning to young adults up to age twenty-five.)[3]

After a spate of bad publicity about financially conflicted researchers, the National Institutes of Health (which includes NIMH) instituted new rules forbidding its employees from taking money from drug or biotech companies. Although at this time the prohibition applies only to those working directly for NIH, and not those like Sackeim who contract with it through grants, there is no logical or ethical reason why grantees should be allowed to be compromised by industry money. And in fact, in 2007 the U.S. Department of Health and Human Services began a review of NIH's conflict-of-interest policies for extramural scientists.[4]

The message of this book that NIMH and the FDA (and much of what passes for scientific research) are rotten to the core has been borne out time and time again, yet the spotlight has been only on drugs, rarely devices, and certainly not on shock.

The parallels to the shock industry are obvious. As will be the differences: shock is "only" a five billion dollar industry compared to the thirty billion drug industry; nearly all the research is funded by NIMH or a couple of private foundations, not by the shock machine companies themselves directly, so it's harder to see how it is financially conflicted; and most importantly, though psychiatric drug use has been normalized to some extent over the years—as long as it's outpatient and is "only" for depression or anxiety—those of us who've had shock are still the pariahs of the mental patient world, thought to have deserved or needed what we got, incapable of being damaged since we had nothing to lose anyway.

Calls for reforms to alleviate the "unprecedented crisis of credibility" caused by financial conflicts in medicine, and in particular in psychiatry, are now unstoppable.[5] Many of these reforms, if implemented—such as giving priority to independent researchers for federal grant money, for medical journal editorship positions, and in practice guidelines groups such as the APA Task Force on ECT—could make it impossible for the shock industry to continue business as usual.

What happened with drugs could happen with shock, following the same script—this is obvious. Whether it will depends on a hundred unpredictable variables such as luck, timing, quirks of place and personality. (For instance, David Healy, who led the crusade against drug industry deceit, is a staunch ally of Max Fink's. The book that Healy co-wrote with Edward Shorter and Fink denies that ECT has ever caused any permanent adverse effects, and doesn't reveal the financial conflicts of any of the ECT promoters.) What's needed, as always, are just a few individuals who care enough to put what's right before everything else, who are willing to make personal sacrifices of time and resources, and who won't give up.

For those individuals, five years from now or fifty, this book will be an invaluable resource. Now that we know this history, now that what mostly hadn't been written is written down in one place, maybe—just maybe—we can keep from repeating it. One thing is for certain: there will continue to be opportunities for the history of electroshock to take a new turn. And though it won't happen in my lifetime, the history will one day be only that—a history and not a present or future; a past our grandchildren will look back on in shame and horror.

Appendix: Letters from FDA Docket No. 82P-0316

The following is a small representative selection from the hundreds of letters sent to the FDA by former ECT patients to assist the agency in assessing the procedure's risks and benefits. FDA Docket No. 82P-0316 is the largest and most detailed public database on ECT's effects.

I was a patient at University Hospital, Denver, Colorado, from early January to March 22, 1989. I was given 12 treatments and allowed to come home. A few days later, I was so desperate to get relief from anxiety and depression that I nearly died by a suicide attempt. I was asked to sign permission for further ECT. . . . I had 20 electroshock treatments and I regret very much my decision to have *any* of the treatments.

I had to retire from part-time work as a paraprofessional in a local high school and I doubt I will ever be able to work again. I have forgotten how to weave, could not concentrate on anything, felt very little pleasure in life and still feel suicidal. I often don't remember people who speak to me, much of my past life is gone from my memory, I have cognitive thinking problems, fear being in any social situation, cannot spell, cannot remember factual information, and lead a rather hermit-like existence.

I believe I have permanent brain damage as a result of ECT and I do not think I will ever again be as intelligent a person as I was before the electroshock treatments. . . .

Sincerely,

Theresa G. Blumen

C450, June 14, 1990

As a former recipient of ECT, I have ongoingly suffered from memory loss. In addition to destruction of entire blocks of pre-ECT memories, I have continued to have considerable difficulty in memory recall with regard to academic pursuits.

To date, of embarrassing necessity, I have been forced to tape-record all education materials that require memorization. This has included basic classes in accounting and word processing materials. . . .

Currently, I am finding it extremely embarrassing and hurtful when fellow classmates (however innocent) refer to my struggles in grasping my study materials, thusly: "You are an AIR-BRAIN!" How can I explain that my struggles are due to ECT?

As far as the loss of my childhood memories, I often feel as though a very vital part of my life "died" as a result of these treatments. In particular, when my family refers to specific earlier experiences, I feel a great sense of loss and grief because I cannot share their memories.

Felicia McCarty Winter

May 23, 1988

Nearly twenty years ago, I underwent 30 shock treatments at the Institute of Living in Hartford, Connecticut. As a result I lost two full years of memory. I have one child, a daughter, and the two years that were wiped out in my memory were the years when she was two and three years old; those memories are irreplaceable. . . . My memories are clear and detailed back to age 2 ¼. But when it comes to those two critical years before I received shock treatments, my mind remains a blank. . . .

As an advocate for over 8000 mental health clients in Maine, I do have contact with many former ECT recipients. I have met many others who have lost over 20 years' worth of memory; I have talked with others who, after shock treatments, were unable to resume their former work and lifestyles because of short term memory damage. I am convinced that brain damage from ECT treatments is not only common, but that it is the rule rather than the exception.

Sincerely,

Sally Clay

November 9, 1987

I had 19 shock treatments. I found out later that they were probably unnecessary and that I had severe thyroid and female hormone deficiencies. Needless to say the electric shocks didn't help my hormone deficiencies!

They did wreck my life however! I suffer severe memory loss which has never returned. It covers 8 to 10 years!

I also have a very deep inability to learn and comprehend things and this has led to problems with my own self understanding. It also has affected my relations with my own family and other people too.

Sincerely,

Dorothy Oimette

C230, January 29, 1988

The 2 years of college I had before the shocks was gone. All I had was a vague memory of my art professor when I looked at the painting I'd done hanging on my wall. So the shock doctors were not only barbaric—they were thieves, robbing me of the one thing in life that brought me the most satisfaction. From day 1 I had dreamed and fantasized of being a teacher—they were my role models. . . . I've been fired and asked to leave job after job in my profession due directly or indirectly to what was forced on me against my will . . . misdiagnosed, mistreated and now unable to perform I exist on less than $300.00 a mo. SS disability. If it weren't for the ECTs I'd have my master's or PhD and still be teaching. ECTs raped and robbed my brain. I'll go to my grave with this—the worst thing that ever happened to me in my whole life.

Betty Scoleri

May 1, 1986

I received over 20 ECTs when I was 17 years old . . . I was told the memories would come back in 6 weeks. I was told the shock treatments were no more powerful than the batteries in a flashlight. . . .

I lost 95% of all my memories before the treatment. They never came back. I went back to high school. I did not remember my fellow students. I could not find my classes. It was awful. To this day I look at the school year books hoping some of the pictures will spark a memory. I used to play the violin. I had won 2nd place in duets in the city of Cleveland. (The only reason I know this is because I have the medal in my drawer.) I could not remember how to play my violin after the first series of treatments. I was devastated. . . . My doctor kept saying that one more series would make me well. . . .

I have trouble with my memory today. I have been told I have permanent brain damage due to the ECT treatment. My IQ was 120 before treatments and it is not anywhere near that now. I have trouble just trying to cook a meal. I do not work. I make lists so that I can try to remember what I need to do.

ECTs changed my life forever—and not for the better. I wish no one would be given ECTs.

Sue Ann Kulcsar

November 9, 2000

Permanent memory loss for the time of the treatments and some time before is usual, not unusual. If a person, even one feeling awful, realizes what this does is to divide life into a present and a past which cannot ever be reconciled psychologically, he or she will realize that ECT is unnatural and wrong.

Yours truly

Mark Fenton

C802, February 1, 1994

I am one of those many people who have been subjected to shock treatments in an attempt to alleviate a severe depression. Had I foreseen the damaging effect that these 24 treatments were to have on my brain, I never would have agreed to undergo them. Because of the subsequent difficulties I have encountered as a result of ECT (including a recurrence of the depression and a suicide attempt), I consider these treatments to have been a setback rather than a help in my recovery.

I was fortunate in that I was able to return to my job but the process of relearning my job and retaining what I learn has been an arduous process. It is extremely stressful for me to cope in many areas of life because of my altered mental capacity. In addition, I have suffered embarrassment because I am unable to remember many people that I had met before the treatment as well as many important events in my life. In school, I have tremendous difficulty recalling what I have read, and, as a consequence, do poorly on essay-type exams. This has limited my coursework in recent years to those subjects that do not use essay exams. I certainly can imagine that unless one has very supportive friends and co-workers, as I do, the effects of ECT would be devastating.

It is most frustrating to experience these changes in my capacity that affect almost everything I do and then listen to a psychiatrist say that it is all in my head.

Sincerely,

Lucinda H. Frend

February 8, 1988

It's been 7–8 years since I had them [shock treatments], the long term damage is there and it's not coming back. At one time I never minded filling out job applications, I loved to read, my goal was to finish high school G.E.D. and become somebody.

I can no longer fill out applications. I'm not able to retain anything I might learn, I read and the next minute it's gone. I can't follow written instructions, I become confused. Just the other day I had to fill out an application for Food Stamps. I couldn't do it. I started to cry Something so simple and it deals with current things, I just couldn't handle it.

At one time I tried to file for Social Security. I could not remember places I worked or years, my mother tells me I was always good with dates, years, etc, not no more. I can't do any math, I've been tutored and helped and it won't sink in. I can read a page in a book and look up and not have any recollection of what I read. I have lost my ability to learn and better myself.

I feel doctors should tell people that are about to have ECT that sometimes, some of the brain is damaged and not all memory might come back. If I had thought for one min. I *might* of lost any of my memory forever, I would *not* of went through with it!

I'd also like to tell you that since the ECT I lost my first husband, I have hardly any memory of him, we were married 10 years.

I can no longer remember from day to day. When I'm lucky enough to find work, it's mass confusion and I usually don't last too long.

Doris Heikila

C140, February 25, 1987

I am one of many ECT patients who cannot help but suspect that ECT caused brain damage. . . .

I am constantly reminded of what I can't do . . . although I could do it once. And what is "it"? I can't remember new information with the ease I could before ECT. Distractions and interruptions seriously interfere with information retention . . . any new bit of information may "cancel out" the bit that preceded it. My auditory and visual memory seem to function episodically . . . enough so I know they exist and how well they functioned before ECT.

How have these deficits, which developed immediately after ECT, affected my life?

1. When I returned to my 6th grade teaching job after ECT I could not remember how to teach. Therefore, 5 months after ECT, I attempted suicide.

2. For two and a half years I worked in a kitchen. The loss in income was dramatic but worse was the total loss of confidence and the perception that I was a complete failure.

3. When I dared to take a college course, even multiple readings of the same material yielded next to nothing.

4. In September of 1987, I matriculated. However, because the information was complex and largely theoretical, and because I found it hard to remember instructions, I withdrew from school. I am very fortunate that I survived the subsequent depression.

5. Why am I not making the $40,000 I would be making if I'd remained in teaching. Why am I praying that I'll find a job that pays me $16,000. Why am I likely to settle for less if it will make few demands on my memory. I'm sure I need not answer "why."

I had a high "B" average in college. I remembered ideas better than facts. I was not a slave to my studies. One year six months later functioning like that was just a bitter memory. If ECT must be used in spite of its damaging effects, can we not develop cognitive retraining programs to help people adapt to their new deficits.

Sincerely,

Pam Maccabee

C323, January 20, 1987

It took me five years of hard work and frustration to restore my reading comprehension to the college level. And I had been a Reading Specialist. For some twenty years I could not play the piano. I doubt I'll ever reach the level I had been before I was subjected to ECT.

It has taken me the past twenty years, and will take me the rest of my life to approximate the education I lost. My career as an Intelligence Officer for the Federal Government was lost forever.

The effects of ECT not only ruined my life, but it nearly destroyed my family and my marriage. . . . My personal belief is that an investigation is in order to prove that ECT is indeed beneficial and not brain damaging. How can I feel differently when that so-called therapy has wrecked a major portion of my life?

Respectfully yours,

Marjorie E. Faeder

C314, January 21, 1988

When I was 19 years old my folks had me in the Hartford Retreat or the Institute of Living to get a series of about 18 shocks. Because of their complete trust in the psychiatrist who recommended I go to that place for my health, I was forced to submit to the hospital's best judgment. It was the hope of my parents that I would be able to resume college and study chemical engineering which I didn't do. . . . Do you believe that I had a fair chance to compete with other college students? Is it not reasonable for our great country to provide that people should be informed of the brain damaging side reaction to ECT before they sign to approve of it as therapy?

Very truly yours,

Monroe Prussack

C201, January 20, 1988

After I'd signed all the papers, including the "formality" of one giving the doctor permission to treat me (the admittance clerk's words), I was taken to the psychiatric ward, given a bed and a sleeping pill. I slept soundly, knowing I was going to get help.

When I awoke the next morning, I met my room-mate. . . . She said, "You know they give you shock treatments, don't you?" Dear God, No! . . .

I tried to run. They caught me and forced me onto the table. I don't remember ever fighting after that. . . .

My family came to see me. I remember none of them, but my oldest son. I will remember that, from what I later learned, till the day I die. At that time, I was so "happy and excited." They had a gift wagon that came by and I had bought four gifts for the kids. Since my oldest son's birthday was Nov. sixteenth, I decided to let him have his pick of the gifts. He turned 13.

He came into the room with his father. He stopped and looked at me, then came in and kissed me. I got out the "gifts" and told him to take his pick and give the other kids the rest. He chose one and said he was going down to the waiting room for a few minutes. I didn't know for some years that he had gone down there to cry, holding the cheap plastic toy that would have been better suited for a five or six year old. He cried for me.

He said he had never been so terrified. I had also not known that he'd been there before. He said I had been very lethargic, eyes vacant. This day, I had seemed happy, but I had acted as though he had been five or six years old. What a hell to put a young boy through. . . .

Soon after that, I was pronounced "well." I could go home. My youngest aunt lived at home, and I asked her a million questions. Where do I live; in a house or an apartment; upstairs or down; what kind of car does my brother-in-law drive; where were the kids, on and on.

I knew nothing of where I kept anything, which bedroom or bed was mine, where did this or that come from.

But the heartbreaking part was my children. They were thirteen, eleven, ten and barely eight. They brought friends in and I would say, "What a nice boy, who is he?" They would look embarrassed and tell me I had known him since we'd moved there.

I don't really remember a lot of what went on in that time, either. I do remember deciding I was going to get a job. I went to a clothing store. They said they didn't need any help then, but would take my number and call me if they needed help. Where had I worked? I told them a dress shop and the town. Name of the shop? Nothing. Who did I work for? Nothing. Who owned the shop? Nothing. I went home, embarrassed and not so enthusiastic.

I remember my sons. They just looked sad or upset, most of the time. I couldn't figure it out. I felt so good, why weren't they happy?

Then, I came down. My problems? Right there, as they had been before the treatments. Only now, the kids were hurting. I couldn't remember things, my family was upset and worried about me. . . .

I felt resentful and so terribly frustrated, and helpless. Because I'd found out the dangers after the fact. I couldn't go back and "un-do" the treatments.

I believe my body, my brain, was violated. By not telling me the type of treatments I would receive; by not telling me of the dangers and the unknown elements involved; by not even telling me of the short term effects, I feel not only myself but my innocent children and family suffered with me.

Cora Lee Ritchey

C124, August 11, 1986

It is 5 and one-half years since my horrifying experience of awaking in a hospital after ECT, not knowing who I was, where I was, who my husband and children were, what were my likes and dislikes, what my family was all about, what classes my children excelled in, what the family liked and disliked, and where I stood in the life I was supposed to be living. . . .

The damage from ECT can be extreme and completely disabling, to a degree inconceivable except by those who have undergone this horror. A diagnosis of organic brain syndrome or senile dementia after ECT through neuropsychological testing is not taken lightly by a person who had once been an intelligent and fully functioning being.

. . . The heartache and striving for health following brain damage is an illness itself after the damage from ECT.

Pat Gabel

C345, January 25, 1990

My doctor informed me that I would experience some short term memory loss, but reassured me that my memory would return to normal within six weeks following the end of the treatments. He pronounced me "cured" and urged me to return to college. I had to drop out of school when I realized I could not remember what I had studied before entering the hospital, and I was totally unable to absorb new material. I suffered for many months from a complete inability to concentrate, and was not even able to read a newspaper or magazine. I have been left with permanent memory loss of events that preceded the ECT by several months. I continue to have difficulty concentrating for extended periods of time, which I believe is the result of ECT. . . .

In my case, it could hardly have been called "informed consent" because I wasn't well informed of the risks involved.

Sharon Heim

November 2, 1990

I had a bunch of them [shock treatments] many years ago and I'm still having problems with my senses and the brain damage it did. . . .

When you come out of this hellish treatment—you sometimes don't know your name—you've forgotten a lot of important events in your life. I forget my children year they were born—I forgot addresses and how to contact people etc.

And years later I'm having the same problems. When I finally got out of the hospital I had to be hand led around on buses, and when I went out.

I have watched many cases of people who had shock treatments and yet am waiting, so far no good results.

Jean Culligan

C420, May 9, 1990

I had no after-care followup in the community. The experience of going back to work was horrendous. I could not remember names of fellow employees, code numbers for the computer department was wiped out of my mind.

Before this hospitalization, I was going to business school for accounting. All that I learned was wiped out of my mind. My vocal studies were brought to an abrupt halt. My repertoire of music was wiped out of my mind.

Followups of each and every patient who have had shock treatment should be a matter of necessity. . . . Rehabilitation should be included after shock treatment.

Elizabeth Plasick

C54, May 20, 1983

Before ECT, I studied math up through calculus. After ECT, I can just barely make change in a store. ECT gives a person a different brain from the one a person had. One never feels sure about this strange new head. Some things come back. A great deal of memory never returns. And one cannot retain new information, so one's future is DEAD.

June Bassett

C51, May 2, 1983

ECT was given to me against my will. . . . Before the ECT I was a college student studying art and a springboard diver in training for the Olympics. After the treatments I tried to resume these things, but I could not remember people who knew me at school and lost my nerve for diving. I feel the shock treatment was responsible.

My parents never would have consented to the treatment if they had been informed it might hurt my memory and damage my brain. . . .

One last thing I want to mention is an example of the effect ECT had on me. I was a young girl, intelligent, athletic, diving, attending college making good grades. I took a trip with my parents after leaving the hospital and I can remember going in the bathroom, coming out carrying a roll of toilet paper. I didn't even realize I had it. I was very embarrassed when I realized I had it and left it sitting in a drinking fountain. That is an example of how I was affected.

Sincerely,

Suza Gaudino

C180, January 24, 1988

I was hospitalized, voluntarily, from January 30 to February 20, 1991, during which I had eight electroshock treatments. The second treatment was with bilateral . . . the others were all unilateral. . . .

ECT did work; it unquestionably saved my life . . .

The ECT got rid of my depression completely for three weeks. After that, my depression began returning intermittently, and by six weeks post-treatment, it was constant again.

The confusion I experienced immediately after each ECT treatment was different enough from routine confusion that it should probably have a different name. I'm not talking about not knowing whether it was morning or afternoon—I'm talking about not even knowing *what* I was, let alone who or where I was. . . .

The "confusion" I continued to experience for about six weeks after my last treatment was another matter. I was unable to organize or conceptualize thoughts and feelings. . . . Everything I thought, said, or wrote was an incoherent stream of consciousness with the result that I was utterly unable to communicate appropriately or effectively. This amounted to a severe occupational and social disability. . . .

"Memory" isn't just a data bank of pieces of information that we might or might not care to use at any given moment. Memory pretty much covers everything we know and feel, and need to know and feel, to function—on every level. I lost knowledge, skills, abilities, and feelings of all kinds, and these losses made it impossible to function in work, routine activities, self-care, relationships, etc.

My memory loss included, at various times for about six weeks following my ECT, not knowing who people were, let alone what their names were; not being able to figure out how to put on my clothes; not having even the most basic job skills necessary to perform my usual work; not being able to drive my car, let alone figure out where I was going; not knowing where anything was in my home; etc.

I found myself wondering such things as: What is that thing (the machine I later recognized as my vacuum cleaner), and what is it for? I wonder if there's any way I can get my floor clean? Is cleaning floors something that normal people do, or am I being strange to want to clean my floor? Who lives in that house across the street? Did I used to know who lives there? Am I the kind of person who *would* have known who lives there? What kind of person am I anyway? What did I used to believe, and would I believe the same things now?

At least a couple of times every day, I found myself screaming and writhing uncontrollably. When there was verbal content to my screams, it consisted of such things as: "What have they *done* to me??" "They've *destroyed* me!" "My *self* is gone!"

I am now living with the deadly depression *and* the debilitating residual effects of the ECT. After the first six weeks post-treatment, my progress in recovering from the adverse effects came to a standstill.

In the six months since my ECT, I have been able to work only a few days altogether. There are still significant gaps in my memory of the past, and I am still often unable to learn and remember in the present. . . .

The content of the information given to me, on the basis of which I was to consent to ECT, was woefully inadequate. . . . I wasn't informed that the debilitating effects I have experienced from ECT were possible outcomes. . . .

I especially wish that I had been forewarned that recuperation from the treatment can be a very difficult and time-consuming process. I wasn't prepared for the possibility that I might be disabled for months by the residual effects of the ECT. . . .

Whenever I reported any of the adverse effects to my attending physician in the hospital, his response was to categorize all my experiences as manifestations of the predictable "memory loss and confusion," and to assure me that they would be of short duration. However, the worst of these effects didn't even become manifest until I left the hospital and tried to return to my life. Since my physician never did any followup on my progress after I left the hospital, he has no way of knowing what the longer-term effects of my ECT have been or how severely they have disabled me. . . .

No one, under any circumstances, should ever be subjected to ECT without his/her fully informed consent. . . . ECT should not be administered without one's consent even if it is known with certainty that suicide will otherwise result. Having been myself in the position of suicide or ECT as the only options available to me, I feel entitled to make that argument. And if I were faced with the choice today, I would unhesitatingly prefer death to ECT.

Karen Rian, Ph.D

Let. 24, September 6, 1991

[Dr. Rian later chose to commit suicide rather than undergo more ECT. This letter has been edited for length from the original seven pages.]

Notes

CHAPTER 2 — EUGENIC CONCEPTIONS I

1. Susan Stefan, *Unequal Rights* (New York: American Psychological Association, 2001), 5.

2. Edward Shorter, quoted in David Hodges, "Shock Therapy's Second Coming," www.medicalpost.com, November 6, 2007 (accessed November 14, 2007).

3. Information about the Coalition for the Abolition of ECT in Texas (CAEST), the only one of these groups which still exists, is at www.endofshock.com (accessed December 10, 2007).

4. www.ect.org/resources/resolution.html (accessed June 25, 2007).

5. Allen Hornblum, *Acres of Skin* (New York: Routledge, 1999).

6. Eileen Welsome, *The Plutonium Files* (New York: Dial Press, 1999), Chapter 37.

7. Ibid., 233–236.

8. I won a favorable ruling against Mecta, holding them potentially liable for damages, but the ruling was reversed at the appellate level. The Court of Appeals (the highest court in New York State) then refused to hear the case. The case against New York Hospital and Julie Hatterer, M.D., could not be tried because Peter Breggin withdrew as my expert witness on the eve of trial.

9. Robert Whitaker, *Mad in America: Bad Science, Bad Medicine, and the Enduring Mistreatment of the Mentally Ill* (Cambridge, Mass.: Perseus Books, 2002), 132.

10. "Treatment Advocacy Center Launches Search for New Executive Director" (press release), Treatment Advocacy Center, Arlington, Va., July 26, 2007.

11. http:www.eurekalert.org/pub_releases/2005–11/plos-afs103105.php (accessed December 31, 2005). In a 2007 publication, Healy disclosed relationships with fifteen drug companies. David Healy, "One Flew over the Conflict of Interest Nest," *World Psychiatry* 6(1) (2007):26–27.

12. Steven Sharfstein, interview on *The Today Show*, NBC-TV, June 27, 2005. "All Fired Up," *People*, July 11, 2005, 87.

13. Mark Graff, interview on *CBS Studio 2*, July 10, 2005.

14. Terry Messman, "Psychiatric Drugs: An Assault on the Human Condition. Interview with Robert Whitaker," *Street Spirit* (Oakland, Calif.), August 2005.

15. Jeffrey Lacasse, Jonathan Leo, "Serotonin and Depression: A Disconnect between the Advertisements and the Scientific Literature," Public Library of Science Medicine 2(12) (2005): e392. DOI:10.1371/journal.pmed.0020392.

16. Loren Mosher, "Community Residential Treatment for Schizophrenia: Two Year Followup," *Hospital and Community Psychiatry* 29(1978):715–723. Susan Matthews, "A Non-Neuroleptic Treatment for Schizophrenia: Analysis of the Two-Year Postdischarge Risk of Relapse," *Schizophrenia Bulletin* 5(1979):332–331.

17. R. J. DeRubeis, L. A. Gelfand, et al., "Medication versus Cognitive Behavior Therapy for Severely Depressed Outpatients: Mega-Analysis of Four Randomized Comparisons," *American Journal of Psychiatry* 156(7) (1999, July):1007–1013. John Read, Loren Mosher, Richard P. Bentall, eds., *Models of Madness: Psychological, Social and Biological Approaches to Schizophrenia* (London: Brunner-Routledge, 2004). Peter Stastny, Peter Lehmann, eds., *Alternatives beyond Psychiatry* (Berlin: Peter Lehmann Publishing, 2007).

18. I. Walker, J. Read, "The Differential Effectiveness of Psychosocial and Biological Causal Explanations in Reducing Negative Attitudes towards 'Mental Illness,'" *Psychiatry* 65 (2002):313–325. J. Read, N. Harre, "The Role of Biological and Genetic Causal Beliefs in the Stigmatization of 'Mental Illness,'" *Journal of Mental Health* 10 (2001):223–235.

19. H. J. Steadman, E. A. Mulvey, et al., "Violence by People Discharged from Acute Psychiatric Inpatient Facilities and by Others in the Same Neighborhoods," *Archives of General Psychiatry* 55 (1998):1–9.

20. U.S. Department of Justice, Bureau of Justice Statistics Special Report, 1994, *Murder in Families.*

21. New York Lawyers for the Public Interest (New York, N.Y.), *Implementation of Kendra's Law Is Severely Biased*, April 7, 2005.

22. Statement of D. J. Jaffe at the NAMI national conference, 1999. http://www.madnation.org/news/IOC/jaffe.htm (accessed February 28, 2005).

23. S. Kisely, L. A. Campbell, N. Preston, "Compulsory Community and Involuntary Outpatient Treatment for People with Severe Mental Disorders," *Cochrane Database of Systematic Reviews*, Issue 3 (2005), Art. No.: CD004408. DOI: 10.1002/14651858. CD004408.pub2.

24. C. W. Colton, R. W. Manderscheid, "Congruencies in Increased Mortality Rates, Years of Potential Life Lost, and Causes of Death among Public Mental Health Clients in Eight States," *Preventing Chronic Disease* 3(2) (2006).

CHAPTER 3 — EUGENIC CONCEPTIONS II

1. John Harvey Kellogg, the inventor of cornflakes, funded "The First National Conference on Race Betterment" in 1914. George Eastman of Eastman Kodak fame contributed to the launch of the American Eugenics Society in 1926. Robert Whitaker, *Mad in America: Bad Science, Bad Medicine, and the Enduring Mistreatment of the Mentally Ill* (Cambridge, Mass.: Perseus Press, 2002), 49, 54.

2. Charles Robinson, ed., *The Science of Eugenics* (W. R. Vansant, 1917), 97.

3. *Eugenical News* 10 (1925, July):27.

4. F. Kallman, "Heredity, Reproduction, and Eugenic Procedure in the Field of Schizophrenia," *Eugenical News* 23 (1938, November-December):105.

5. William J. Robinson, as cited in D. J. Kevles, *In the Name of Eugenics: Genetics and the Uses of Human Heredity* (New York: Knopf, 1985), 93–94.

6. Whitaker, *Mad in America*, 59.

7. Alexis Carrel, *Man the Unknown* (New York: Harper and Brothers, 1935), 318–319.

8. Foster Kennedy, "The Problem of Social Control of the Congenital Defective: Education, Sterilization, Euthanasia," *American Journal of Psychiatry* 99 (1942):13–16.

9. Leo Kanner, "Exoneration of the Feebleminded," *American Journal of Psychiatry* 99 (1942):17–22.

10. Anonymous, "Euthanasia," *American Journal of Psychiatry* 99 (1942):141–143.

11. Jay Joseph, "The 1942 'Euthanasia' Debate in the *American Journal of Psychiatry*," *History of Psychiatry*; 16(2) (2005):171–179.

12. Letter from Dr. Abraham Brill to W. A. White, October 31, 1936, cited in G. N. Grob, *Mental Illness and American Society 1975–1940* (Princeton, N.J.: Princeton University Press, 1983).

13. Julius Wagner van Jauregg won for malarial fever therapy in 1927, Egas Moniz for leucotomy, the earliest form of psychosurgery, in 1949. Elliott Valenstein, *Great and Desperate Cures: The Rise and Decline of Psychosurgery and Other Radical Treatments for Mental Illness* (New York: Basic Books, 1986), 30 and 225.

14. Valenstein, *Great and Desperate Cures*, 47.

15. Lucie Jessner, V. Gerard Ryan, *Shock Treatment in Psychiatry: A Manual* (New York: Grune and Stratton, 1941), 55–56.

16. Valenstein, *Great and Desperate Cures*, 57.

17. "Insulin for Insanity," *Time,* January 25, 1937; "Death for Sanity," *Time,* November 20, 1939; "Bedside Miracle," *Reader's Digest* 35 (1939, November).

18. Valenstein, *Great and Desperate Cures*, 59.

19. R. M. Mowbray, "Historical Aspects of Electric Convulsive Therapy," *Scottish Medical Journal* 4 (1959):375.

20. Eugene Ziskind, Esther Somerfeld-Ziskind, "Loss of Recently Acquired Learning Due to Metrazol Therapy," *Journal of the Los Angeles Neurological Society*, 1939.

21. Rankine Good, "Some Observations on Psychological Aspects of Cardiazol Therapy," *Journal of Mental Science* 86 (1940):491–501.

22. Good, "Some Observations," 493. Solomon Katzenelbogen, "A Critical Appraisal of the Shock Therapies in the Major Psychoses and Psychoneuroses, III—Convulsive Therapy," *Psychiatry* 3 (1940):419.

23. Michael Burleigh, *Death and Deliverance: Euthanasia in Germany 1900–1945* (London: Pan Books, 2002), 91.

24. Lawrence Geeslin, "Anomalies and Dangers in the Metrazol Therapy of Schizophrenia," *American Journal of Psychiatry* 96 (1939):183. Simon Kwalwasser, "Report on 441 Cases Treated with Metrazol," *Psychiatric Quarterly* 14 (1940):527–546. Katzenelbogen, "A Critical Appraisal," 409–420. Leon Reznikoff, "Evaluation of Metrazol Shock in Treatment of Schizophrenia," *Archives of Neurology and Psychiatry* 43 (1940):318–325. Richard Whitehead, "Pharmacologic and Pathologic Effects of Repeated Convulsant Doses of Metrazol," *American Journal of the Medical Sciences* 199 (1940):352–359. P. A. Davis, W. Sulzbach, "Changes in the Electroencephalogram during Metrazol Therapy," *Archives of Neurology and Psychiatry* 43 (1940):341–355.

25. A. Kennedy, "Critical Review: The Treatment of Mental Disorders by Induced Convulsions," *Journal of Neurology & Psychiatry* 3 (1940):49–82.

26. Jessner and Ryan, *Shock Treatment*, 99; Whitaker, *Mad in America*, 93.

27. Ladislas J. Meduna, "The Convulsive Treatment: A Reappraisal," in Felix Marti-Ibanez et al., eds., *The Great Physiodynamic Therapies in Psychiatry* (New York: Hoeber-Harper, 1956), 84.

28. Ibid., 92.

29. Ugo Cerletti, "Old and New Information about Electroshock," *American Journal of Psychiatry* 15(1950):191–217.

30. Ugo Cerletti, "Electroshock Therapy," in Marti-Ibanez et al., *The Great Physiodynamic Treatments*, 93.

31. Ugo Cerletti, Lucio Bini, "Le Alterazioni Istopatologiche del Sistema Nervoso in Seguito all'E.S.," *Rivista Sperimentale di Freniatria* 64 (1940).

32. Ugo Cerletti, "Electroshock Therapy," 93–94.

33. Cited in F. J. Ayd, "Guest Editorial: Ugo Cerletti M.D. 1877–1963," *Psychosomatics* 4 (1963):A6–A7.

34. David Healy, Edward Shorter, *Shock Therapy: A History of Electroconvulsive Treatment in Mental Illness* (New Brunswick, N.J.: Rutgers University Press, 2007), 43.

35. L. Kolb, V. H. Vogel, "The Use of Shock Therapy in 305 Mental Hospitals," *American Journal of Psychiatry* 99 (1942):90–93.

36. Valenstein, *Great and Desperate Cures*, 52.

37. Edwin Black, *War against the Weak: Eugenics and America's Campaign to Create a Master Race* (New York: Thunders Mouth Press, 2003), 283–285.

38. Burleigh, *Death and Deliverance*, 120.

39. Gotz Aly, Peter Chroust, Christian Pross, *Cleansing the Fatherland: Nazi Medicine and Racial Hygiene* (Baltimore: Johns Hopkins University Press, 1994), 23–26.

40. Ibid., 38.

41. Ibid., 204–205.

42. Fredric Wertham, *A Sign for Cain* (New York: Macmillan, 1966). This is also the estimate made by the Czech War Crimes Commission and repeated at Nuremberg.

43. Richard Abrams, "Interview with Lothar Kalinowsky, M.D.," *Convulsive Therapy* 4(1)1988:24–39.

44. Ibid.

45. http://www.nyspi.cpmc.columbia.edu/Kolb/index.htm (accessed December 14, 2005).

46. Abrams, "Interview with Lothar Kalinowsky."

47. S. E. Pulver, "The First Electroconvulsive Treatment Given in the United States," *American Journal of Psychiatry* 117 (1961):845–846.

48. Between 1972 and 1977, Gracie Square administered 88 percent of the ECT in New York City and 22 percent of all treatments administered in the entire state. "Through selective referral and attraction of organically-oriented psychiatrists, these specialized hospitals [which I have referred to by their colloquial name of shock mill] account for the vast majority of patients administered ECT in American psychiatric facilities." J. P. Morrissey, N. M. Burton, et al., "Developing an Empirical Base for Psycho-Legal Policy Analyses of ECT: A New York State Survey," *International Journal of Law and Psychiatry* 2(1)(1979, January):99–111.

49. Richard Abrams, "An Appreciation. Lothar Kalinowsky, M.D., 1899–1992," *Convulsive Therapy* 8(3)(1992):218–220.

50. Thomas Roder, Volker Kubillus, Anthony Burwell, *Psychiatrists—The Men behind Hitler* (Los Angeles: Freedom Publishing, 1995), 276–277.

51. Ladislas J. Meduna, "The Carbon Dioxide Treatment: A Review," in Marti-Ibanez et al., *The Great Physiodynamic Treatments*, 138–152.

52. Ugo Cerletti, "Electroshock Therapy," in Marti-Ibanez et al., *The Great Physiodynamic Treatments*, 109–115.

53. Ibid., 94.

54. J. S. Madden, "Euthanasia in Nazi Germany," *Psychiatric Bulletin* 24 (2000):347.

55. William J. Cole, "Doctor Implicated in Nazi Atrocities Dies," Associated Press, December 22, 2005; http://news.yahoo.com/s/ap/20051222/ap_on_re_eu/obit_nazi_doctor (accessed December 23, 2005).

56. Aly et al., *Cleansing the Fatherland*, 2.

CHAPTER 4 — A LITTLE BRAIN PATHOLOGY

1. Lucio Bini, "Experimental Researches on Epileptic Attacks Induced by the Electric Current," *American Journal of Psychiatry* 94(6) (Supp.) (1938):172–174.

2. Bernard J. Alpers, "The Brain Changes Associated with Electrical Shock Treatment: A Critical Review," *Journal-Lancet* 66 (1946):363–369.

3. S. Eugene Barrera, Nolan D. C. Lewis, et al., "Brain Changes Associated with Electrically Induced Seizures," *Transactions of the American Neurological Association* 68 (1942 June):31–35.

4. Armando Ferraro, Leon Roizen, Max Helfand, "Morphologic Changes in the Brain of Monkeys Following Electrically Induced Convulsions," *Journal of Neuropathology and Experimental Neurology* 5 (1946):285–308. Armando Ferraro, Leon Roizen, "Cerebral Morphologic Changes in Monkeys Subjected to Large Numbers of Electrically Induced Convulsions," *American Journal of Psychiatry* 106 (1949):278–284.

5. Hans Hartelius, "Cerebral Changes Following Electrically Induced Convulsions," *Acta Psychiatrica Neurologica Scandinavica* 77 (Supp.) (1952):1–128.

6. Jules Masserman, Mary Grier Jacques, "Effects of Cerebral Electroshock on Experimental Neuroses in Cats," *American Journal of Psychiatry* 104 (1947):92–99.

7. J. L. McGaugh, T. A. Williams, "Neurophysiological and Behavioral Effects of Convulsive Phenomena," in Max Fink et al., eds., *Psychobiology of Convulsive Therapy* (New York: Wiley, 1974), 85–97.

8. J. Quandt, H. Sommer, "Zur Frage der Hirngewebsschadigungen nach electrischer Krampfbehandlung," *Zeitschrift für Neurologie und Psychiatrie* 34 (1966):513.

9. M. M. Aleksandrovskaya, R. I. Krugilov, "Influence of Electroshock on Memory Function and Glial-Neuronal Relationship in the Rat Brain," *Proceedings of the Academy of Science (USSR)* 197 (1971):1216–1218.

10. E. J. Colon, S. L. H. Notermans, "A Long-Term Study of the Effects of Electro-Convulsions on the Structure of the Cerebral Cortex," *Acta Neuropathologica* 32 (1975): 21–25.

11. Bernard J. Alpers, Joseph Hughes, "The Brain Changes in Electrically Induced Convulsions in the Human," *Journal of Neuropathological and Experimental Neurology* 1 (1942):172–177.

12. Leo Madow, "Brain Changes in Electroconvulsive Therapy," *American Journal of Psychiatry* 113 (1956):337–347.

13. W. Riese, "Report of Two New Cases of Sudden Death after Electric Shock Treatment with Histopathological Findings in the Central Nervous System," *Journal of Neuropathology and Experimental Neurology* 7 (1948):98–100.

14. David Impastato, "Prevention of Fatalities in ECT," *Diseases of the Nervous System* 18 (Sec. 2) (1957):34–75.

15. F. Patrick McKegney, Anthony F. Panzetta, "An Unusual Fatal Outcome of Electro-convulsive Therapy," *American Journal of Psychiatry* 120 (1963):398–400. J. R. Matthew, E. Constan, "Complications Following ECT over a Three Year Period in a State Institution," *American Journal of Psychiatry* 120 (1964):1119–1120. J. Gomez, "Death after ECT," *British Medical Journal* 2 (1974):45.

16. R. R. Grinker, N. A. Levy, H. M. Serota, "Disturbances in Brain Function Following Convulsive Therapy," *Archives of Neurology and Psychiatry* 47 (1942):1028–1029.

17. Abraham Myerson, "Borderline Cases Treated with Electric Shock," *American Journal of Psychiatry* 100 (1943):355.

18. Max Fink, "Effect of Anticholinergic Agent, Diethazine, on EEG and Behavior: Significance for Theory of Convulsive Therapy," *Archives of Neurology and Psychiatry* 80 (1958):380–384.

19. Abraham Myerson, in "Discussion of Franklin G. Ebaugh et al., Fatalities Following Electric Convulsive Therapy: A Report of 2 Cases with Autopsy Findings," *Transactions of the American Neurological Association* 68 (1942):39.

20. Paul Hoch, "Discussion and Concluding Remarks (Round Table on ECT)," *Journal of Personality* 17 (1948):48.

21. Bernard L. Pacella, "Sequelae and Complications of Convulsive Shock Therapy," *Bulletin of the New York Academy of Medicine* 20 (1944):575–585.

22. Barrera et al., "Brain Changes."

23. Leon Salzman, "An Evaluation of Shock Therapy," *American Journal of Psychiatry* 103 (1947):676.

24. Calvin Stone, "Losses and Gains in Cognitive Functions as Related to Electro-Convulsive Shocks," *Journal of Abnormal Psychology* 42 (1947):206–214.

25. S. M. Cannicott, "Unilateral Electro-convulsive Therapy," *Postgraduate Medical Journal* 38 (1962):451–459. He cites the following: E. Schildge, *Zur Erlebnisseite der Elektrokrampfbehandlung* (Tuebingen, Germany: Bericht, 1947). E. Stengel, "Intensive ECT," *Journal of Mental Science* 97 (1951):139. E. W. A. Anderson, *Mental Disease: Physical Methods of Treatment, Medical Annual* (Bristol, U.K.: John Wright, 1951), 173. E. W. A. Anderson, *Mental Disease: Physical Methods of Treatment, Medical Annual* (rev. ed.) (Bristol, U.K.: John Wright, 1953), 234. R. W. Russell, *Brain Memory Learning* (London: Oxford University Press, 1959), Chapters 5, 6, 7. Borje Cronholm, Lars Molander, "Memory Disturbances after Electro-Convulsive Therapy," *Acta Psychiatrica Scandinavica* 32 (1957):280. C. P. Stone, *American Psychologist* 1 (1946):254.

26. Lucie Jessner, V. Gerard Ryan, *Shock Treatment in Psychiatry* (New York: Grune and Stratton, 1941), 109.

27. *Report No. 1: Shock Therapy* (New York: Group for the Advancement of Psychiatry, 1947).

28. A. Z. Barhash, in "Discussion of Theodore R. Robie, Is Shock Therapy on Trial?" *American Journal of Psychiatry* 106 (1950):909.

29. Jules Masserman, "Experimental Neurosis," *Scientific American* (1950, March), 249.

30. Jules Masserman, *Principles of Dynamic Psychiatry* (Philadelphia: W. B. Saunders, 1961), 160.

31. Manfred J. Sakel, "Sakel Shock Treatment," in F. Marti-Ibanez et al., eds., *The Great Physiodynamic Therapies in Psychiatry* (New York: Hoeber-Harper, 1956), 30.

32. Emerick Friedman, Paul H. Wilcox, "Electro-stimulated Convulsive Doses in Intact Humans by Means of Unidirectional Currents," *Journal of Nervous and Mental Disease* 96 (1942):56–63.

33. W. T. Liberson, Paul H. Wilcox, "Electric Convulsive Therapy: Comparison of 'Brief Stimuli Technique' with Friedman-Wilcox-Reiter Technique," *Digest of Neurology and Psychiatry* 8 (1945):292–302.

34. Paul Hoch, "Discussion and Concluding Remarks. The Effects of Electric Convulsive Therapy on the Functioning of Mental Patients: A Symposium," *Journal of Personality* September 17(1) (1948):48–51.

35. Liberson and Wilcox, "Electric Convulsive Therapy."

36. Barbara S. Kendall, Warren B. Mills, Thomas Thale, "Comparison of Two Methods of Electroshock in Their Effect on Cognitive Functions," *Journal of Consulting Psychology* 20 (1956):423–429.

37. D. Impastato, S. Berg, A. R. Gabriel, "The Molac-II—An Alternating Current Electroshock Therapy Machine Incorporating a New Principle," *Journal of Nervous and Mental Disease* 125 (1957):380–384.

38. W. T. Liberson, "Time Factors in Electric Convulsive Therapy," *Yale Journal of Biology and Medicine* 17 (1945):571–578. W. T. Liberson, "Brief Stimulus Therapy," *American Journal of Psychiatry* 105 (1948):28–39.

39. Leo Alexander, "Modified Electroconvulsive Therapy with Unidirectional Currents," *Diseases of the Nervous System* 16 (1955):1–4.

40. Liberson and Wilson, "Electric Convulsive Therapy."

41. Borje Cronholm, Jan-Otto Ottoson, "Ultrabrief Stimulus Technique in Electroconvulsive Therapy I. Influence on Retrograde Amnesia of Treatments with the Elther ES Electroshock Apparatus, Siemens Konvulsator III and of Lidocaine-Modified Treatment," *Journal of Nervous and Mental Disease* 137 (1963):117–123. Borje Cronholm, Jan-Otto Ottoson, "Ultrabrief Stimulus Technique in Electroconvulsive Therapy II. Comparison Studies of Therapeutic Effects and Memory Disturbances in Treatment of Endogenous Depression with the Elther ES Electroshock Apparatus and the Siemens Konvulsator III," *Journal of Nervous and Mental Disease* 137 (1963):268–276. M. Valentine, K. M. Keddie, D. Dunne, "A Comparison of Techniques in Electroconvulsive Therapy," *British Journal of Psychiatry* 14 (1968):989–996.

42. Sibile Morency, "Electroshock Therapy Gets a Makeover," *ABC News*, July 20, 2007. http://abcnews.go.com/Technology/story?id=3397685&page=51 (accessed July 23, 2007). Here Dr. Harold Sackeim says the recycled technique "does away with life-long memory loss" (his first and only admission that there is ever any lifelong memory loss).

43. Richard J. Kohlman, "Medical Malpractice: Electroconvulsive Therapy," *44 American Jurisprudence Proof of Facts 2d.* (New York: Lawyers Co-Operative Publishing, 1986).

44. Deposition of Harold Sackeim, Ph.D., Case No. 01069713, Atze Akkerman and Elizabeth Akkerman v. Joseph Johnson, Santa Barbara Cottage Hospital, and Does 1–20, Court of the State of California for the County of Santa Barbara, Anacapa Division, March 14, 2004, 180: "I was going to say that the reason that people are oxygenated, started all of this, is to provoke seizures in people who one couldn't provoke seizures in, was to assist in provoking seizures, and in making them longer in particular, and in having the seizures longer."

45. J. C. Barker, J. A. Baker, "Deaths Associated with Electroplexy," *Journal of Mental Science* 105 (1959):339–348. J. R. Novello, ed., *A Practical Handbook of Psychiatry* (Springfield, Ill.: Charles C. Thomas, 1974). Lothar Kalinowsky, "The Danger of Various Types of Medication during Electric Convulsive Therapy," *American Journal of Psychiatry* 112 (1956):745–746. David Impastato, "Prevention of Fatalities in Electroshock Therapy," *Diseases of the Nervous System* 18 (Sec. 2) (1957):34–75. See also *John Bolam v. Friern Hospital Management Committee*, Queens Bench Division, U.K., 1957; http://www.oxcheps.new.ox.ac.uk/casebook/Resources/BOLAMV_1%2ODOC.pdf (accessed January 10, 2006).

46. Hartelius, "Cerebral Changes," 78–83.

47. Kitty Dukakis, Larry Tye, *Shock: The Healing Power of Electroconvulsive Therapy* (New York: Avery, 2006), 174.

48. M. B. Brody, "Prolonged Memory Defects Following Electro-Therapy," *Journal of Mental Science* 90 (1944):777–77.

49. Irving L. Janis, "Psychologic Effects of Electric Convulsive Treatments (I. Post-Treatment Amnesias)," *Journal of Nervous and Mental Disease* 111 (1950):359–381.

50. R. K. Davies, T. P. Detre, et al., "Electroconvulsive Therapy Instruments: Should They Be Reevaluated?" *Archives of General Psychiatry* 25 (1971):97–99.

51. For instance, neuroscientist Dr. Peter Sterling proposed a replication of the Janis study to the assembly of the state of New York in public hearings on ECT on July 18, 2001.

52. "The Isolation, Description, and Treatment of the Pathological Behavior of ECT-Damaged Patients," in Robert Morgan, ed., *Electric Shock* (Toronto: IPI Publishing, 1985), 17–18.

53. "Relationship of Ethnic Background, Religion, Diagnosis, Memory and Other Variables to Presence of Shock Therapy. History for a Sample of Hospitalized Mental Patients: Preliminary Investigation of the Lasting Effects of Shock Treatment on Behavior," in Morgan, *Electric Shock*, 21–26.

54. Robert J. Grimm, Statement to APA Task Force on ECT, May 7, 1976, in Leonard Roy Frank, *The History of Shock Treatment* (San Francisco, 1978), 119–120.

CHAPTER 5 — INFORMED CONSENT AND THE DAWN OF THE PUBLIC RELATIONS ERA

1. David Impastato, "Prevention of Fatalities in ECT," *Diseases of the Nervous System* 18 (Sec. 2) (1957):51.

2. Dr. Manfred Guttmacher, statement before a Senate subcommittee, "Constitutional Rights of the Mentally Ill: Part 1, Civil Aspects" (March 28–30, 1961) (Washington, D.C.: U.S. Government Printing Office, 1961), 155.

3. Bruce Ennis, Loren Siegel, *The Rights of Mental Patients: An American Civil Liberties Union Handbook* (New York: Richard W. Baron, 1973), 69.

4. Jean Dietz, "Shock Therapy Lacks Scientific Study, Law," *Boston Globe*, July 25, 1972. Jean Dietz, "ECT Study Reveals Disparity between Public and Private Units," *Psychiatric News*, August 6, 1975.

5. A. Harris, "Wiswall Hospital: Shock Therapy Abuse," *Boston Phoenix*, November 14, 1972. P. Cowen, "Mental Health Department Probes Hospital's Shock Treatment," *Boston Globe*, December 6, 1972.

6. Fred Frankel, "Electro-convulsive Therapy in Massachusetts: A Task Force Report," *Massachusetts Mental Health Journal* 4 (1973):3–29.

7. Edward L. Bernays, "The Engineering of Consent," *Annals of the American Academy of Political and Social Science* 250 (1947, March):113–120.

8. "ECT Use in Mass. Found Down after State Regulation," *Psychiatric News*, April 6, 1984.

9. Doris Pearsall, "An Eleven-Year Trend Study on the Use of Electroconvulsive Therapy in Massachusetts Public and Private Hospitals," Division of Research and Evaluation, Division of Policy and Planning, Massachusetts Department of Mental Health, November 1, 1984.

10. G. H. Grosser et al., "The Regulation of Electroconvulsive Treatment in Massachusetts: A Follow-up," *Massachusetts Journal of Mental Health* 5 (1975):12–25.

11. Full-page advertisement for the IPAAE, *Psychiatric News*, May 2, 1980.

12. Max Fink, letter to H. C. Tien of December 26, 1974, in *American Journal of Electrotherapy* 1(1) (1976, January).

13. *New York City Health and Hospitals Corporation v. Stein*, 70 Misc. 2d 944, 335 N.Y.S.2d 461 (Sup. Ct. 1972).

14. New York Mental Hygiene Law Section. 15.03 (b) (4) (McKinney Supplement 1976), today incorporated into Section 33.03. Delaware Code Annotated, Title 16, Section 5161(2)(d) (Supplement 1975). Florida Statutes Annotated, Section 394.459(3)(b) (1975). Connecticut General Statutes Annotated, Section 17–206(d) (1975). Michigan Compiled Laws Annotated, Section 330.1716 (1975).

15. *Wyatt v. Stickney*, 325 FS 781 (M.D. Ala., 1971).

16. *Wyatt v. Hardin*, Civ. Action No. 3195-N (M.D. Ala., Feb. 28, 1975).

17. *Price v. Sheppard*, 307 Minn 250, 239 N.W.2d 905 (1976).

18. *Gundy v. Pauley*, 619 S.W.2d 730 (Ky. App. 1981).

19. Ames Fischer, "Analysis of Impact of Assembly Bill 4481 (Vasconcellos)—with Concurrence by the Council of the Northern California Psychiatric Society," in Leonard Roy Frank, *The History of Shock Treatment* (San Francisco, 1978), 148.

20. Aden earned the sobriquet "Doctor of Desire" from Scott Winokur of the *San Francisco Examiner*, in "An Examiner Special Report: Surveys Indicate Big Problem of Abuse by Psychotherapists," August 4, 1991. Also see Rex Dalton, "Psychiatrist's Former Patient Tells Story of Abuse," *San Diego Union*, January 1, 1989.

21. *Aden v. Younger*, 57 C.A.3d 662 (1976); 129 Cal. Rptr. 535.

22. Gary Aden, "The International Psychiatric Association for the Advancement of Electrotherapy: A Brief History," *American Journal of Social Psychiatry* IV(4) (1984, Fall):9–10.

23. Frazier was later reappointed as a staff psychiatrist at McLean Hospital, without regaining his faculty position at Harvard. Allison Bass, "McLean Hires Back Doctor Ordered to Quit," *Boston Globe*, February 10, 1989. Morton Hunt, "Did the Penalty Fit the Crime?" *New York Times*, May 14, 1989.

24. P. H. Blachly, D. Gowing, "Multiple Monitored Electroconvulsive Treatment," *Comprehensive Psychiatry* 7 (1966, April):100–109. Even the American Psychiatric Association now says this technique is "not recommended," but it is still in use.

25. Full-page advertisement for the IPAAE, *Psychiatric News*, May 2, 1980.

26. Food and Drug Administration, Dockets Management Branch, Docket No. 82P-0316, C00088; March 21, 1984 (letter from Dr. Gary Aden).

27. California Assembly Bill No. 1032, Section 5325f (1976), Welfare & Institutions Code.

28. Carol A. B. Warren, "Electroconvulsive Therapy: 'New' Treatment of the 1980s," *Research in Law, Deviance and Social Control* 8 (1986):41–55.

29. Max Fink, "The Impact of the Antipsychiatry Movement on the Revival of Electroconvulsive Therapy in the United States," *Psychiatric Clinics of North America* 14(4) (1991):793–801.

30. *Price v. Sheppard* at 910.

31. M. H. Shapiro, "Legislating the Control of Behavior Control: Autonomy and the Coercive Use of Organic Therapies," 47 *S. Cal. Law Review* 237, 262 (1974).

32. M. Greenblatt, "Editorial Introduction: Electroconvulsive Therapy, a Problem in Social Psychiatry," *American Journal of Social Psychiatry* IV(4) (1984, Fall):3–5.

33. "It Was More than a Game," *Psychiatric News*, November 4, 1983.

CHAPTER 6 — THE AMERICAN PSYCHIATRIC ASSOCIATION TASK FORCE

1. Max Fink, "Convulsive Therapy Today," *Fair Oaks Hospital Psychiatry Letter* IV(2) (1986, February):7–11.

2. American Psychiatric Association. Task Force Report 14, *Electroconvulsive Therapy* (Washington, D.C.: American Psychiatric Association, 1978), iii.

3. Fink, "Convulsive Therapy Today."

4. Peter Breggin, *Electroshock: Its Brain-Disabling Effects* (New York: Springer Publishing, 1979), 15.

5. M. McDonald, "The ECT Debate: Con," *Psychiatric News*, July 16, 1976.

6. Robert J. Grimm, Statement to APA Task Force on ECT, May 7, 1976, in Leonard Roy Frank, *The History of Shock Treatment* (San Francisco, 1978), 119–120.

7. Max Fink, "Myths of 'Shock Therapy,'" *American Journal of Psychiatry* 134(9) (1977, September):991–996.

8. H. Goldman, F. E. Gomer, D. I. Templer, "Long-term Effects of Electroconvulsive Therapy upon Memory and Perceptual-Motor Performance," *Journal of Clinical Psychology* 28 (1972):32–34.

9. D. Templer, C. Ruff, G. Armstrong, "Cognitive Functioning and Degree of Psychosis in Schizophrenics Given Many Electro-convulsive Treatments," *British Journal of Psychiatry* 123 (1973):441–443.

10. Irving L. Janis, paper presented at "The Effects of Electric Convulsive Therapy on The Functioning of Mental Patients: A Symposium," Temple University, Philadelphia, Pa., April 17, 1948.

11. S. E. Barrera, N. D. C. Lewis, et al., "Brain Changes Associated with Electrically Induced Seizures," *Transactions of the American Neurological Association* 68 (1942, June): 31–35. J. H. Globus, A. van Harreveld, C. A. G. Wiersma, "The Influence of Electric Current Application on the Structure of the Brain of Dogs," *Journal of Neuropathology and Experimental Neurology* 2 (1943):263–276. W. L. Lidbeck, "Pathologic Changes in the Brain after Electric Shock: An Experimental Study on Dogs," *Journal of Neuropathology and Experimental Neurology* 3 (1944):81–85. K. T. Neuberger, R. W. Whitehead, et al., "Pathologic Changes in the Brains of Dogs Given Repeated Electric Shocks," *American Journal of Medical Science* 204 (1942):381–387.

12. Mary Midgley, *Can't We Make Moral Judgments?* (New York: St. Martin's Press, 1993), 55.

13. American Psychiatric Association, Task Force Report 14, *Electroconvulsive Therapy* (Washington, D.C.: American Psychiatric Association, 1978), x.

14. Max Fink, *Electroshock: Restoring the Mind* (New York: Oxford University Press, 1999), back cover.

15. Edward L. Bernays, "Engineering of Consent," *Annals of the American Academy of Political and Social Science* 250 (1947, March):113–120.

16. Peter Stevens, David J. Harper, "Professional Accounts of Electroconvulsive Therapy: A Discourse Analysis," *Social Science and Medicine* 64 (2007):1475–1486.

17. Ibid.

18. Arthur Rifkin, "Shock Therapy: A History of Electroconvulsive Treatment in Mental Illness (book review)," *New England Journal of Medicine* 358(2) (2008, January 10):204–205.

19. G. Sheppard, S. Ahmed, "A Critical Review of the Controlled Real vs. Sham ECT Studies in Depressive Illness," paper presented at the First European Symposium on ECT, Graz, Austria, March 1992.

20. Colin Ross, "The Sham ECT Literature: Implications for Consent to ECT," *Ethical Human Psychology and Psychiatry* 8(1) (2006):17–28.

21. H. A. Sackeim, R. F. Haskett, et al., "Continuation Pharmacotherapy in the Prevention of Relapse Following Electroconvulsive Therapy," *Journal of the American Medical Association* 285 (10) (2001, March 14):1299–1307.

22. "Consensus Conference: Electroconvulsive Therapy," *Journal of the American Medical Association* 254 (15) (1985, October 18):2103–2108. Service User Research Enterprise (SURE), Institute of Psychiatry, *Review of Consumers' Perspectives on Electroconvulsive Therapy* (London: SURE, January 2002).

23. David Healy, Edward Shorter, *Shock Therapy: A History of Electroconvulsive Treatment in Mental Illness* (New Brunswick, N.J.: Rutgers University Press, 2007), 3.

24. Shafica Karagulla, "Evaluation of Electric Convulsion Therapy as Compared with Conservative Methods of Treatment," *Journal of Mental Science* 96 (1950):1060–1091.

25. (1) D. W. Black, G. W. Winokur, et al., "Does Treatment Influence Mortality in Depressives? A Follow-up of 1076 Patients with Major Affective Disorders," *Annals of Clinical Psychiatry* 1(3) (1989):166–173. (2) D. A. Avery, G. W. Winokur, "Mortality in Depressed Patients Treated with Electroconvulsive Therapy and Antidepressants,"

Archives of General Psychiatry 33 (1976):1029–1037. (3) H. M. Barbigian, L. B. Guttmacher, "Epidemiologic Considerations in Electroconvulsive Therapy," *Archives of General Psychiatry* 41 (1984):246–253. (4) D. Koessler, B. S. Fogel, "Electroconvulsive Therapy for Major Depression in the Oldest Old: Effects of Medical Co-Morbidity on Post-treatment Survival," *American Journal of Geriatric Psychiatry* 1(1) (1993):30–37. (5) D. A. O'Leary, A. S. Lee, "Seven Year Prognosis in Depression: Mortality and Readmission Risk in the Nottingham ECT Cohort," *British Journal of Psychiatry* 169(4) (1996):423–429.

26. Trine Munk-Olsen, Poul Videbech, et al., "All-Cause Mortality among Recipients of Electroconvulsive Therapy," *British Journal of Psychiatry* 190 (2007):435–439.

27. V. Milstein, J. G. Small, et al., "Does Electroconvulsive Therapy Prevent Suicide?" *Convulsive Therapy* 2(1) (1986):3–6.

28. Sue E. Kemsley, "ECT: Life-Saving Treatment?" *The Survivor* (Bury St. Edmonds, Suffolk, U.K.), April 18, 2000, 51–59.

29. Max Fink, *Electroshock: Restoring the Mind* (New York: Oxford University Press, 1999), 20.

30. For example, Lothar Kalinowsky: "Even during the many years when ECT was used without oxygenation, prolonged seizures or neurological dysfunction were not observed." Lothar Kalinowsky, "Is Multiple-Monitored ECT Safe? Letter to the Editor," *American Journal of Psychiatry* 138 (1981):701–702.

31. Deposition of Harold Sackeim, Ph.D., Case No. 01069713, *Atze Akkerman and Elizabeth Akkerman v. Joseph Johnson*, Santa Barbara Cottage Hospital, and Does 1–20, Court of the State of California for the County of Santa Barbara, Anacapa Division, March 14, 2004, 173–188.

> Q: You always oxygenate during the procedure? At Payne-Whitney [the psychiatric arm of New York Hospital]?
>
> A: No.
>
> Q: If you find any [anesthesiologists] that are doing it incorrectly by not oxygenating you teach them to do it?
>
> A: See, I don't think that it's going to matter, I don't think it's going to make a bit of difference . . . during the period of the seizure, they simply, you know, they don't turn blue.
>
> Q: Why do you give oxygen to patients if you don't think it's necessary during the seizure?
>
> A: There's more than one reason. One is like why do you wear seat belts if you haven't been in a car accident? Because if you're going to get into a car accident, if you, for instance you have difficulty ventilating a patient, if the patient is going to go into a prolonged seizure post status, you would like to have as much oxygen on board as you can. Does that mean for the routine treatment it makes much difference?
>
> Q: Are you aware of any studies done indicating that there's no need to give oxygen during an ECT seizure?
>
> A: Yes . . . Holmberg essentially found that you got a little bit longer seizure, but it didn't look like you had much other consequence for patients.

Q: You are not an expert on this issue though, are you?

A: I would say so.

Q: If indeed Max Fink said oxygenation is necessary during a seizure to prevent memory loss, and indeed often the problem historically with extensive memory loss from ECT arises out of failure to oxygenate, would you disagree with that?

A: Disagree.

Q: And you disagree with his assertion that you should always oxygenate to prevent memory loss?

A: Yes.

32. N. Motohashi, S. Awata, T. Higuchi, "A Questionnaire Survey of ECT Practice in University Hospitals and National Hospitals in Japan," *Journal of ECT* 20(1) (2004):21–23.

33. Healy and Shorter, *Shock Therapy*, 105.

34. Edward Coffey told his students in 1991, "The indication for anesthetic is simply that it reduces the anxiety and the fear and the panic that are associated with the treatment. OK? It doesn't do anything beyond that. . . . There are, however, significant disadvantages in using an anesthetic during ECT. . . . The anesthetic elevates seizure threshold. . . . Very, very critical." "Practical Advances in ECT: 1991," Continuing Medical Education course given at the Marriott Marquis Hotel, New York City, April 20–21, 1991.

35. Jan-Otto Ottoson, "Convulsive Therapy," in H. M. van Praag et al., eds., *Handbook of Biological Psychiatry* (New York: Marcel Dekker, 1981), 421.

36. Testimony of Richard D. Weiner, M.D., *Atze Akkerman vs. Mecta Corporation*, United States District Court, Central District of California. Case No. CV 01–10362 RSWL(RZx), October 27, 2005, 17–36. Deposition of Harold Sackeim, Ph.D., *Akkerman v. Johnson*, 63–78. Deposition of Harold Sackeim Ph.D, *Imogene Lori Rohovit et al. v. Mecta Corporation*, State of Iowa, Edward Sathoff M.D. et al., Iowa District Court for Johnson County, No. 52489, April 12, 1996, 38–39.

37. Harold A. Sackeim, "Are ECT Devices Underpowered? (Editorial)," *Convulsive Therapy* 7(4) (1991):233–236. A. D. Krystal, M. D. Dean, et al., "ECT Stimulus Intensity: Are Present ECT Devices Too Limited?" *American Journal of Psychiatry* 157 (2000):963–967. Handout from the Mecta Corporation salesmen at the American Psychiatric Association conference, 2004.

38. Charles Kellner, "Electroshock with Susan Spencer" (TV interview), 48 Hours, C. Lasiewicz, producer. New York, CBS-TV, February 2, 1994.

39. Continuing Medical Education seminar sponsored by the Association for Convulsive Therapy at the American Psychiatric Association annual meeting, 1996.

40. Douglas G. Cameron, "ECT: Sham Statistics, the Myth of Convulsive Therapy, and the Case for Consumer Misinformation," *Journal of Mind and Behavior* 15(1–2) (1994):177–198.

41. Ibid. To calculate the maximum output of the devices, Cameron uses these formulas: For sine wave devices, joules = volts × current × duration, or joules = current squared × impedance × duration. For brief pulse devices, it is joules = volts × current × (hz × 2) × wave length × duration. By these formulas, the Somatics Thymatron DG

put out 250 joules or watts of electricity, while the Mecta SR and JR put out 256 joules. These machines, in use circa 1985–1995, have now been replaced by even more powerful models.

42. The U.K. ECT Review Group, "Efficacy and Safety of Electroconvulsive Therapy in Depressive Disorders: A Systematic Review and Meta-analysis," *The Lancet* 361 (2003, March 8):799–805.

43. For instance, N. P. Lancaster, R. R. Steinert, I. Frost, "Unilateral Electroconvulsive Therapy," *Journal of Mental Science* 104 (1958):221–227. C. G. Costello, G. P. Belton, et al., "The Amnesic and Therapeutic Effects of Bilateral and Unilateral ECT," *British Journal of Psychiatry* 116 (1970):69–78.

44. Richard Abrams, "Stimulus Titration and ECT Dosing," *Journal of ECT* 18(1) (2002):3–9.

45. Deposition of Harold Sackeim, Ph.D., *Akkerman v. Johnson*, 135.

46. Abrams, "Stimulus Titration."

47. Max Fink, "Move On!" *Journal of ECT* 18(1) (2002):11–13.

48. http://www.wired.com/news/print/0.1294.394.87.00.html (accessed September 20, 2000).

CHAPTER 7 — THE MAKING OF AN AMERICAN ACTIVIST

1. Letter, Marilyn Rice to Leonard Frank, March 29, 1975.

2. Letter, Marilyn Rice to Berton Roueché, November 20, 1973.

3. Marilyn Rice, "The Rice Papers," in Leonard Roy Frank, *The History of Shock Treatment* (San Francisco, 1978), 96.

4. Ibid., 95.

5. Berton Roueché, "As Empty as Eve," *New Yorker*, September 4, 1974.

6. Letter, Marilyn Rice to Berton Roueché, November 2, 1974.

7. Letter, Marilyn Rice to Linda Andre, August 12, 1988.

8. Letter, Marilyn Rice to Leonard Frank, February 16, 1975.

9. National Institute of Mental Health, *Facts About: Electroshock Therapy* (Pamphlet 0470–547) (Washington, D.C.: U.S. Government Printing Office, 1972).

10. Memo, Marilyn Rice to Dr. Peter Mendelis, October 8, 1973.

11. Barry M. Maletzky, *Multiple-Monitored Electroconvulsive Therapy* (Boca Raton, Fla.: CRC Press, 1981), 186.

12. Roueché, "As Empty as Eve."

13. Letter, Marilyn Rice to Berton Roueché, September 22, 1974.

14. Letter, Marilyn Rice to Berton Roueché, November 2, 1974.

15. Letter, Marilyn Rice to John Friedberg, July 31, 1980.

16. Letter, Marilyn Rice to Leonard Frank, February 16, 1975.

17. Letter, Marilyn Rice to Leonard Frank, undated, circa February 1977.

18. *Marilyn Rice vs. Dr. John Nardini and Psychiatric Institute*, Superior Court, District of Columbia, Civil Action No. 703–74.

19. Letter, Peter Mendelis to Lothar Kalinowsky, August 14, 1974. Letter, Lothar Kalinowsky to Peter Mendelis, August 22, 1974. Letter, Peter Mendelis to Lothar Kalinowsky, August 30, 1974.

20. Letter, Marilyn Rice to Leonard Frank, September 28, 1976. Letter, Marilyn Rice to Leonard Frank, November 22, 1978.

21. Letters, Marilyn Rice to Leonard Frank, February 28, 1976, May 28, 1977. Letter, Marilyn Rice to Peter Breggin, September 5, 1978. Trial transcript, *Rice vs. Nardini.*

22. Letter, Marilyn Rice to Fred Hapgood, undated, circa May 1980.

23. Letter, Marilyn Rice to Springer Publishing Co., January 16, 1981. Letter, Marilyn Rice to Hank Mallory, September 12, 1978. The experts who weren't heard were Dr. Joseph deVeaugh-Geiss, Dr. Peter Sterling, and Dr. Stephan Chorover.

24. Letter, Marilyn Rice to Leonard Frank, undated.

25. Letter, Marilyn Rice to Leonard Frank, February 25, 1977.

26. Letter, Marilyn Rice to Springer Publishing Co., January 16, 1981. Letter, Marilyn Rice to Christopher Gadsden, May 8, 1981.

27. *Rice vs. Nardini,* Plaintiff's Response to Defendant Nardini's Opposition to Plaintiff's Motion for Reconsideration, June 1981.

28. Letter, Marilyn Rice to Springer Publishing Co., January 16, 1981.

29. Letter, Marilyn Rice to Leonard Frank, March 17, 1975.

30. Letter, Marilyn Rice to Hank Mallory, May 1, 1979.

31. J. P. Morrissey, N. M. Burton, H. J. Steadman, "Developing an Empirical Base for Psycho-Legal Policy Analyses of ECT: A New York State Survey," *International Journal of Law and Psychiatry* 2(1) (1979):99–111.

32. Letter, Marilyn Rice to Arthur Ochs Sulzberger, June 27, 1979.

CHAPTER 8 — THE ECT INDUSTRY COWS THE MEDIA

1. "An Important Message from the APA President," *Psychiatric News*, October 7, 1977.

2. American Psychiatric Association, Addendum to Public Affairs Guidelines. Part III: Radio and Television. Adopted by the Board of Trustees, March 13, 1982.

3. Ronald McMillen, "Psychiatry in the Mass Media," *Psychiatric News*, December 7, 1979.

4. Letter, Marilyn Rice to Charles D. Farris, chairman of the FCC, December 12, 1977.

5. John Wykert, "NY Psychiatrists to Use PR Firm for 'Image Problem,'" *Psychiatric News*, April 18, 1980.

6. Marilyn Rice, "ECT: A Life-Saving Treatment—for Psychiatry," unpublished paper, February 1982.

7. Maggie Scarf, "Shocking the Depressed Back to Life," *New York Times Magazine*, June 17, 1979.

8. Ann Landers's syndicated column, various media outlets, 1979. *Prime Time Sunday,* NBC-TV, October 28, 1979. *Parade,* December 1979. *Reader's Digest,* August 1978. *Newsweek,* November 12, 1979. *Time,* November 19, 1979.

9. McMillen, "Psychiatry in the Mass Media."

10. Letter, Fred Hapgood to Marilyn Rice, April 30, 1980.

11. Fred Hapgood, "Electroshock: The Unkindest Therapy of All," *Atlantic Monthly*, January 1980.

12. Letter, Fred Hapgood to Marilyn Rice, May 11, 1980.

13. The National News Council (1973–1983) was an independent media oversight organization. Its only powers were to investigate complaints against the media and, if warranted, to draw public attention to unethical journalism.

14. Letter, Marilyn Rice to Sue Bradshaw, June 25, 1980.

15. McMillen, "Psychiatry in the Mass Media."

16. Robert Mendelsohn, *The People's Doctor* (syndicated newspaper column), April 19, 1980.

17. Letter, Marilyn Rice to Robert Mendelsohn, M.D., April 30, 1980.

18. L. R. Squire, P. C. Slater, "Electroconvulsive Therapy and Complaints of Memory Dysfunction: A Prospective Three-Year Follow-up Study," *British Journal of Psychiatry* 142 (1983):1–8.

19. Quoted in Mark Cohen, "Not with My Hippocampus You Don't!" *GQ*, December 1994.

20. G. H. Grosser, D. T. Pearsall, et al., "The Regulation of Electro-Convulsive Treatment in Massachusetts: A Follow-up," *Massachusetts Journal of Mental Health* 5 (1975):12–25. Extrapolation by Peter Breggin, *Electroshock: Its Brain-Disabling Effects* (New York: Springer Publishing, 1979), 3.

21. J. P. Morrissey, N. M. Burton, H. J. Steadman, "Developing an Empirical Base for Psycho-Legal Policy Analyses of ECT: A New York State Survey," *International Journal of Law and Psychiatry* 2 (1979):99–111. Extrapolation is by Breggin, *Electroshock*, 4.

22. R. W. Thompson, R. D. Weiner, C. P. Meyers, "Use of ECT in the United States in 1975, 1980, and 1986," *American Journal of Psychiatry* 151 (1994):1657–1661.

23. J. W. Thompson, J. D. Blaine, "Use of ECT in the United States in 1975 and 1980," *American Journal of Psychiatry* 144 (1987):557–562.

24. Colleen O'Connor, "The Return of Electroshock," *Washington Post*, December 1, 1985.

25. Jean Dietz, "Shock Therapy: Advocates Giving a Jolt to Villainous Hollywood Image," *Boston Globe*, January 21, 1985.

26. Dietz caught a big fish here, but one that, in the prevailing political climate, would be thrown back and left out of the decades of comeback articles to come. This was the first time Fink admitted his financial ties to the shock machine companies; he's steadfastly denied or hidden them ever since (even in contexts where disclosure is mandatory). He's only been caught once, in 1996, in Sandra Boodman, "Shock Therapy: It's Back," *Washington Post*, Health section, September 24, 1996.

CHAPTER 9 — LONG STRANGE TRIP

1. Patrice Weil, "From Toothbrush to Pacemaker: The F.D.A. Is Moving In," *New York Times*, December 31, 1978.

2. Bruce Ingersoll, "Amid Lax Regulation, Medical Devices Flood a Vulnerable Market," *Wall Street Journal*, March 24, 1992.

3. Ibid.

4. Utah Biomedical Test Laboratory. Final Report (Revision A), "A Study of Safety and Performance Requirements for Electroconvulsive Therapy Devices," TR 226–011, December 15, 1977.

5. Summary minutes, Diagnostic and Monitoring Instruments and Devices Subcommittee, Neurological Devices Classification Panel, November 5, 1976, Washington, D.C.

6. Remarks of Harold Stevens at the November 5, 1976, meeting of the Neurological Devices Classification Panel, quoted in C09, Docket No. 78N-1103 (comments of Public Citizen).

7. *Federal Register*, Vol. 43, No. 220, November 28, 1979, 55729, Classification of Electroconvulsive Therapy Devices.

8. Minutes of the third meeting of the Neurological Section, Respiratory and Nervous Systems Devices Panel, Food and Drug Administration, Washington, D.C., May 29, 1979.

9. Testimony of Richard D. Weiner, M.D., *Atze Akkerman v. Mecta Corporation*, United States District Court, Central District of California. Case No. CV 01–10362 RSWL(RZx), October 27, 2005, 17–36.

10. *Federal Register*, Vol. 44, No. 172, September 4, 1979, 51776, Neurological Devices: Classification of Electroconvulsive Therapy Devices. Final Rule.

11. Letter, Marilyn Rice to James Veale, October 23, 1979.

12. Marilyn Rice, notes of a telephone conversation with Mr. Burdette of the FDA, April 12, 1988.

13. Letter, Marilyn Rice to James Veale, May 12, 1980.

14. J. M. Davis, "Official Actions: The Council on Research," *American Journal of Psychiatry* 138(4) (1981):572.

15. Jeanne Lindsay, "FDA Hearings on Electroshock, a Personal Report," *Madness Network News*, Spring 1983.

16. Docket No. 82N-0316, CP0002, Food and Drug Administration, October 19, 1982.

17. Testimony of Marilyn Rice at the FDA hearing on the APA petition to reclassify the electroconvulsive therapy device, November 4, 1982.

18. Comments of Susan B. Foote, Docket No. 82P-0316, C69, June 2, 1983.

19. Testimony of Richard Weiner at the FDA hearing on the APA petition to reclassify the electroconvulsive therapy device, November 4, 1982.

20. Marilyn Rice, "The Industry Wins (letter)," *New York Times*, November 25, 1982.

21. *Federal Register*, Vol. 48, No. 66, April 5, 1983, 14758. Reclassification of Electroconvulsive Therapy Device. Notice of Intent.

CHAPTER 10 — THE COMMITTEE FOR TRUTH IN PSYCHIATRY

1. Letter, Marilyn Rice to Leonard Frank, May 3, 1985.

2. The founding members were Marilyn Rice, Joy Rose, Marge Faeder, Elizabeth Plasick, June Ray, Joanne Marcellus, June Bassett, Ellen Field, Pam Maccabee, Margaret Gill, Lynn Sorlie, Carol Terry, Patricia Calder, Betty Scoleri, Mary Dietrich, Connie Neil, and Janet Gotkin.

3. FDA Docket No. 84P-0430, dated December 17, 1984.

4. Petition for reconsideration, Docket No. 84P-0430, December 14, 1985.

5. Letter, FDA to Marilyn Rice re Docket No. 84P-0430, June 3, 1986.

6. American Psychiatric Association, Petition to Reclassify ECT Devices, FDA Docket No. 82P-0316, F3.

7. "ECT Patients Petition for Animal CT Scans," *Dickinson's FDA* 1(8) (1985, September 15).

8. "CT-scan Pressure on FDA Grows," *Dickinson's FDA*, 2(5) (1986, March 1).

9. Marilyn Rice, "FDA's Proposal to Reclassify the ECT Device: A Review and Critique," (unpublished paper,) undated (September 1990).

10. Peter Breggin, Abstract, "Neuropathology and Cognitive Dysfunction from ECT," Program and Abstracts book, NIMH Consensus Development Conference on ECT, June 10–12, 1985.

11. Freeman quoted his own study. C. P. L. Freeman, R. E. Kendell, "ECT I: Patients' Experiences and Attitudes," *British Journal of Psychiatry* 137 (1980):8–16. For a critique of this study, see L. Johnstone, H. Frith, "Discourse Analysis and the Experience of ECT," *Psychology and Psychotherapy: Research and Practice* 78 (2005):1–16.

12. "Consensus Conference: Electroconvulsive Therapy," *Journal of the American Medical Association* 254 (15) (1985, October 18): 2103–2108.

13. L. R. Squire, P. C. Slater, "Electroconvulsive Therapy and Complaints of Memory Dysfunction: A Prospective Three-Year Follow-up Study," *British Journal of Psychiatry* 142 (1983):1–8.

14. Press release, Ad Hoc Committee for a Moratorium on Electroshock, June 12, 1985.

15. *Today Show*, NBC-TV, June 12, 1985.

16. Letter, Marilyn Rice to Leonard Frank, July 20, 1985.

17. FDA Docket No. 86P-0016, December 28, 1985.

18. Decision letter on Docket No. 86P-0016, FDA to Linda Andre, May 22, 1986.

19. Decision letter on Docket No. 86P-0016/PRC, FDA to Linda Andre, October 31, 1986.

20. FDA Docket No. 86P-0253.

21. Letter, Marilyn Rice to petitioners for CAT scans, September 7, 1987.

CHAPTER 11 — ANECDOTE OR EVIDENCE?

1. FDA Docket No. 82P-0316, C543, October 18, 1990.

2. FDA Docket No. 82P-0316, C88, March 21, 1984.

3. FDA Docket No. 82P-0316, Sup. 1, Vol. 8, May 7, 1984; Let. 11, April 30, 1984; C90, April 19, 1984.

4. FDA Docket No. 82P-0316, C543, October 18, 1990.

5. FDA Docket No. 82P-0316, Let. 13 (letter from Iver Small, May 8, 1984). The patient letters on stationery from Larue D. Carter Memorial Hospital in Indianapolis, a state facility, are C110 (February 20, 1984) and C112 (February 28, 1984).

6. Letter, U.S. Representative Charles Rangel to Frank Young of the FDA, December 14, 1987.

7. FDA Docket No. 82P-0316, C10, Rex Hiatt, November 14, 1982.

8. FDA Docket No. 82P-0316, C635, Robin Nicol, November 16, 1990.

9. FDA Docket No. 82P-0316, C01, Harry Feinstein of Hittman Medical Systems, September 16, 1982. Hittman was the parent company of Medcraft, the third U.S. manufacturer of shock machines and the only one that still manufactures sine wave devices.

10. FDA Docket No. 82P-0316, Comments 55, 66, 70, 71, 72, 82, 519, 527, 539, 625, Sup. 4, 728.

11. FDA Docket No. 82P-0316, C04, Herbert Pardes, October 14, 1982.

12. FDA Docket No. 82P-0316, C71, Conrad Swartz, June 1, 1983.

13. This example is from Malcolm Spector and John I. Kitsuse, eds., *Constructing Social Problems* (New Brunswick, N.J.: Transaction Publishers), 2001, 146.

14. Some examples: Phyllis Chesler, *Women & Madness* (New York: Doubleday, 1972); Patients' Rights Office, Sacramento, Calif., statistics on the statewide use of ECT 1994–1996; New York State Office of Mental Health, selected statistics released in 2004.

15. Among the small number of women with a career interest in ECT are Laura Fochtmann, Joan Prudic, Teresa Rummans, Sarah Holly Lisanby, and Joyce Small.

16. M. F. Belenky, B. M. Clinchy, N. R. Goldberger, J. M. Tarule, eds., *Women's Ways of Knowing: The Development of Self, Voice, and Mind* (New York: Basic Books, 1986), Chapter 6.

17. Ibid. The quote is from Peter Elbow, *Writing without Teachers* (London: Oxford University Press), 1973, 173.

18. Personal communication with Beth Gundelach, patient of Dr. Max Fink; personal communication with Selma Lanes, patient and research subject of Harold Sackeim, Ph.D.; letter, Lanes to Sackeim, November 5, 1991.

19. Belenky et al., *Women's Ways*, 104.

20. M. Philpot, C. Collins, et al., "Eliciting Users' Views of ECT in Two Mental Health Trusts with a User-Designed Questionnaire," *Journal of Mental Health* 13(4) (2004):403–413.

21. Anne B. Donahue, testimony at the public hearing of the Vermont (U.S.) Health and Welfare Committee on electroconvulsive therapy, March 12, 1999. Jonathan Cott, *On the Sea of Memory* (New York: Random House), 2005.

22. Marilyn Rice, Message to CTIP Members and Supporters, July 17, 1988.

23. ECT Task Force of the American Psychiatric Association, *The Practice of Electroconvulsive Therapy: Recommendations for Treatment, Training, and Privileging* (Washington, D.C.: American Psychiatric Association), 1990.

24. "APA Report: A Report from the Medical Director, Melvin Sabshin, M.D.," *Psychiatric News*, January 5, 1990.

25. *Federal Register*, Vol. 55, No. 172, Wednesday, September 5, 1990, p. 36578: Neurological Devices; Proposed Rule to Reclassify the Electroconvulsive Therapy Device Intended for Use in Treating Severe Depression.

26. Marilyn Rice, "FDA's Proposal to Reclassify the ECT Device: A Review and Critique," (unpublished paper) September 1990.

27. D. R. Weinberger, E. F. Torrey, et al., "Lateral Cerebral Ventricular Enlargement in Chronic Schizophrenia," *Archives of General Psychiatry* 36 (1979):735–739. S. P. Calloway, R. J. Dolan, et al., "ECT and Cerebral Atrophy: A Computed Tomographic Study," *Acta Psychiatrica Scandinavica* 64 (1981):442–445. R. J. Dolan, S. P. Calloway, et al., "The Cerebral Cortical Appearance in Depressed Subjects," *Psychological Medicine* 16(4) (1986, November):775–779.

28. L. R. Squire, P. C. Slater, "Electroconvulsive Therapy and Complaints of Memory Dysfunction: A Prospective Three-Year Follow-up Study," *British Journal of Psychiatry* 142 (1983):1–8.

29. L. R. Squire, J. A. Zouzounis, "Self-Ratings of Memory Dysfunction: Different Findings in Depression and Amnesia," *Journal of Clinical and Experimental Neurology* 10(6) (1988):727–738.

30. L. R. Squire, P. C. Slater, P. L. Miller, "Retrograde Amnesia Following ECT: Long-Term Follow-up," *Archives of General Psychiatry* 32 (1981):89–95.

31. D. I. Templer, C. F. Ruff, G. Armstrong, "Cognitive Functioning and Degree of Psychosis in Schizophrenics Given Many ECT," *British Journal of Psychiatry* 123 (1973):441–443.

32. Herbert Goldman, Frank E. Gomer, Donald I. Templer, "Long-term Effects of Electroconvulsive Therapy upon Memory and Perceptual-Motor Performance," *Journal of Clinical Psychology* 28 (1972):32–35.

33. David Avery, George Winokur, "Mortality in Depressed Patients Treated with Electroconvulsive Therapy and Anti-Depressants," *Archives of General Psychiatry* 33 (1976):1029–1037.

34. L. Brunschwig, J. Strain, T. G. Bidder, "Issues in the Assessment of Post-ECT Memory Changes," *British Journal of Psychiatry* 119 (1973):73–74.

35. This is known as the Columbia autobiographical memory inventory (AMI) because it was created by the Sackeim team. I have examined this questionnaire closely and found that approximately 60 percent of the questions are irrelevant to the type of amnesia experienced after shock. They test very old, overlearned information, which we know people don't forget, such as the names of their grandparents. The questionnaire is not designed to assess memories more than one year old.

36. R. D. Weiner, H. J. Rogers, et al., "Effects of Stimulus Parameters on Cognitive Side Effects," *Annals of the New York Academy of Sciences* 462 (1986):315–325.

37. C. P. L. Freeman, D. Weeks, R. E. Kendell, "ECT II: Patients Who Complain," *British Journal of Psychiatry* 137 (1980):17–25.

38. FDA Task Force on ECT (James McCue, Chairman), "Review of Literature and Other Articles on Electroconvulsive Therapy, 1982 to 1988."

39. Marilyn Rice, "FDA's Proposal to Reclassify the ECT Device: A Review and Critique" (unpublished paper), September 1990.

40. Letter, Elaine Johnson, FDA Freedom of Information Staff, Office of Standards and Regulations, Center for Devices and Radiological Health, to Marilyn Rice, November 8, 1990.

41. Letter, Hugh Cannon, FDA Associate Commissioner for Legislative Affairs, to Senator Alan Cranston, December 21, 1985.

CHAPTER 12 — SHAMING SCIENCE

1. Certificate of incorporation of the International Association for Psychiatric Research, Inc., on file with the Department of State of New York; amended to reflect a name change to Scion Natural Science Association, Inc., St. James, New York. The officers are Drs. Jonathan and Rachel Fink. The foundation gave a $34,000 grant to the authors (including Fink himself, according to the Web site of the Department of Psychiatry at the State University of New York/Stony Book) of *Shock Therapy: A History of Electroconvulsive Treatment in Mental Illness* (New Brunswick, N.J.: Rutgers University Press, 2007).

2. Eliot Marshall, "Gene Therapy on Trial," *Science* 288 (2000):951–957. A series of articles by Sheryl Gay Stolberg ran in the *New York Times*, including "Teenager's Death Is Shaking Up Field of Human Gene-Therapy Experiments," January 27, 2000.

3. University Science, "Study Shows Journals Report Few Conflicts of Interest." http://www.unisci.com/stories/20012/0523014.htm, May 23, 2001 (accessed March 24, 2006). Meryl Nass, "Can Medical Research Findings Be Trusted?" http:www.red-flagsweekly.com/ nasspubhlth.html (accessed February 13, 2002). Sue McGreevey, "Almost Half of All Faculty on Institutional Review Boards Have Ties to Industry," http://www.academicmedicine.org/cgi/content/full/78/8/831, August 14, 2003 (accessed September 20, 2003). Sheryl Gay Stolberg, "Study Says Clinical Guides Often Hide Ties of Doctors," *New York Times*, February 6, 2002. Ted Agres, "NIH Ethics Investigation. Cash Gifts from Grantees Prompt Congressional Investigation of NIH Officials," *The Scientist*, June 30, 2003. David Willman, "Stealth Merger: Drug Companies and Government Medical Research," *Los Angeles Times*, December 7, 2003.

Rick Weiss, "NIH Scientists Broke Rules, Panel Says; Deals with Companies Went Unreported, Probe of Potential Conflicts of Interests Finds," *Washington Post,* June 23, 2004.

4. Marcia Angell, "Is Academic Medicine for Sale?" *New England Journal of Medicine* 342 (2000, May 18):1516–1518.

5. "Is Academic Medicine for Sale?" Talk by Marcia Angell at the Third National Ethics Conference, sponsored by Friends Research Institute, November 4, 2000, Baltimore, Md. Quoted in Robert Whitaker, *Mad in America: Bad Science, Bad Medicine, and the Enduring Mistreatment of the Mentally Ill* (Cambridge, Mass.: Perseus Books, 2002), 65.

6. Fred Gardner, "Eli Lilly's Bitch: The NIMH," *Counterpunch*, September 11–12, 2004. http://www.counterpunch.org/gardner09112004.html (accessed September 14, 2004).

7. This according to the 1978 APA ECT Task Force Report, referencing "Research in the Science of Mental Health: Report of Research Task Force of NIMH," DHEW Publication (ADM) 75–236, 1975, Chapter 12.

8. National Institute of Mental Health, response to a Freedom of Information request for the grant files of NIMH Grant No. 35636, January 25, 2001. The information that is publicly disclosable includes the grant award letters that state the amount of money awarded.

9. Harold A. Sackeim, (1) "Self-Deception, Self-Confrontation, and Personality," Master's thesis, 1975, University of Pennsylvania, Department of Psychology. (2) "On

Self-Deception," Presentation at the 15th Annual Meeting of the Rappaport-Klein Study Group, Austin-Riggs Center, Stockbridge, Mass., 1976. (3) "Self-Deception: Motivational Determinants of the Non-Awareness of Cognition." Ph.D.diss., 1977, University of Pennsylvania, Department of Psychology. (4) "Self-Deception: A Concept in Search of a Phenomenon," *Journal of Personality and Social Theory* 34 (1979):147–169 (with co-author R. C. Gur). (5) "Self-Deception, Other-Deception, and Self-Reported Psychopathology," *Journal of Consulting and Clinical Psychology* 47 (1979):213–215 (with co-author R. C. Gur). (6) "Self-Deception: A Synthesis." In J. S. Lockard and D. Paulhus, eds., *Self-Deception: An Adaptive Mechanism?* (New York: Prentice Hall, 1988), 146–165.

10. Edward Bernays, quoted in Stewart Ewen, *PR! A Social History of Spin* (New York: Basic Books, 1996), 11.

11. Deposition of Max Fink, Cause No. 992–00167, *Raymond A. Chiodini v. Deaconess Health Services Corporation et al.*, Circuit Court for St. Louis City, Missouri, April 12, 2001.

12. Deposition of Harold Sackeim Ph.D., *Imogene Lori Rohovit et al. v. Mecta Corporation, State of Iowa, Edward Sathoff M.D. et al.*, Iowa District Court for Johnson County, No. 52489, April 12, 1996, 35. Deposition of Harold Sackeim Ph.D., Case No. 01069713, *Atze Akkerman and Elizabeth Akkerman v. Joseph Johnson*, Santa Barbara Cottage Hospital, and Does 1–20, Court of the State of California for the County of Santa Barbara, Anacapa Division, March 14, 2004, 63 et seq.

13. Robin Nicol has a Master's degree in English and her co-owner husband, Gorham, an MBA. Mecta is simply one of their investments. The extent to which the Nicols, neither of whom has any medical training, rely entirely on the shock doctors they hire for information on ECT was illustrated in Gorham Nicol's 2005 testimony to a California jury.

> MR. NICOL: I was buying another company for an investor, and Mecta was in the same building, and they were bankrupting it. . . . When I walked through their building, the engineer that had built it said—you know, I was just asking, "What is that?" And they said, "It's electroconvulsive therapy equipment and we are bankrupting it." And I said, "Well, is it good equipment or—" He said, "Here. Look at the list of doctors that want it."
>
> Q: You never actually learned whether or not the machines were actually harming patients, did you, when you bought the company?
>
> A: I have never had a doctor come up to me and say that he had a patient that had been injured. . . . So I had no indication that the machine could harm anyone.
>
> Q: I want to know if you have done any safety studies on humans to see if it is safe to use on human beings?
>
> A: Those studies are done by the experts in the field, and we take the results of their expertise.
>
> Q: So the answer is no, Mecta has never done any safety studies of its own?
>
> A: Mecta is a machine manufacturer, and we make what we think is the best piece of equipment in the world, and we don't do tests on humans in our plant.
>
> Q: Has Mecta ever commissioned anyone to do any tests on humans to make sure your machine is safe to actually use on human beings?

A: No.

Q: In the past 25 years Mecta has never conducted any research of its own into the safety and efficacy of its ECT machines, has it?

A: We've relied on the experts for that information.

Q: The answer is no?

A: That event needs to take place in the industry, and we have had it supplied to us and have not had to create it. So we have used what the experts have found to be true.

Q: You take no interest or responsibility in the creation of the shock machines; correct?

A: I have interest, but I don't take the design responsibility. . . . The doctors in research centers provide the medical requirements and information we need to build the equipment because our function is strictly as a manufacturer.

Q: Over time has one of those experts included Dr. Weiner?

A: Yes, sir. It has.

Q: And have you relied upon the advice of experts like Dr. Weiner as to the medical effects of the therapy?

A: Yes, we have.

Q: Is there anybody that is employed at the company that is capable of conducting scientific studies, clinical studies with human beings with respect to the effects of ECT?

A: Absolutely not.

Testimony of Gorham Nicol, *Atze Akkerman v. Mecta Corporation,* United States District Court, Central District of California, Case No. CV 01–10362 RSWL(RZx). October 12, 2005, 182, 193–194. October 14, 2005, 76–77, 80–81, 98–100.

14. U.S. Department of Health and Human Services, Public Health Service, "Responsibility of Applicants for Promoting Objectivity in Research for Which PHS Funding Is Sought," 42 CFR Subpart F, Sec. 50.601 et seq., 60 FR 35815, July 11, 1995; 60 FR 39076, July 31, 1995.

15. As an employee and officer of the State of New York, Harold Sackeim is required to make financial disclosure of any amounts over $1,000 to the New York State Ethics Commission. The records of the commission are public, and they show that as of 2001, Sackeim made no disclosure of funds from Mecta or Somatics, although he does disclose funding from companies that make magnetic therapy devices. As a grantee of the National Institute of Mental Health, Sackeim is required to make the same financial disclosure to his institution, New York State Psychiatric Institute (P.I.). This information can be obtained by a Freedom of Information request, since P.I. is a public institution. Records of such requests show that, as of 2005, Sackeim had never made any financial disclosures. Private institutions, like Duke University, do not make financial disclosures public.

16. Abstract, NIMH Grant No. 1R01MH035636, Sidney Malitz, Principal Investigator, written for the funding period December 1, 1981, to November 30, 1984.

17. Abstract, NIMH Grant No. 5R37MH035636, Harold Sackeim, Principal Investigator, written for the funding period 1992–1995.

18. Harold A. Sackeim, "Memory Loss and ECT: From Polarization to Reconciliation," *Journal of ECT* 16(2) (2000):87–96.

19. Abstract, NCRR Grant No. 5M01RR000030–320448, Richard Weiner, Principal Investigator, written for Fiscal Year 1993.

20. Abstract, NIMH Grant No. 5R37MH030723, Richard Weiner, Principal Investigator, written for the funding period 1991–1994.

21. C. D. Frith, M. Stevens, et al., "Effects of ECT and Depression on Various Aspects of Memory," *British Journal of Psychiatry* 142 (1983):610–617.

22. S. H. Lisanby, D. P. Devanand, et al., "Exceptionally High Seizure Threshold: ECT Device Limitations," *Convulsive Therapy* 12(3) (1996, September):156–164.

23. R. D. Weiner, C. E. Coffey, "Electroconvulsive Therapy in the United States," *Psychopharmacology Bulletin* 27(1) (1991):9–15. M. C. Webb, C. E. Coffey, et al., "Cerebrovascular Response to Unilateral Electroconvulsive Therapy," *Biological Psychiatry* 28(9) (1990, November 1): 758–766. C. E. Coffey, G. S. Figiel, R. D. Weiner, W. B. Saunders, "Caffeine Augmentation of ECT," *American Journal of Psychiatry* 147(5) (1990):579–585.

24. Testimony of Richard D. Weiner, M.D., *Akkerman v. Mecta*, October 27, 2005, 17–36.

25. Mecta Model SR and JR Instruction Manual, Mecta Corporation, undated (circa 1985). Richard Abrams and Conrad Swartz, ECT Instruction Manual, Somatics, Inc., June 1989.

26. *The Phil Donahue Show*, April 1996.

27. Sandra Boodman, "Shock Therapy: It's Back," *Washington Post*, Health section, September 24, 1996.

28. T. Whitney, "Doctoring of Science," *Bangor News* (Maine), December 10, 2003.

29. U.S. Patent No. 5,626,627, filed July 27, 1995.

30. American Psychiatric Association, *The Practice of Electroconvulsive Therapy: Recommendations for Treatment, Training, and Privileging* (Washington, D.C.: American Psychiatric Association, 2001), viii.

31. Deposition of Harold Sackeim Ph.D., *Rohovit v. Mecta*, 59. Deposition of Harold Sackeim Ph.D., *Akkerman v. Johnson*, 207.

32. C. Edward Coffey, Richard D. Weiner, et al., "Effects of ECT on Brain Structure: A Pilot Prospective Magnetic Resonance Imaging Study," *American Journal of Psychiatry* 145(6) (1988):701–706.

33. C. Edward Coffey, Richard D. Weiner, et al., "Brain Anatomic Effects of Electroconvulsive Therapy: A Prospective Magnetic Resonance Imaging Study," *Archives of General Psychiatry* 48 (1991):1013–1021.

34. Richard D. Weiner, "Does Electroconvulsive Therapy Cause Brain Damage?" *Behavioral and Brain Sciences* 7 (1984):1–53.

35. D. P. Devanand, H. A. Sackeim, et al., "Does ECT Alter Brain Structure?" *American Journal of Psychiatry* 151 (1994):957–970.

36. G. Walter, "ECT Literature: Frequently Cited Papers and Their Impact on the Field (Letter to the Editor)," *Journal of ECT* 18(2) (2002, June):107–109.

37. C. Tavris, C. Wade, *Psychology,* 6th ed. (Upper Saddle River, N.J.: Prentice Hall, 2000), 623.

38. Deposition of Harold Sackeim Ph.D., *Rohovit v. Mecta,* 7–8, 20.

39. Ibid., 22.

40. Ibid., 14–17.

41. Barbara Seaman, *The Greatest Experiment Ever Performed on Women* (New York: Hyperion, 1977), 70.

42. Abstract, NIMH Grant No. 5K07MH01090 to William V. McCall, funding period 1995–2000.

43. Abstract, NIMH Grant No. 3K07MH000821 to Charles Kellner, funding period 1989–1992.

44. "Disclosure of Significant Relationships with Relevant Commercial Companies," handout at Electricity and Behavior meeting of the American Neuropsychiatric Association, New York, May 5, 1996.

45. "Welcome Our Newest Member to the ECT Hall of Shame," http://www.ect.org/shame/kellner.html (accessed January 22, 2008).

46. Drugs and ECT: Combined Treatment and Maintenance Treatment, workshop at "Advanced Clinical Issues in ECT: The Certificate Course", Continuing Medical Education course given at the Marriott Marquis Hotel, New York City, April 1992.

47. American Psychological Association, ethics complaint against Dr. Harold Sackeim, March 9, 1993.

48. U.S. Patent No. 4,870,969, "Thymapad" (TM) disposable electrodes. The "ECT accessory" market includes electrodes, jelly, and mouthguards, all discarded after one use.

49. Dennis Cauchon, "Shock Therapy," *USA Today,* December 6 and 7, 1995.

50. The mandatory financial disclosures are printed in the Program and Abstracts book of the American Psychiatric Association conferences. The program of the 2004 conference, where Swartz presented, reflects that Swartz made no disclosure.

51. Jonathan Cott, *On the Sea of Memory* (New York: Random House, 2005).

52. David Healy, *Let Them Eat Prozac* (Toronto: James Lorimer and Co. 2004), 401.

53. "Study Shows Journals Report Few Conflicts of Interest," Psychiatry-Research email alert, May 23, 2001, citing G. A. Fava, "Conflict of Interest and Special Interest Groups," *Psychotherapy and Psychosomatics* 70 (2001):1–5; S. Krimsky, "Journal Policies on Conflict of Interest: If This Is the Therapy, What's the Disease?" *Psychotherapy and Psychosomatics* 70 (2001):115–117. At http://www.unisci.com/stories/20012/0523014.htm, University Science Web site (accessed May 23, 2001).

54. Giovanni Fava, "Conflict of Interest and Special Interest Groups," *Psychotherapy and Psychosomatics* 70 (2001):1–5.

55. Vera Hassner Sharav, Director, Association for Human Research Protection, "Why Did OHRP Shred Informed Consent Documents?" Infomail (email alert) from AHRP to electronic mailing list. http://www.ahrp.org/infomail/03/10/25.php (accessed October 13, 2003).

CHAPTER 13 — THE LIE THAT WON'T DIE

1. Brent Cunningham, "Re-Thinking Objectivity," *Columbia Journalism Review*, July–August 2003.

2. Timothy Gower, "Crackling," *Boston Phoenix*, April 24, 1992.

3. "The Return of Shock Therapy," *Providence Journal Bulletin*, September 18, 1990.

4. The story by FAIR's Jeff Cohen and Norman Solomon was sent out by Creators Syndicate in June 1995 and ran in various outlets with different titles, for instance, "Shock Therapy Stories Lack Opponents' Views," *Register-Guard* (Eugene, Ore.), June 4, 1995. It is available online at http://www.mentalhelpnet.com/electro.htm (accessed April 5, 2005.)

5. "A New Image for Shock Therapy," *Los Angeles Times*, September 15, 1992; "Taking the Shock out of Electroshock," *U.S. News and World Report*, January 24, 2000; "Shock Therapy Loses Some of Its Shock Value," *New York Times*, September 19, 2006.

6. Dorothy Nelkin, *Selling Science: How the Press Covers Science and Technology*, rev. ed. (New York: W. H. Freeman and Co., 995), 88.

7. Ibid.

8. Jennifer Hughes, "Electroshock Treatments Can Ease Depression but Still Face Sharp Criticism," *The Record* (Bergen County, N.J.), October 25, 2005.

9. "Electrical Safety for Laboratory Workers" by Dr. Dale Karweik of Ohio State University Department of Chemistry, http://www.chemistry.ohio-state.edu/ehs/electric.htm (accessed November 29, 2007.)

10. Brent Cunningham, "Across the Great Class Divide," *Columbia Journalism Review*, May–June 2004.

11. Daniel Smith, "Shock and Disbelief," *Atlantic Monthly*, February 2001.

12. Daniel Smith, author response in Letters to the Editor column, *Atlantic Monthly*, May 2001.

CHAPTER 14 — ERASING HISTORY

1. Alfred A. Fusco, "Federal Government Must Listen to Electroshock Patients' View," *Syracuse Post Standard*, October 9, 1998.

2. Letter, Bernie Arons to Committee for Truth in Psychiatry, March 28, 1997. Capitalization his.

3. See, for instance, Anne C. Mulkern, "More than 100 Top Regulatory Officials Represented Industry as Lobbyists, Lawyers," *Denver Post*, May 24, 2004.

4. Giovanni Fava, "Conflict of Interest and Special Interest Groups," *Psychotherapy and Psychosomatics* 70 (2001):1–5.

5. "Setting the Stage for the Surgeon General's Report: Report of the Fifteenth Annual Rosalynn Carter Symposium on Mental Health Policy," November 1999, 30.

6. Erica Goode, "Federal Report Praising Electroshock Stirs Uproar," *New York Times*, October 6, 1999. Michelle Beaulieu, "Patient Groups Criticize Federal Report on Shock Therapy," Reuters, October 7, 1999. J. Ciment, "Consumer Group Criticizes Surgeon General on ECT," *British Medical Journal* 319 (1999, October 23):1092. Reports also appeared in the *Newark Star Ledger* and *Minneapolis Herald Tribune*.

7. Matthew Rudorfer, William Z. Potter, "Electroconvulsive Therapy: A Modern Medical Procedure," *New England Journal of Medicine* 328(12) (1993):882–883. Matthew Rudorfer, editorial praising ECT as "lifesaving," *Washington Post*, Health section, June 5, 1985, 6. Matthew Rudorfer, presentation and handout at the annual NAMI New York State conference, September 12, 1992.

8. Ciment, "Consumer Group Criticizes Surgeon General on ECT."

9. Leye Chzanowski, "ECT Document Reverberates over the Internet," *Disability News Service*, October 13, 1999.

10. http://www.surgeongeneral.gov (accessed December 1, 1999).

11. Letter from Ruth Ralph (coordinator of consumer contributions), signed by Thomas Arthur, Jean Campbell, Larry Fricks, J. Rock Johnson, Jean Risman, and Laura van Tosh, to David Satcher, October 18, 1999.

12. "Setting the Stage for the Surgeon General's Report," 60, 63.

13. Ibid., 62.

14. I was not taking notes during our conversation, so these quotes are not verbatim. However, they accurately reflect what was said.

15. So vicious and mean spirited is ECT politics that there were those who claimed Loper faked her seizures to gain political advantage.

16. Anne B. Donahue, "Electroconvulsive Therapy and Memory Loss: A Personal Journey," *Journal of ECT* 16(2) (2000):133–143.

17. Ibid.

18. *Counterpoint* (publication of Vermont Psychiatric Survivors, Rutland, Vt.), Winter 1999.

19. Vermont Department of Mental Health (formerly the Vermont Department of Developmental and Mental Health Services), records of the 1999–2001 ECT study committees. Anne Donahue, "What Makes Up True 'Informed' Consent?" December 15, 2000.

20. Anne Donahue vs. Dartmouth Hitchcock Medical Center et al., Docket No. 235–5–99, Superior Court, Washington County, Vermont.

21. Vermont Department of Mental Health, letter, Anne Donahue to William McMains, May 13, 1999.

22. Vermont Department of Mental Health, email, Anne Donahue to Harold Sackeim, August 29, 1999.

23. Vermont Department of Mental Health, letter, Cindy Haggett to Jennifer Myka, July 28, 2000.

24. Transcript of the session of the Vermont House Health and Welfare Committee hearing on H.12 (comments of Anne Donahue), January 20, 2000.

25. Vermont Department of Mental Health, email, Anne Donahue to William McMains, Rod Copeland, and Wendy Beinner, January 21, 2000.

26. Vermont Department of Mental Health, letter, Anne Donahue to Jennifer Myka, June 26, 2000.

27. Vermont Department of Mental Health. Some titles of her missives to the committees were: "What Makes Up True 'Informed' Consent?"; "ECT Research Data: Available Resources"; "Overview of Some Key Information Tidbits."

28. Vermont Department of Mental Health, "ECT Consent Forms and Procedure Guidelines," undated submission by Anne Donahue.

29. Vermont Department of Mental Health, letter from William McMains, Medical Director of DDMHS, November 9, 2001.

30. Vermont Department of Mental Health, memo from Anne Donahue, November 6, 2000.

31. Personal communication, William Sullivan, November 13, 2004.

32. Vermont Department of Mental Health, materials submitted by Anne Donahue, December 15, 2000.

33. Harold A. Sackeim, "Memory and ECT: From Polarization to Reconciliation," *Journal of ECT* 16(2) (2000):87–96.

34. Richard Abrams, "Does Brief-Pulse ECT Cause Persistent or Permanent Memory Impairment? Guest Editorial," *Journal of ECT* 18(2) (2002):71–73.

CHAPTER 15 — THE TRIUMPH OF PUBLIC RELATIONS OVER SCIENCE

1. Yvette I. Sheline, Milan Sanghavi, et al., "Depression Duration but Not Age Predicts Hippocampal Volume Loss in Medically Healthy Women with Recurrent Major Depression," *Journal of Neuroscience* 19 (1999):5034–5043. Yvette I. Sheline, Po W. Wang, et al., "Hippocampal Atrophy in Recurrent Major Depression," *Proceedings of the National Academy of Sciences* 93 (1996):3908–3913.

2. Yvette I. Sheline, "Neuroimaging Studies of Mood Disorder Effects on the Brain," *Biological Psychiatry* 54 (2003):338–352.

3. As McEwen explained to me, current research shows, "When the brain is subjected to serious trauma like in stroke or seizures, stress hormones do make the damage, the cell loss, worse." Personal communication, April 23, 2001. Sapolsky calls this "worsening the neurotoxicity of seizure." Robert Sapolsky, "The Possibility of Neurotoxicity in the Hippocampus in Major Depression: A Primer on Neuron Death," *Biological Psychiatry* 48 (2000):755–765.

4. T. C. Neylan, J. D. Canick, et al., "Cortisol Levels Predict Cognitive Impairment Induced by Electroconvulsive Therapy," *Biological Psychiatry* 50(5) (2001):331–336.

5. Bruce McEwen, personal communication, April 23, 2001.

6. Email from Robert Sapolsky, June 11, 2001.

7. Sheline et al., "Depression Duration."

8. P. J. Shah, M. F. Glabus, et al., "Chronic, Treatment-Resistant Depression and Right Fronto-Striatal Atrophy," *British Journal of Psychiatry* 180 (2002):434–440.

9. V. W. Swayze, N. C. Andreasen, et al., "Subcortical and Temporal Structures in Affective Disorder and Schizophrenia: A Magnetic Resonance Imaging Study," *Biological Psychiatry* 31 (1992):221–240. D. Velakoulis, C. Pantelis, et al., "Hippocampal Volume in First-Episode Psychoses and Chronic Schizophrenia," *Archives of General Psychiatry* 56 (1999):133–140. E. Mervaala, J. Fohr, M. Kononen, et al., "Quantitative MRI of the Hippocampus and Amygdala in Severe Depression," *Psychological Medicine* 30 (2000): 117–125. M. Ashtari, B. S. Greenwald, et al., "Hippocampal/Amygdala Volumes in Geriatric Depression," *Psychological Medicine* 29 (1999):629–638. D. A. Axelson, P. M. Doraiswamy, et al., "Hypercortisolemia and Hippocampal Changes in Depression," *Psychiatry Research* 47 (1993):180–186.

10. T. M. Madsden, P. E. Kristjansen, et al., "Increased Neurogenesis in a Model of Electroconvulsive Therapy," *Biological Psychiatry* 47 (2000):1043–1049. L. Santarelli et al., "Requirement of Hippocampal Neurogenesis for the Behavioral Effects of Antidepressants," *Science* 301 (2003):805–809. T. D. Perrera, J. D. Coplan, et al., "Antidepressant-Induced Neurogenesis in the Hippocampus of Adult Nonhuman Primates," *Journal of Neuroscience* 27(18) (2007):4894–4901.

11. A. C. Chen, K. H. Shin, et al., "ECS-Induced Mossy Fiber Sprouting and BDNF Expression Are Attenuated by Ketamine Pretreatment," *Journal of ECT* 17(1) (2001):27–32.

12. Benedict Carey, "Shock Therapy and the Brain," *Los Angeles Times,* November 17, 2003.

13. "Brain Stimulation: New Treatments for Mood Disorders." Panel presented at the American Psychiatric Association annual meeting, May 3, 2004.

14. Bruce McEwen, personal communication, April 23, 2001.

15. Douglas Montero, "Dad's Rights Zapped by the Shock Docs," *New York Post,* June 17, 2001. Wade Harkavy, "Watts Up: More New Yorkers Getting Zapped by Court Order," *Village Voice,* May 22, 2001.

16. New York State Commission on the Quality of Care for the Mentally Disabled. Survey of the Provision of Electro-Convulsive therapy (ECT) at New York State Psychiatric Centers, August 2001. During the time period studied, two patients in five were given ECT via a court order.

17. Robert Kalani, testimony at trial, *Matter of Pilgrim Psychiatric Center, Petitioner, v. Paul Henri Thomas, an Alleged Mentally Ill Patient.* Supreme Court, Suffolk County, IAS Part 34, Index No. 11807/83, April 2, 2001.

18. Price v. Sheppard, 307 Minn. 250, 239 N.W.2d 910 (1976).

19. Missouri Circuit Court, 22nd Judicial Circuit, Probate Division, St. Louis City, No.3–00–536-P-CC, May 16, 2000.

20. Amicus brief, New York State Psychiatric Association and Healthcare Association of New York State, matter of Paul Henri Thomas, dated June 6, 2001, submitted by Seth P. Stein and Robert L. Schonfeld, attorneys for NYSPA and HANYS.

21. Email from Robert Sapolsky, March 2, 2005.

22. Memorandum by W. Bromley Hall, *Pilgrim Psychiatric Center v. Thomas,* April 16, 2001.

23. Zachary Dowdy, "Judge Continues Electroshock," *Newsday,* April 17, 2001.

24. Testimony of Harold Sackeim, Ph.D., before the Mental Health Subcommittee of the New York State Assembly, hearings on electroconvulsive therapy, May 18, 2001.

25. This is based on his statement that shortly after making his offer he had received seventy-five, and my collection of at least a hundred that were sent to him after that.

26. Deposition of Harold Sackeim Ph.D., Case No. 01069713, *Atze Akkerman and Elizabeth Akkerman v. Joseph Johnson,* Santa Barbara Cottage Hospital and Does 1–20, Court of the State of California for the County of Santa Barbara, Anacapa Division, March 14, 2004, 45–63.

CHAPTER 16 — SHOULD ECT BE BANNED?

1. Marilyn Rice, personal communication, June 10, 1985.

2. P. M. Haddad, S. M. Benbow, "Electroconvulsive Therapy-Related Psychiatric Knowledge among British Anesthesiologists," *Convulsive Therapy* 9(2) (1993):101–107.

3. For instance, at the May 2004 APA conference during the presentation by Conrad Swartz, co-owner of Somatics. Fink has literally grabbed the microphone away from me at meetings when I tried to speak.

4. Harold Sackeim and the New York State Office of Mental Health's proposed informational materials for ECT, beginning in 2001.

5. "Advocate Laura J. Fochtmann, M.D., Works to Stop Limitations of Availability of Electroconvulsive Therapy," in promotional daily newspaper of the 2004 APA conference, Issue No. 4, May 5–6, 2004.

6. Personal communication with Jennifer Burson of Harold Sackeim's research team, December 11, 2001.

7. Testimony of Gorham Nicol, co-owner of Mecta Corp., Case No. 01069713, *Atze Akkerman and Elizabeth Akkerman v. Joseph Johnson*, Santa Barbara Cottage Hospital and Does 1–20, Court of the State of California for the County of Santa Barbara, Anacapa Division, October 13–14, 2005, 196. Nicol didn't know the answer to how many times his company had been sued; he said "numerous," then guessed seven.

8. Letter, Dr. Peter Mendelis to Berton Roueché, October 9, 1974.

9. Letter, Marilyn Rice to Berton Roueché, November 20, 1973.

10. American Psychiatric Association, *The Practice of Electroconvulsive Therapy: Recommendations for Treatment, Training, and Privileging* (Washington, D.C: American Psychiatric Association, 2001), 59, 324.

11. David Impastato, "Prevention of Fatalities in Electroshock Therapy," *Diseases of the Nervous System* 18 (Supp.) (1957):34–75. Dennis Cauchon, "Patients Aren't Informed of Full Danger," *USA Today*, December 6, 1995.

12. J. Prudic, M. Olfson, et al., "Effectiveness of Electroconvulsive Therapy in Community Settings," *Biological Psychiatry* 55(3) (2004, February 1):301–312.

13. Deposition of Harold Sackeim, Ph.D., *Akkerman v. Johnson*, 228–231. Specifically asked to provide the one-year followup data, he refused. In a memorandum to Dr. John Oldham, director of the New York State Psychiatric Institute, Sackeim claimed to have followed up ECT patients three and five years after shock, and to be in the process of publishing the results. That was November 12, 1992. No such results have ever been published. The research protocol signed by Selma Lanes specified that subjects in her study would be followed up for the purpose of memory assessment one year after shock. No such assessment occurred.

14. S. H. Lisanby, J. H. Maddox, et al., "The Effects of Electroconvulsive Therapy on Memory of Autobiographical and Public Events," *Archives of General Psychiatry* 57(6) (2000):581–190. C. Sobin, H. A. Sackeim, et al., "Predictors of Retrograde Amnesia Following ECT," *American Journal of Psychiatry* 152 (1995):995–1001.

15. Erick H. Turner, Annette M. Matthews, et al., "Selective Publication of Antidepressant Trials and Its Influence on Apparent Efficacy," *New England Journal of Medicine* 358 (3) (2008, January 17):252–260.

16. H. A. Sackeim, J. Prudic, et al., "The Cognitive Effects of Electroconvulsive Therapy in Community Settings," *Neuropsychopharmacology* 32 (2007):244–254.

17. Lucy Johnstone, "Adverse Psychological Effects of ECT," *Journal of Mental Health* 8(1) (1999):69–85.

18. D. I. Templer, D. M. Veleber, "Can ECT Permanently Harm the Brain?" *Clinical Neuropsychology* 4(2) (1982):62–66.

19. D. I. Templer, "ECT and Permanent Brain Damage," in D. I. Templer, L. C. Hartlage, W. G. Cannon, eds., *Preventable Brain Damage* (New York: Springer Publishing, 1992).

20. Andrew Reisner, "The Electroconvulsive Therapy Controversy: Evidence and Ethics," *Neuropsychology Review* 13(4) (2003):199–219.

21. Bernard L. Pacella, "Sequelae and Complications of Convulsive Shock Therapy," *Bulletin of the New York Academy of Medicine* 20 (1944):575–585.

22. Paper presented at the 129th annual meeting of the American Psychiatric Association, May 10–14, 1976, Miami Beach, Fla.

23. Max Fink, Jan-Otto Ottoson, *Ethics in Electroconvulsive Therapy* (New York: Brunner-Routledge, 2004), 111–112, 47, 45.

24. Fink recounted the incident at a similar workshop a year later: "Drugs and ECT: Combined Treatment and Maintenance Treatment," workshop at the Continuing Medical Education course "Advanced Clinical Issues in ECT: The Certificate Course," Marriott Marquis Hotel, New York City, April 1992.

25. Martha Manning, *Undercurrents* (New York: Harper San Francisco, 1994), 166.

26. Martha Manning, "Exploring Wellness," talk given at the 15th annual conference of the Depression and Bipolar Support Alliance, Orlando, Fla., August 2002.

27. Anne B. Donahue, "Electroconvulsive Therapy and Memory Loss: A Personal Journey," *Journal of ECT* 16(2) (2000):133–143.

28. Anne B. Donahue, "Riding the Mental Health Pendulum: Mixed Messages in the Era of Neurobiology and Self-help Movements," *Social Work* 45(5) (2000, October):427–438.

29. Sylvia Caras, Ph.D., "On Gratitude." http://www.peoplewho.org/readingroom/caras.gratitude.htm (accessed April 30, 2003).

30. Max Fink, Jan-Otto Ottoson, *Ethics in Electroconvulsive Therapy* (New York: Brunner-Routledge, 2006).

31. C. Gilligan, J. V. Ward, J. M. Taylor, *Mapping the Moral Domain* (Cambridge, Mass.: Harvard University Press, 1988).

32. Deposition of Julie Hatterer, M.D., in the matter of *Linda Andre v. Somatics Inc., Mecta Corp., The New York Hospital, Julie Hatterer, and Thomas Kramer*, Supreme Court of the State of New York, 9220/87, October 14, 1988.

33. Max Fink, "Complaints of Loss of Personal Memories after Electroconvulsive Therapy: Evidence of a Somatoform Disorder?" *Psychosomatics* 48 (2007):290–293. Most of the statements Fink makes about Rice here are false—his account of her dental problems, his portrayal of her health and life thereafter, his claim that she had repeatedly attempted suicide (she never did), and so on.

34. David Healy, Edward Shorter, *Shock Therapy: A History of Electroconvulsive Treatment in Mental Illness* (New Brunswick, N.J.: Rutgers University Press, 2007), 186, 207.

35. Sonja Brisbee Wulff, "Fort Collins Psychiatrist Loses License," *Fort Collins Coloradoan*, December 1, 1999. Sally Bridges, "Court Reinstates Hageseth's License," *Fort Collins Coloradoan*, February 17, 2001. Barbara Feder Ostrov, "Parents Sue Online Pharmacy, Doctor," *San Jose Mercury News*, March 14, 2006. "Doctor Extradited to Face Charges in Patient's Suicide," *Fort Collins Coloradoan*, December 1, 2007.

36. L. Hocksander, "Victims of 1950s Mind-Control Experiments Settle with CIA," *Washington Post*, October 5, 1988. L. Rubenstein, "The CIA and the Evil Doctor," *New York Times*, November 7, 1988.

37. Max Fink, "The Impact of the Antipsychiatry Movement on the Revival of ECT in the United States," talk given at State University of New York at Stony Brook, 1992.

CHAPTER 17 — WHERE DO WE GO FROM HERE?

1. FDA Docket No. 02N-0434.

2. The cite is 515(i) (21 U.S.C. 360e(i)). April 19, 1994, memorandum from FDA Acting Director, Office of Device Evaluation, to ODE Division Directors, re Preamendments Class III Strategy.

3. *Federal Register*, Vol. 60, No. 156, 41986–41989. Monday, August 14, 1995, Docket No. 94N-0417.

4. I am aware that Richard Abrams, in his textbook, 2002 edition, 12, claims the manufacturers made submissions to the FDA. But all the evidence shows that nothing was ever submitted. Letter from Kathy Bradford, FOI staff, Center for Devices and Radiological Health, FDA, September 4, 1997; numerous personal communications with attorney Joseph Sheehan, CDHR Office of Regulations, between 2000 and 2004; conversations with Steve Hinckley, FDA device evaluator, in 2000. FDA Docket No. 94N-0417 shows no submissions.

5. Section 502(t) of the FDCA (21 USC 352(t)), Sections 301(a) and (q) of the FDCA (21 USC 331(a) and (q)). Conversation with Joseph Sheehan, March 26, 2003: "Theoretically, they shouldn't be marketing the device" after ignoring 515(i); this "could lead to serious action like criminal prosecution."

6. Letter, Linda Andre to Steve Hinckley, August 10, 2000.

7. Personal communication with Joseph Sheehan, March 26, 2003.

8. Letter from Linda Kahan, Deputy Director, FDA Center for Devices and Radiological Health, to Linda Andre, September 3, 2004.

9. Royal College of Psychiatrists, U.K., *Fact Sheet on ECT* (London: Royal College of Psychiatrists, 1995).

10. ECT Anonymous, *Questionnaire Results: March 1999* (Riddlesden, Keighsley, West Yorks, U.K.: ECT Anonymous, 1999). M. Peddler, *Shock Treatment: A Survey of People's Experience of Electroconvulsive Therapy (ECT)* (London: MIND, 2000). UKAN (United Kingdom Advocacy Network), *ECT Survey: The National Experience* (Sheffield, U.K.: UKAN, 1996).

11. Service User Research Enterprise (SURE), Institute of Psychiatry, *Review of Consumers' Perspectives on Electroconvulsive Therapy* (London: SURE, January 2002).

12. Diana Rose, Pete Fleischmann, et al., "Patients' Perspectives on Electroconvulsive Therapy: Systematic Review," *British Medical Journal* 326(7403) (2003, June 21):1363–1367.

Diana Rose, Til Wykes et al., "Information, Consent and Perceived Coercion: Patients' Perspectives on Electroconvulsive Therapy," *British Journal of Psychiatry* 186 (2005):54–59.

13. M. Philpot, C. Collins, et al., "Eliciting Users' Views of ECT in Two Mental Health Trusts with a User-Designed Questionnaire," *Journal of Mental Health* 13(4) (2004, August):403–413.

14. National Institute for Clinical Excellence, *Guidance on the Use of Electroconvulsive Therapy: Technology Appraisal 59* (London: NICE, April 2003).

15. W. V. McCall, A. Dunn, P. B. Rosenquist, "Quality of Life after Electroconvulsive Therapy," *British Journal of Psychiatry* 185 (2004):405–409. The discussion continued in a subsequent issue: see "Quality of Life and ECT (letters)," *British Journal of Psychiatry* 186 (2005):264–265.

16. A. I. F. Scott, ed., *The ECT Handbook, 2d ed.* (Council Report CR128) (London: Royal College of Psychiatrists, 2005).

17. Harold Robertson, Robin Pryor, "Memory and Cognitive Effects of ECT: Informing and Assessing Patients," *Advances in Psychiatric Treatment* 12 (2006):228–238.

18. Maeve A. Mangaong, Jim V. Lucey, "Cognitive Rehabilitation: Assessment and Treatment of Persistent Memory Impairments Following ECT," *Advances in Psychiatric Treatment* 13 (2007):90–100.

19. A. I. F. Scott, "College Guidelines on Electroconvulsive Therapy: An Update for Prescribers," *Advances in Psychiatric Treatment* 11 (2005):150–156.

20. Brochure, ECT Accreditation Service, Royal College of Psychiatrists, circa 2004.

21. Scott, "College Guidelines on Electroconvulsive Therapy."

EPILOGUE

1. Thomas Goldsmith, "Electroshock Reborn as Valid Therapy," *News & Observer* (Raleigh, N.C.), January 13, 2008.

2. David Armstrong, "Medical Journal Editor to Quit in Wake of Disclosure Oversight," *Wall Street Journal*, August 25, 2006.

3. Benedict Carey, "F.D.A. Expands Suicide Warning on Drugs," *New York Times*, May 3, 2007.

4. R. Beamish, "HHS Watchdog to Re-Check Ethics Cases," Associated Press, March 29, 2007.

5. Giovanni Fava, "Financial Conflicts of Interest in Psychiatry," *World Psychiatry* 6 (2007):19–24.

Resources

If you have had ECT, are considering it, or just want to know more about it, far and away the most comprehensive and unbiased source of information is www.ect.org. The site has been in operation since 1995. You will find, among other things, journal articles, legal information, updates on forced shock cases, and the opportunity to interact with others in the forums pages.

The Committee for Truth in Psychiatry (CTIP), a nonprofit organization made up entirely of persons who have received ECT, has advocated for truthful informed consent since 1984. A newsletter, *Shockwaves*, is available on request. CTIP can be reached at P.O. Box 1214, New York, NY 10003 and (917) 642–4625. Membership forms and other information are also available via link from the www.ect.org site.

The Web site of the Law Project for Psychiatric Rights (www.psychrights.org), whose mission is "bring fairness and reason into the administration of legal aspects of the mental health system, particularly unwarranted court ordered psychiatric drugging and electroshock," maintains a bibliography on ECT and is currently the only place on the Web where you can obtain important hard-to-find, full-text journal articles on ECT free of charge, including many articles cited in this book.

Index

Italicized page numbers refer to figures.

Abrams, Richard, 41, 105, 145, 175, 252; authorship of ECT textbook, 208–209; nondisclosure of financial conflict, 208; ownership of Somatics Inc., 103, 132, 162, 175, 208–209; patents on ECT accessories, 208

Aden, Gary, 76–78, 86, 170, 283

Aden v. Younger, 75–78, 83

Ad-Hoc Committee for a Moratorium on Electroshock, 164–165

Alabama, legislation on shock treatment, 74–75, 113

Alexander, Leo, 41

Alpers, Bernard, 45, 48

Alternatives '99, 239

American Medical Association, 111, 119

American Psychiatric Association (APA): consent form for shock treatment, 93, 149–150, 156, 159, 203, 247–248, 296; denial of brain damage from shock treatment, 91–92, 148–149, 275; denial of permanent memory loss from shock treatment, 89–91, 148–149; influence on the media, 124–128, 129–130, 133, 135–136, 213, 225; opposition to regulation of shock treatment, 88, 92–93; opposition to safety investigation of shock treatment, 144–146, 170, 175, 197; opposition to statistics on shock treatment use, 136, 214, 268; petition to the FDA to reclassify ECT devices, 146, 148–155, 287; as stand-in for shock machine manufacturers, 144–145, 146, 153, 189; Task Force on ECT (1974–1978), 86–88; Task Force Report on ECT (1978), 86, 88–93, 125, 128–129, 134, 144, 148, 192; Task Force on ECT (1988–2001), 131, 268, 290; Task Force Report on ECT (1990), 122, 182, 199, 203, 208, 226, 250; Task Force Report on ECT (2001), 199, 204; use of public relations tactics, 83–85, 86–87, 107, 124–126, 127–128, 133, 135, 136, 137, 213, 253

American Society for Electrotherapy (ASE), 78. *See also* International Psychiatric Association for the Advancement of Electrotherapy (IPAEE)

AMI (Autobiographical Memory Inventory), 185, 273, 335n35

amnesia: anterograde in ECT patients, 264–265, 272; in metrazol shock, 32–33; permanent in ECT patients, 58–63, 89, 112–113, 115, 149, 150, 156–157, 184, 185, 186, 210, 216, 226, 235, 244, 251, 272, 273, 274, 282, 293, 296, 297; in shocked animals, 48

anesthesia, 49, 56–57, 99–101, 133, 328n34

Angell, Marcia, 191

animal studies, 48, 202, 257–258. *See also under* autopsy studies

"antipsychiatry," 16, 107, 207

Arons, Bernie, 233–234

As Empty as Eve (Roueché), 112–113, 269

Association for Convulsive Therapy (ACT), 79, 171

Atlantic Monthly, 128–130, 227–230

Austwick, Lucille, 233, 260, 264

autopsy studies: animal, 44–48, 91, 99, 159, 202; human, 48–51, 91–92, 99

Azemar, Andre, 261–262

ban on shock treatment, 80–81, 155, 224, 226, 227, 228, 243–244, 245, 284–286, 302; in Berkeley (Calif.), 80, 285, 302; in Europe, 285

Barhash, Abraham, 53

Barrera, S. Eugene, 91

Bayh-Dole Law, 199

believing game, 180

Benson, James, 141

Berkeley (California), 80, 155, 285, 302

Bernays, Edward, 70, 95

Bernstein, Joel, 224–227, 258

Binding, Karl, 37

Bini, Lucio, 34, 44

Blachly, Paul, 78, *79*, 103, 120–121, 123, 194

brain damage: acceptability for mental patients, 50–51, 54, 91, 275; as cause of improvement in shock patients, 49–51, 98, 157, 164; denial of in shock treatment, 57–58, 88, 91–92, 148–149, 166, 202, 206, 219, 237, 242, 253–254, 259;

brain damage (*Continued*)
  depression and, 253–258, 265; from ECT,
  8–12, 44, 82, 87, 99–100, 117, 143, 187,
  200–202, 226, 229, 235, 257–258, 267,
  274–275; from insulin shock, 31; from
  metrazol shock, 33; in human autopsy
  studies, 48–51; professional warnings
  about, 45, 48–51, 52–54, 55, 59–60, 65,
  275; in shocked animals, 44–48, 91
brain scans, 23, 44, 117, 202, 205–206, 253,
  255, 256, 265, 275. *See also* CAT scan;
  MRI
Breggin, Peter, 115–118, 122, 131, 135,
  162–163, 225–226, 249
brief pulse shock treatment: as element of
  public relations campaign, 79, 101–104,
  133; false claims of less electricity,
  100–101, 237; false claims of less memory
  loss, 104, 151, 205; machine modifications
  to increase electrical output, 103–104;
  1940s–1950s experiments, 54–56, 103,
  151; recommended by FDA, 142
Brody, M. B., 58–60

CAEST (Coalition for the Abolition of
  Electroshock in Texas), 17
California: legislation on shock treatment,
  75–78, 80; statistics on shock treatment,
  133
Cameron, Douglas, 103–104, 243
Cameron, Ewen, 283
Canadian Psychiatric Association, 183–184
Cannicott, S.M., 52
Caras, Sylvia, 280
Carnegie, Andrew, 28
Carrel, Alexis, 29
Carter, Rosalynn, 239
Carter Center, 231–232, 239–240
CAT scan (computerized axial tomogra-
  phy), 44, 67–68, 84, 117–118, 142, 143,
  151–152; animal study proposed by ex-
  patients to the FDA, 160–161; human
  study proposed by ex-patients to the
  FDA, 166–168; human study proposed
  to NIMH, 268; in persons who have
  had shock treatment, 117–118, 143, 184
Cauchon, Dennis, 208
Center for Mental Health Services
  (CMHS), 231, 232, 233–235, 236, 242,
  239, 243; "Background Paper on
  Electroconvulsive Therapy," 231,
  233–235, 236, 242, 243
Cerletti, Ugo, 34–36, 42–42, 44
Chabasinski, Ted, 122

"chemical imbalance" theory, 22–23, 95
Chicago Medical School, 41, 175, 209
coercion in psychiatry, 3–5, 16, 228, 277,
  280, 293–294
Coffey, Edward, 200–201, 202, 213
cognitive deficits in shock treatment,
  51–52, 89, 184, 185, 186, 237, 242, 256,
  268, 273, 295–299; author's experience
  of, 1, 8–11; documented by neuropsychological testing, 8–11, 181, 244, 248
cognitive rehabilitation, 66, 298–299
Coleman, Lee, 163
Colorado, reporting system in, 133–134
Columbia University, 40–41, 175, 193
commitment, civil, 3–5, 21, 27. *See also*
  outpatient commitment
Committee for Truth in Psychiatry
  (CTIP), 169, 171, 227–230, 233–234, 239,
  246, 269, 286, 291; animal CAT scan
  petition to FDA, 160–161; founding of,
  157–159, 333n2 (chap.10); informed
  consent petition to FDA, 159; informed
  consent statement, 156–157, 159; mission of, 158–159, 227; participation in
  NIMH Consensus Conference, 164–166
Communicate (U.K.), 294
competent patients, 74, 75, 76, 80, 83, 243,
  253, 261
conflict of interest: in medicine, 190–192,
  194, 210–211, 304; in psychiatry, 191,
  303–305; in shock treatment, 131,
  144–145, 162, 191–192, 194–196,
  198–200, 204, 206, 208–209
connected knowing, 178
Connecticut, 74
Consensus Development Conference on
  ECT (NIMH), 161–166, 271
consent forms for shock treatment: APA,
  93, 149–150, 156, 159, 203, 247–248,
  296; CTIP, 156–157, 159; New York, 83;
  Texas, 243; Vermont, 246–251
Continuing Medical Education (CME),
  206–207
Cott, Jonathan, 181, 210
Counterpoint, 245

Davenport, Charles, 28, 37
death rates. *See* mortality
depression, 74, 96, 184, 186, 187, 242, 277,
  285, 295, 296; "chemical imbalance"
  theory of, 22–23; claims of brain damage in, 253–258, 265; proposed reclassification of ECT devices for, 155, 183,
  186

Dietz, Jean, 68, 72, 135–136

discourse analysis, 95

Donahue, Anne, 181, 244–252, 279, 280, 281, 286, 302

Donahue, Phil, 223–224

doubting game, 178–180, 241, 253

drugs, psychiatric: development of, 23; effects of, 15, 125; forced, 18, 20; industry, 210, 303–305; vs. shock treatment, 72, 95, 96, 97; studies on, 272–273; and violence, 24; in young people, 303

Duke University, 12, 175, 196, 199–200, 205, 206, 213

ECT (electroconvulsive therapy). *See* shock treatment

ECT Accreditation Service (ECTAS) (U.K.), 300

ect.org, 225

ECT Review Group (U.K.), 104

EEG (electroencephalogram), 33, 49, 79

efficacy of shock treatment: brief pulse vs. sine wave, 55; claims of, 53, 92, 176, 271; as an effect of organic brain syndrome/brain damage, 49–51, 96, 98, 157, 164, 271; FDA on, 141–142, 186; lack of evidence for, 69, 76, 97–98, 148, 153, 165, 246, 291; outweighed by adverse effects, 295, 299; short-term duration of, 97–98, 157, 163, 165, 271, 293, 295; studies of, 97, 271–272; unilateral vs. bilateral, 299–300

Eisenberg, Leon, 240

electricity: amount used in contemporary shock treatment, 4, 103–104, 217–218, 328n41; amount used in first shock machines, 36; amount used in unilateral shock treatment, 105; attempts to reduce amount used in shock treatment, 55–56; false claims of reduced in contemporary shock treatment, 101–103, 237, 242, 243; shock industry calls for more, 101–103; in research devices, 97, 198, 270; as therapeutic agent in shock treatment, 103

Electroconvulsive Therapy (Abrams), 208–209, 252

electroconvulsive therapy (ECT). *See* shock treatment

electroshock. *See* shock treatment

Electroshock: The Unkindest Therapy of All (Hapgood), 128–130

electroencephalogram. *See* EEG

ElectroLoveTherapy, 78

Ellingson, Lei, 239–240

England. *See* United Kingdom (U.K.)

eugenics movement: in Germany, 37–38; in the United States, 28–30

"euthanasia" of mental patients: advocacy of in the United States, 28–30; in Germany, 37–39, 42

Facts About: Electroconvulsive Therapy (NIMH), 112

Fairness and Accuracy in Reporting (FAIR), 213–214

Fairness Doctrine, 126–127, 220

Federal Register, 140, 143, 144, 155, 288

Ferraro, Armando, 45

financial conflict of interest. *See* conflict of interest

Fink, Max, 41, 73, 80, 99, 110, 179, 190, 277, 284, 302; admission of brain damage from shock treatment, 49–50; on the APA ECT Task Force, 86–88; denial of permanent amnesia from shock treatment, 99, 136, 179, 280, 282; dismissal of unilateral shock treatment, 106; on ethics of shock treatment, 280–281; financial ties to shock machine manufacturers, 145, 331n26; and Scion foundation, 87, 190; as source of false statistic on permanent amnesia, 121

Florida, 74, 285

Fochtmann, Laura, 263, 290–291, 302

Food and Drug Administration (FDA), 35, 44, 101, 119, 137, 156, 262, 268, 285; Class I devices, 139; Class II devices, 139, 287; Class III devices, 139, 287, 288; classification of the ECT device, 145; hearings on the ECT device, 142–143, 144–145, 150–155; letters from Congresspeople, 173–174; letters from ECT device manufacturers, 174–175; letters from former ECT patients, 171–173, 177–178, 181, 187–188, 306–315; letters from the general public, 173; letters from Protection and Advocacy agencies, 173–174; letters from psychiatrists, 170, 175–176, 187; lobbied for safety investigation of ECT device, 171, 173–174, 187–188; lobbied to prevent safety investigation of ECT device, 170–172, 174–176, 177, 187; Medwatch program, 288; Neurological Devices panel, 141, 142, 147, 290–291; performance standard for devices, 139, 287; performance standard for ECT devices, 149,

Food and Drug Administration (*Continued*) 183; petition to adopt patient-written ECT consent form (Docket No. 84P-0430), 159; petition for animal CAT scans (Docket No. 85P-0422), 160–161; petitions for human CAT scans, 166–168; petition to maintain the ECT device in Class III (Docket No. 2003P-0555), 291; petition to reclassify the ECT device (Docket No. 82P-0316), 146, 148–155, 287; premarket approval applications (PMAs) for devices, 139, 140, 145, 169, 288; premarket approval applications (PMAs) for ECT devices, 145, 146, 153–154, 288, 289, 291; proposed reclassification of the ECT device, 154–155, 161–162, 183–188, 287; regulation of medical devices, 138–140; reports on ECT, 141–142, 186–187; Safe Medical Devices Act of 1990 (SMDA), 287–288; special controls for devices, 287–288; substantial equivalence (510(k)), 140, 289

Foote, Susan, 152–154

forced shock treatment, 17, 25, 68, 97, 233, 259–264, 267, 269, 277, 280; court decisions on, 74–76, 80, 82–83; in England, 293–294; in New York State, 260

forced treatment, 17–18, 20–21, 25, 27, 81–82

Frank, Leonard Roy, 113–114, 122, 157, 163, 282

Frankel, Fred, 69, 86, 87, 88

Frazier, Shervert, 78, 124, 162

Freeman, C. P. L. (Chris), 162, 163, 186, 292, 295

Friedberg, John, 87, 113, 244, 275

Frith, Chris, 198

Garrett, Kathleen, 260, 263, 264

Gatto, Laurie, 264

Gelsinger, Jesse, 190

gender differences: in ECT usage, 177; in moral orientation, 281–282; in ways of knowing, 178–180

Glasscote, Raymond, 129–130

Globus, Joseph, 91

Gluck, Michael, 152–153, 154, 162

Gotkin, Janet, 163, 166

Gracie Square Hospital, 41, 319n48

Greenblatt, Milton, 69, 71, 84, 87, 135

Grimm, Robert, 65, 87–88

Grinker, Roy, 49

Group for the Advancement of Psychiatry (GAP), 53

Gundy v. Pauley, 75

Hageseth, Christian, 283

Haggett, Cindy, 248

Hall, W. Bromley, 263

Hapgood, Fred, 128–129

Hartelius, Hans, 46–48

Healy, David, 22, 210, 303, 305

Hernandez, Dina, 260

Hiatt, Rex, 174

Hinckley, Steve, 289–290

hippocampus: effect of seizures on, 255; in persons formerly depressed, 257; in persons with depression, 255; in persons who have had ECT, 256–257; in shocked animals, 257

Hippocratic oath, 275, 276, 280

Hoch, Paul, 50

Hoche, Alfred, 37

Hughes, Jennifer, 217–218

Hughes, Joseph, 48

Illinois, 214, 233

Impastato, David, 40

incompetent patients, 73–74, 83, 243, 245, 259–262

informed consent: American Psychiatric Association on, 93, 149–50; doctrine of, 68; lack of in shock treatment, 17, 165, 262, 286, 293–294; lawsuits, 9, 74, 76, 77, 80, 82, 115, 118–119, 279; as right of mental patients, 16, 67; for shock patients in Vermont, 246–251; truthful for shock treatment, 156–159, 286, 297–298

Insane Liberation Front, 14

Institute of Psychiatry (U.K.), 292

insulin shock treatment, 31–32, 33, 37, 39, 44, 113, 265

intelligence, effects of shock treatment on, 50, 52, 181, 210, 254, 265, 292, 294, 298. *See also* IQ

International Association for Psychiatric Research, 86. *See also* Scion Natural Science Association

International Association of Psychosocial Rehabilitation Services, 239

International Psychiatric Association for the Advancement of Electrotherapy (IPAAE), 78, 86, 124, 162, 170–171

involuntary shock. *See* forced shock

IQ, effects of shock treatment on, 8–9, 12, 181, 244, 247, 252. *See also* intelligence

Jaffe, D. J., 25

Janis, Irving, 60–63, 89, 149, 202, 242

Joan T., 260
Joseph, Jay, 30
Johnstone, Lucy, 274
journalism: accountability in, 220–224, 223; "balance" in, 130, 136, 214–216; bias towards shock treatment, 136, 213–219; class bias in, 218–219; cronyism in, 221–222; fact-checking in, 219–220; "fairness" in, 131, 214–215; free speech in, 220–221, 230; "hit and run," 222–223; "objectivity" in, 136, 214–216; press releases as, 220

Kaiser Wilhelm Institute for Psychiatry, 37
Kalani, Robert, 262
Kalinowsky, Lothar, 40–41, 45, 51, 115, 117
Kanner, Leo, 30
Kellner, Charles, 101, 206, 218
Kelly, Michael, 230
Kemsley, Sue, 99
Kendell, R. E., 186
Kendra's Law, 26
Kennedy, Foster, 29–30
Krystal, Andrew, 206

Lake, Celinda, 235–236
Lanes, Selma, 209–210
Lawrence, Juli, 225
lawsuits: against shock machine companies, 19, 268, 316n8; against state officials, 74–77, 82–83; by individuals, 19–20, 114–119, 247, 316n8
Lebensohn, Zigmund, 41
leucotomy, 50
Liberson, W. T., 55–56
Lidbeck, William, 91
Lindsay, Jeanne, 150–152, 154
Lisanby, Sarah Holly, 258, 302
lobotomy, 21, 30–31, 50–51, 63–64, 94
long-term studies of shock treatment. *See* research: long-term studies of shock treatment; Sackeim, Harold: unpublished long-term studies
Loper, Diann'a, 224, 226, 243–244
Lucey, Jim, 298

MacArthur Research Network on Mental Health, 24
Madness and Medicine, 122–123, 124, 126, 127
Madness Network News, 14–15, 114
Malitz, Sidney, 193, 195
Mangaong, Maeve, 298

Manning, Martha, 277–279
Margolis, Lester, 170
Massachusetts: regulation of shock treatment, 71, 92; reporting system, 71; shock treatment abuses in, 68; statistics on shock treatment, 133; survey of shock use, 134; task force on ECT, 69–71; use of shock treatment for children, 71–72
Masserman, Jules, 47, 53
Matthews, Michael, 260
McCall, W. Vaughn, 205, 295
McEwen, Bruce, 255–256, 258–259
McGaugh, James, 48
Mecta Corporation, 78–79, *102*, 337n13; lawsuits against, 19, 316n8, 345n7
Medcraft Corporation, 144, 175
media: author's personal experiences with, 130–132, 136, 166, 216–218, 219–220, 222, 224–230; bias toward shock treatment, 213–219; coverage of conflict of interest in medical research, 190–192; coverage of shock treatment, 37, 112–113, 122–123, 128–136, 166, 182, 223–230, 237, 303; influence of American Psychiatric Association, 124–128, 129–30, 137, 182, 213. *See also individual media*
medical model, 21–23
Meduna, Ladislas, 32, 34, 40, 41
memory disability in shock treatment, 64, 90, 109, 131–132, 164, 184–186, 256, 297–298
memory loss in shock treatment, 49, 51, 55–56, 82, 90–91, 143, 145, 160, 172, 192, 210, 235, 239, 246, 247, 251, 282; denial of permanent, 104, 121, 184–185, 226, 237, 252, 254, 263, 268, 292; descriptions of permanent, 1–2, 5–6, 11, 59, 63, 109, 244, 306–315; extent of permanent, 58–63, 156–157, 163–164, 185–186, 210, 228, 243, 244, 245, 274, 293, 302–303; incidence of permanent, 156–157, 164, 228, 274, 293, 294, 296, 302–303; in metrazol shock, 32–33; studies of permanent, 58–63, 89, 163–164, 185, 273, 293, 294, 302–303
Mendelis, Peter, 115, 117, 269–270
Menninger, Karl and William, 53
mental patients: acceptability of brain damage for, 50–51, 54, 91, 275; attitudes towards, 13, 18–21, 43, 231–232; deprivation of human and civil rights of, 13, 16, 17, 18, 25–27; forced sterilization of,

mental patients (*Continued*)
28–29; forced treatment of (*see* forced
treatment); killing ("euthanasia") of,
28–30, 37–39, 42; legal rights of, 67–68,
73–74, 82–83; mortality rate, 26; movement for human and civil rights, 13–17,
113–114, 121–122; names for, 16, 292;
and violence, 24–25
Mental Patients' Liberation Front, 14
Mental Patients' Liberation Project, 14
metrazol shock treatment, 32–33, 37, 42
Michigan, 74
MIND (U.K.), 294
MindFreedom International (formerly
Support Coalition International), 17
Minnesota, 75, 83
Moench, Louis, 141, 172, 182
Moniz, Egas, 50
moral aspects of shock treatment, 267–286;
assessing help vs. harm, 270–274; ban,
moral argument for, 284–286; brain damage as treatment, 274–275; choices made
by industry, 267–269; gender perspectives
on, 281–282; "lifesaving" argument,
98–99, 269–271; listening as moral
choice, 280–283; lying to patients, 119,
144, 276–279, 286; paternalism of practitioners, 284–285
Morgan, Robert, 63
Moritsugu, Kenneth, 240
Morrissey, Joseph P., 121–122
mortality: from ECT, 49, 57, 243, 268,
271; from insulin shock, 31; rate in
mental patients, 26
mossy fiber sprouting, 258
MRI (magnetic resonance imaging), 44,
200–201, 206, 262
muscle paralyzers/relaxants: 49, 56–57, 133
multiple monitored ECT (MMECT), 79
Myerson, Abraham, 49, 50

Nakamura, Richard, 237–238, 241, 242, 282
Nardini, John, 78, 116
National Alliance on Mental Illness
(NAMI), 21, 25
National Association of Protection and
Advocacy Systems, 239
National Center on Research Resources, 197
National Council on Disability (NCD),
26–27
National Institute for Clinical Excellence
(NICE) (U.K.), 294–295
National Institute of Mental Health
(NIMH), 23–24, 162, 166, 191–192, 234,

304; brochure on shock treatment,
111–112; conflict of interest in research
(*see* conflict of interest); Consensus
Development Conference (*see*
Consensus Development Conference
on ECT); estimates of shock treatment
use, 134; grants for shock treatment
research, 189–190, 192–198, 200, 202,
204, 206, 209, 237, 271, 295; grants for
training shock practitioners, 205–206;
rules on conflict of interest, 194, 304
National Mental Health Association
(NMHA), 238, 239
National Mental Health Consumers' Self-
Help Clearinghouse (formerly National
Mental Health Consumers'
Association), 236, 239
National News Council, 129–130, 220
Network Against Psychiatric Assault, 76,
114, 122
Neuberger, Karl, 91
Neufeld, Victor, 132
neurogenesis, 257–258
neuropsychological testing: explained,
8–10; of former shock patients, 66,
89, 177, 180–181, 229, 242, 244,
297, 298
New Hampshire, 285
New York: forced shock in, 260; law on
consent to ECT, 74; proposed ECT
legislation, 121, 264
*New York City Health and Hospitals
Corporation v. Stein*, 74
New Yorker, 112–113, 114, 157, 269
New York State Psychiatric Association,
127, 263
New York State Psychiatric Institute. *See*
Psychiatric Institute
Nicol, Gorham, 194, 337n13
Nicol, Robin, 174–175, 337n13
Nobler, Mitchell, 206
Nowakowski, Richard, 257–258

Objectivity in Research rule, 194
One Flew Over the Cuckoo's Nest, 67, 93–94,
100, 101, 106, 123, 133, 225
On the Sea of Memory (Cott), 181
Operation T-4, 38–39
Opton, Edward, 163
Ottoson, Jan-Otto, 100
outpatient commitment, 20–21, 25–26, 27
Oxford University Press, 208–209
oxygenation, 56–57, 58, 99–100, 237,
323n44, 327n30, 327n31

Pacella, Bernard, 51

Pardes, Herbert, 175–176, 182

"Parker, Natalie" (pseudonym for Marilyn Rice), 113

Permission for the Destruction of Lives Unworthy of Life (Binding and Hoche), 37

Potter, William Z., 162

Preventable Brain Damage (Templer et al.), 275

Price v. Sheppard, 75, 82, 262

private psychiatric hospitals, use of shock treatment in, 37, 68, 72

Protection and Advocacy agencies (P&As), 173–174, 207, 245

Pryor, Robin, 297–298

Psychiatric Institute (P.I.) (New York City), 40–41, 45, 51, 175, 193

Psychiatric Institute (Washington, D.C.), 109

psychosurgery, 27, 30–31, 50, 74, 82

public relations: campaign to promote psychiatry, 124–128; campaign to sell shock treatment, 43, 65, 67, 84–85, 86–88, 90, 93–95, 106, 107, 124–126, 127–128, 135, 136, 146, 211, 253, 262–263; effects on journalism, 213; principles of, 70, 95, 193

Reisner, Andrew, 275

REJECT (Responsible Education and Judgment on ECT), 17

research, 189–190; animal studies, 48, 202, 257–258; conflict of interest in (*see* conflict of interest); funding for, 189–190, 194; long-term studies of shock treatment, 58–63, 89, 131–132, 163–164, 184, 185, 186, 271–273, 292–293; on shock treatment, 97, 192–198, 200, 209–210; systematic review of literature on "consumers' perspectives" on ECT (SURE), 292–294; systematic review of efficacy of ECT (ECT Review Group), 104. *See also* autopsy studies; National Institute of Mental Health: grants for shock treatment research

review articles on shock treatment: selective as substitute for original research, 201–203; systematic, 104, 292–294

Rice, Marilyn, 107–122, *108*, 155, 165, 166, 244, 269, 279, 280, 281; authorship of ECT consent form, 156–157; on banning shock, 157, 286; criticism of media coverage of ECT, 127, 130; and the

FDA, 140–141, 143–148, 150–152, 160, 161, 168, 171, 173, 182, 183; founding of Committee for Truth in Psychiatry, 158–159

Rice v. Nardini, 114–119

right (of mental patients) to refuse (treatment), 17, 67, 68, 73, 74, 76, 80, 253, 262; court decisions on, 74–76, 82–83

Robertson, Harold, 297–298

Rockefeller, John D., 28

Rogers, Joseph, 236–238, 239, 242

Rogers, Susan, 238, 239–240, 242

Roizen, Leon, 45

Rose, Diana, 294

Rose, Robert, 166

Roueché, Berton, 112–113, 114, 125, 269

Royal College of Psychiatrists (U.K.), 183–184, 291–292, 293, 295, 296, 297, 299–300

Rudin, Ernst, 37

Rudorfer, Matthew, 237–238, 242

Sabshin, Melvin, 130

Sackeim, Harold, 103, 162, *193*, 204, 209–210, 242, 245; admission of permanent substantial memory loss in shock treatment, 251, 273, 302–303; on APA ECT Task Force, 182, 203, 204; attacked by Abrams, 252; authorship of AMI (Autobiographical Memory Inventory), 185, 273, 335n35; denial of brain damage in shock treatment, 200–204, 226, 253, 258; denial of permanent memory loss in shock treatment, 179, 226, 253–254; early career, 192–193; on depression and brain damage, 253–255; financial ties to shock machine manufacturers, 131, 145, 162, 194–196, 203, 226–227, 303; grantsmanship, 192, 194; influence on Vermont consent form, 249–250; influence on Vermont shock legislation, 245–248; later career, 203–204; lying to students, 207–208; in the media, 131, 225–226, 228, 229; NIMH grant, 195–196, 198; nondisclosure of financial conflicts, 249–250, 338n15; proposed evaluation of amnesia in shock patients, 264–266; research articles, 203, 210, 271–273, 302–303; as reviewer of articles and grants, 204; unpublished long-term studies, 272–273

Sakel, Manfred, 31–32, 54

Salzman, Leon, 51, 87

Sapolsky, Robert, 255–256, 263
Scion Natural Science Association, 86, 190
Seaman, Barbara, 204
seizures: attempts to induce with minimal
    electricity, 54–56; effects of, 4, 96; in
    experimental animals, 34–35; first
    experiments with electrical induction,
    36–37; first use as "therapy," 32; harm-
    fulness of, 47, 87–88, 255, 256, 263–264;
    induced by camphor, 32; induced by
    insulin, 31; induced by metrazol, 32–33;
    measuring, 199; multiple, 79; oxygena-
    tion and, 57; physical injury caused by,
    32, 56; prolonging with caffeine, 198;
    spontaneous, 224; as therapeutic agent
    in shock treatment, 56, 103
seizure threshold: amount exceeded in
    shock treatment, 103, 105, 195–196;
    and anesthesia, 57, 101
separate knowing, 178–179
Service User Research Enterprise (SURE)
    (U.K.), 292–294
Shah, P. J., 257
Sham ECT, 97
Sharav, Vera, 303
Sheline, Yvette, 254–257
Sheppard, Graham, 97
shock machines: amount of electricity
    used, 4, 103–104, 217–218, 328n41; APA
    petition to reclassify, 146, 148–155, 287;
    design modifications to increase electri-
    cal output, 103–104; FDA regulation of,
    141–146; FDA classification of, 145;
    modified for research, 97, 198; profits
    from, 208–209. *See also* Mecta
    Corporation; Medcraft Corporation;
    Somatics Inc.
shock treatment (electroconvulsive ther-
    apy, ECT): and ability to work, 51, 54,
    59–60; 232; amnesia in (*see under* amne-
    sia); ban on (*see* ban on shock
    treatment); brain damage (*see under*
    brain damage); in children, 71, 72, 80,
    243, 285; cognitive deficits in (*see* cogni-
    tive deficits in shock treatment);
    "comeback" of, 132, 133–135, 213–214,
    219, 225, 302; consent for, 68, 71, 74–76,
    93; cost of, 3; death rate (*see* mortality:
    from ECT); effects on intelligence (*see*
    intelligence, effects of shock treatment
    on); effects on IQ (*see* IQ, effects of
    shock treatment on); efficacy (*see* effi-
    cacy of shock treatment); estimates of
    use, 3, 134; euphoria caused by, 4, 157,

164; forced (*see* forced shock); informed
    consent for (*see under* informed con-
    sent); invention of, 34–37; legislation
    on (passed), 76–78, 80, 245–249; legisla-
    tion on (proposed), 76, 121, 243, 264,
    285, 302; maintenance, 4, 58, 242, 295;
    mechanisms of action, 4, 49–51, 98,
    103, 157; in the media (*see under*
    media); memory disability in (*see* mem-
    ory disability in shock treatment);
    memory loss (*see* memory loss in shock
    treatment); modified, 49, 56–57; moral-
    ity of (*see* moral aspects of shock treat-
    ment); in Nazi Germany, 39; "new and
    improved" claim made for, 94–95, 101,
    104, 105, 132–133, 140; "one in two
    hundred" (false estimate of permanent
    memory loss), 121–122, 216; patents on
    accessories, 208; patents on techniques,
    199–200; regulation by states, 71,
    72–73, 74–75, 76, 92–93, 250; reporting
    systems, 71, 76, 133–134, 214, 243;
    research (*see under* research); sham vs.
    real compared, 97; statistics on, 37,
    133–134, 143, 271; and suicide, 25,
    98–99, 185; "taming effect," 7; "ultra-
    brief," 56; unilateral, 105–106, 237, 263,
    299–300; unmodified, 100
Shock Treatment in Psychiatry (Jessner and
    Ryan), 52–53
Shock Treatment Is Not Good For Your Brain
    (Friedberg), 87, 113
Shockwaves (newsletter), 234
sine wave shock treatment, 55, 104, 142
60 Minutes II, 224–227, 258
Small, Iver, 99, 171–172, 182
Small, Joyce, 99, 162
Smith, Daniel, 227–230
Somatics Inc. (now Somatics LLC), 103,
    104, 132, 175, 198–199, 208–209
Soteria House, 23–24
square wave. *See* brief pulse shock treatment
Squire, Larry, 86, 89–91, 113, 131–132,
    163–164, 184, 192, 242
Stefan, Susan, 13
Sterling, Peter, 144
Stone, Calvin, 52
Stony Brook (State University of New
    York), 175
suicide: in shock treatment patients, 25,
    98–99, 185; in young people using psy-
    chiatric drugs, 304
Support Coalition International. *See*
    MindFreedom International

Surgeon General (David Satcher), 231, 235, 238, 239, 242
Surgeon General's Report on Mental Health, 203, 231, 232, 235–243, 249
Swartz, Conrad, 103, 171, 175; ownership of Somatics Inc., 208–209; nondisclosure of financial conflict, 209
Syszko, Adam, 260

Templer, Donald, 184, 274–275
Texas, 214, 243, 246, 285
Thomas, Paul Henri, 260–264
Tien, H.C., 78, 283
Today show, 166
Torrey, E. Fuller, 123
Treatment Advocacy Center (TAC), 21
Truth in Psychiatry letters, 119–121, 158
20/20, 130–133, 135, 226

"ultrabrief" shock treatment, 56
United Kingdom (U.K.): ban on psychiatric drugs for children, 302; ECT patient surveys, 292–294; forced shock in, 293–294; ECT Review Group, 104; Institute of Psychiatry, 292; National Institute for Clinical Excellence (NICE) Report on ECT, 294–295; oversight of shock treatment, 300; patient ("user") advocacy groups, 292, 294; Royal College guidelines on ECT, 295–296; Service User Research Enterprise (SURE), 292–294. *See also* Royal College of Psychiatrists
University of Iowa, 175
Utah, 285

Valenstein, Elliott, 31
Veale, James, 143, 145, 147, 150

Veleber, David, 274–275
Vermont, 181, 214, 231, 244, 245, 252, 301; ECT consent form, 246, 250–251, 252; ECT informed consent materials, 247–249; ECT legislation, 245–247; ECT study committees, 246–247, 249–250; proposed ban on shock treatment, 243, 285
Villforth, John, 141

Washington Post, 199, 331n26
waveforms, electrical. *See* brief pulse shock treatment; sine wave shock treatment
Weeks, D., 186
Weiner, Richard: advocacy of shock treatment at the FDA, 144–145, 150–154, 170, 202; on the APA ECT Task Force, 131, 182, 199; financial ties to shock machine manufacturers, 131, 144–145, 198–200; media appearances, 131, 199, 224; patents, 199–200; research grants, 196–198, 200–202; research studies, 185, 198, 200–201; review article on brain damage, 202
West Virginia, 285
Wheaton, Pat, 164
Whitaker, Robert, 20, 22–23
World Association of Electroshock Survivors, 17
Wyatt v. Hardin, 74–75
Wyatt v. Stickney, 74

Ziegler, Laura, 207–208

About the Author

Linda Andre writes and surfs in New York City. She is the director of the Committee for Truth in Psychiatry, a national nonprofit organization of ECT survivors that advocates for truthful informed consent. She has published numerous articles in general interest and scholarly journals, has presented workshops at conferences in the United States and Europe, and frequently appears in the media. She is a longtime advocate for the rights of people with psychiatric labels.